Praise for *Blind Eye*

"*Blind Eye* is a remarkable piece of reporting." —Scott McLemee, *Newsday*

"Swango's odyssey is so compelling that I became riveted. I needed to know when and how he would be caught, and what ultimately happened to him."—Dr. Robert B. Daroff, *The Plain Dealer* (Cleveland)

"Stewart has produced an extraordinary book."—Steve Twedt, *Pittsburgh Post-Gazette*

"James B. Stewart's *Blind Eye* is a persuasive case against Dr. Michael Swango."—R. Z. Sheppard, *Time* magazine

"The facts gathered by Stewart are compelling. [He] . . . persuasively dissects the medical establishment."—Steve Weinberg, *Chicago Tribune*

"Is *Blind Eye* worth reading? Yes, Jim Stewart's books always are." —Joseph Nocera, *Fortune*

"Stewart tells a story that both grips and enrages. . . . Throughout *Blind Eye*, [he] shows how the medical establishment took the path of least resistance when it came to Swango. They didn't want to know."—Ray Locker, *The Tampa Tribune*

"If Swango is guilty—and author James B. Stewart builds a persuasive case against him—Stewart also makes a strong argument that he must share responsibility with a medical establishment that let him move freely from state to state, from hospital to hospital, without warning or punishment."—Dale Singer, *St. Louis Post-Dispatch*

"Best-selling author Stewart brings us inside the life of a killer who thrived in a medical establishment where doctors typically cover up for other doctors, where hospital administrators live in constant fear of litigation, and where regulatory agencies don't share crucial information. . . . Stewart writes skillfully."—*Kirkus Reviews*

ALSO BY JAMES B. STEWART

Follow the Story

Blood Sport

Den of Thieves

The Prosecutors

The Partners

BLIND EYE

*The Terrifying
Story of a Doctor
Who Got Away
with Murder*

JAMES B. STEWART

*A Touchstone Book
Published by Simon & Schuster
New York   London   Toronto   Sydney   Singapore*

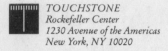

TOUCHSTONE
Rockefeller Center
1230 Avenue of the Americas
New York, NY 10020

10 9 8 7 6 5 4 3 2 1

The Library of Congress has cataloged the Simon & Schuster edition as follows:
Stewart, James B.
    Blind eye: how the medical establishment let a doctor get away with
murder / James B. Stewart
        p.   cm.
    Includes index.
    1. Swango, Michael.   2. Serial murderers—United States Biography.
3. Physicians—United States Biography.   4. Serial murders—United States
Case studies.   5. Serial murders—Zimbabwe Case studies.   I. Title.
HV6248.S76S78   1999
364.15'23'0973—dc21   99-37044
                                                                                              CIP

ISBN 0-684-85484-8
      0-684-86563-7(Pbk)

The author and the publisher gratefully acknowledge permission
to reprint an excerpt from "Twelve Songs," from W. H. Auden:
Collected Poems, by W. H. Auden, edited by Edward Mendelson.
Copyright © 1940 and renewed 1968 by W. H. Auden.
Reprinted by permission of Random House, Inc.

PHOTO CREDITS
1, 2, 3, 4   Family Collection
5   SIU Yearbook
6, 7   The Ohio State University Photo Archives
8, 11   Argus Leader, Sioux Falls, South Dakota
9, 10, 13   Cooper Family Collection
12   J. R. Romanko
14, 15, 16   James B. Stewart
17   Newsday, Inc. © 1997

CAST OF CHARACTERS

Michael Swango, M.D.

MURIEL SWANGO, his mother
JOHN VIRGIL SWANGO, his father
ROBERT SWANGO, his brother
JOHN SWANGO, his brother
RICHARD KERKERING, his half brother
RUTH MILLER, his aunt
LOUISE SCHARF, his aunt

At Southern Illinois University

JAMES ROSENTHAL, medical student
KEVIN SWEENEY, medical student
DAVID CHAPMAN, medical student
DR. MARK ZAWODNIAK, medical resident
DR. KATHLEEN O'CONNOR, medical resident
DR. JOHN MURPHY, professor of pathology and toxicology
DR. LYLE WACASER, part-time professor of neurosurgery
DR. WILLIAM RODDICK, chairman, department of obstetrics and
    gynecology
RICHARD MOY, dean of the School of Medicine

At Ohio State University

EDWARD JENNINGS, president
DR. MANUEL TZAGOURNIS, university vice president, health
  services, and dean of the College of Medicine
RICHARD JACKSON, university vice president, business and finance
DR. MICHAEL WHITCOMB, medical director, Ohio State
  University Hospitals
DR. LARRY CAREY, chief, department of surgery
DR. WILLIAM HUNT, director, department of neurosurgery
DR. JOSEPH GOODMAN, professor of neurosurgery
DR. REES FREEMAN, chief resident, neurosurgery
DONALD CRAMP, executive director, Ohio State University
  Hospitals
DONALD BOYANOWSKI, associate executive director, business and
  finance
CHARLES GAMBS, assistant vice president, university public safety
JAN DICKSON, R.N., associate executive director/nursing
AMY MOORE, R.N., head nurse
ANNE RITCHIE, R.N.
RITA DUMAS, R.N.
KAROLYN TYRRELL BEERY, student nurse
JOE RISLEY, nurse's aide
IWONIA UTZ, patient
RENA COOPER, patient

ROBERT HOLDER, associate attorney general, State of Ohio
ALPHONSE CINCIONE, partner, Butler, Cincione, DiCuccio, and
  Barnhart

In Quincy, Illinois

MARK KRZYSTOFCZYK, paramedic
GREG MYERS, paramedic
BRENT UNMISIG, paramedic
LONNIE LONG, chief paramedic
DENNIS CASHMAN, judge, Eighth Judicial Circuit

CAST OF CHARACTERS   9

CHET VAHLE, assistant state's attorney, Adams County
ROBERT NALL, sheriff
CHARLES GRUBER, chief of police
WAYNE JOHNSON, coroner
DAN COOK, attorney

In Columbus, Ohio

MICHAEL MILLER, prosecuting attorney, Franklin County
EDWARD MORGAN, assistant prosecuting attorney
PETER HERDT, chief of police, Ohio State University
BRUCE ANDERSON, police officer
RICHARD HARP, police officer
CHARLES ELEY, investigator, Ohio State Medical Board
JAMES MEEKS, dean of the College of Law, Ohio State University

In Newport News, Virginia

KRISTIN KINNEY, R N
SHARON COOPER, her mother
AL COOPER, her stepfather

In Sioux Falls, South Dakota

DR. ROBERT TALLEY, dean of the University of South Dakota
    School of Medicine
DR. ANTHONY SALEM, professor of internal medicine and director
    of the residency program
LISA FLINN, R.N.
VERN COOK, hospital administrator

At the State University of New York–Stony Brook, Long Island

DR. JORDAN COHEN, dean of the School of Medicine

DR. ALAN MILLER, professor of psychiatry, director of the
    psychiatric residency program
BARRON HARRIS, patient
ELSIE HARRIS, his wife
DOMINIC BUFFALINO, patient
TERESA BUFFALINO, his wife

In the Republic of Zimbabwe

HOWARD MPOFU, director of hospitals, Evangelical Lutheran
    church
DR. DAVIS DHLAKAMA, medical director, Midlands province
DR. NABOTH CHAIBVA, superintendent, Mpilo Hospital,
    Bulawayo
DR. IAN LORIMER, resident
DR. CHRISTOPHER ZSHIRI, director, Mnene Mission Hospital
KENEAS MZEZEWA, patient
VIRGINIA SIBANDA, patient
P. C. CHAKARISA, superintendent, Zimbabwe Republic police
DAVID COLTART, attorney, Webb, Low & Barry, Bulawayo
LYNETTE O'HARE, landlady
MARY CHIMWE, her servant
ELIZABETH KEREDO, her servant
JOANNA DALY, housewife

I observe the physician with the same
diligence as he the disease.
—JOHN DONNE (1572–1631)

PROLOGUE

KENEAS MZEZEWA *had dozed off for a nap that May afternoon, but was awakened at about two P.M. when he felt someone removing his loose-fitting pajama trousers. He lifted his head, still a bit groggy from sleep, and saw that it was Dr. Mike. The handsome American doctor had a syringe in his hand, and seemed about to give him an injection, so Mzezewa, eager to help, pulled down his trousers and turned on his side. Then the doctor plunged the unusually large needle into his right buttock. Mzezewa saw that after he finished the injection, the doctor concealed the used syringe in the pocket of his white medical coat.*

"Good-bye," Dr. Mike said softly, pausing briefly to look back at Mzezewa.

Then he left the hospital ward.

HOWARD MPOFU, the director of hospitals for the Evangelical Lutheran Church in Zimbabwe, liked the new doctor the minute he met him, in November 1994, when he picked him up at the Bulawayo city airport. Michael Swango looked like the American athletes Mpofu had seen on television. He was blond and blue-eyed, taller than Mpofu, with a ready smile. According to the résumé the church had received, he was forty years old, but he looked younger. Mpofu tried to help Swango with his duffel bags, but the doctor wouldn't hear of it. He quickly hoisted the heavy bags and insisted on carrying them to the car himself.

On the ride into the city, Swango was garrulous, flushed with excitement at his new assignment. Mpofu asked why Swango had wanted to come to Zimbabwe to take up a post that would pay him a small fraction of what he could earn in the United States. After all, Swango was an honor student; he'd graduated from an American medical school and had completed an internship at the prestigious Ohio State University Hospitals, which meant he could go anywhere. "All my life," Swango told him, "I have dreamed of helping the poor and the disadvantaged." He said America had plenty of doctors, but in Africa, he would be truly needed. Mpofu couldn't argue with that.

When they reached the Lutheran church headquarters in central Bulawayo, they walked up one flight of stairs to the church offices, and Mpofu introduced Swango to the Lutheran bishop of Zimbabwe. To the amazement of the church officials, Swango knelt before the bishop and kissed the floor. He said he was so grateful to have been hired and to be in Zimbabwe at last.

The bishop seemed equally delighted. Indeed, he and Mpofu were overjoyed simply to have succeeded in recruiting an American doctor for one of their mission hospitals, let alone one willing to kiss the ground at their feet. Before Swango, the only European or American doctors the church had succeeded in bringing to Zimbabwe were Evangelical Lutherans from church headquarters in Sweden, and none of them stayed more than a few years.

Not many foreign doctors—even from places like Eastern Europe and Asia—wanted to come to Zimbabwe, the former British colony of Rhodesia, which lies between Mozambique and Botswana, just north of South Africa. Before the end of the white supremacist regime of Ian Smith and the holding of supervised elections in 1980, the country had endured a prolonged civil war. And after independence came the consolidation of dictatorial power by the mercurial Robert Mugabe, who, among other controversial pronouncements, has denounced homosexuals as "perverts" who are "worse than dogs and pigs." Since independence, the country has experienced the suppression of human rights, the collapse of its currency, a steep decline in the standard of living, and the emigration of much of its white population. Fully 25 percent of the adult population of Zimbabwe is estimated to be infected with HIV, the highest infection rate in the world. At times the country's hospital system has been plunged into turmoil, and there is a critical shortage of doctors.

With a population of about 650,000, Bulawayo is Zimbabwe's second-largest city, the capital of the province of Matabeleland, once a powerful African nation in its own right. For the most part, the local population speaks Ndebele, a linguistic cousin of Zulu, whereas the Zimbabwean majority speaks Shona. A debilitating civil war between the two ethnic groups broke out almost immediately after Zimbabwe gained independence, and though a truce was reached, simmering tensions persist.

Bulawayo residents complain that the city has been neglected by the national government because of continuing ethnic discrimination against the Ndebele. But a result of that neglect has been that the colonial-era architecture and city plan have been largely unmarred by the building boom that has swept Harare, the nation's capital. Even the cars generally date from the fifties and sixties, owing to years of international economic embargo during white-supremacist rule and the collapse of the Zimbabwean dollar following independence. Many people in Bulawayo seem to prefer the atmosphere of faded gentility, especially the fifty thousand or so remaining whites, most of British descent. These days few live lavishly; there is little conspicuous wealth. But they praise the city's unhurried pace (nearly all businesses seem to close by three P.M.); the nearly ideal climate of the high African veldt, in which even summer temperatures almost never reach ninety degrees; the gracious residential neighborhoods of walled villas and jacaranda-lined streets. Most white people still return home for a lunch prepared by black servants. They congregate at the Bulawayo Golf Club, the oldest club in Zimbabwe, with manicured fairways and a swimming pool, and the Bulawayo Club, an imposing beaux-arts mansion downtown.

By contrast, the orderly grid of colonial Bulawayo is surrounded by scores of "settlements," in which thousands of black people live crowded into small houses and shanties along dirt roads that seem to have been laid down at random. Many commute into the city on aging, diesel-fume-spewing buses, and the central bus terminal is a colorful and chaotic mass of shouting passengers, piles of goods and luggage, buses, taxis, bicycles, and handcarts. There is an almost eerie sense of a time warp in Bulawayo. In the award-winning 1988 film *A World Apart*, it stood in for 1960s Johannesburg.

Swango spent his first night in Zimbabwe at the Selborne, a

colonial-era hotel whose wide verandah overlooks the city's bustling central square. The next morning, Mpofu picked him up for the drive to the church's mission hospital at Mnene. Mpofu had made the six-hour drive many times, and he was accustomed to the dismay of first-time visitors as the pavement gave way to a dirt road so rough that a four-wheel-drive vehicle or truck is required. Yet Swango voiced no complaints as they ventured ever farther from what most Americans would consider civilization.

Mnene—a cluster of buildings—can't be found on many maps. It lies in the region of Mberengwa in south-central Zimbabwe, in what in colonial times were known as the tribal lands of Belingwe, in the heart of the bush. Inhabitants identify themselves by the name of their tribal chief; the land is still owned communally, and the local people's life of subsistence farming has changed little for generations. There are no towns to speak of, scant electricity, almost no telephones. Most people live in extended family units in clusters of mud-walled buildings with thatched roofs. The landscape is often stunningly beautiful: verdant valleys give way to distant panoramas of mountain ranges. Drought and malaria are constant threats, in part because the lower elevation makes the climate more tropical than it is on the high plateau where most of the white population lives.

The region is served by three hospitals, one of them also called Mnene, all founded in the early part of the century by Evangelical Lutheran missionaries. Mnene Mission hospital, a cluster of one-story whitewashed buildings with corrugated metal roofs and wide verandahs, is set atop a hill with distant views and refreshing breezes. The buildings look much the same as they do in a photograph taken in 1927, when the hospital was built.

When Mpofu and Swango finally arrived, Dr. Christopher Zshiri, the hospital director, hurried out to greet them. He introduced Swango to Dr. Jan Larsson, a Swedish missionary doctor who was the other member of Mnene's medical staff, and showed Swango to his quarters, a spacious bungalow with a verandah, adjacent to the hospital. Zshiri is a native Zimbabwean. Under the country's system of socialized health care, he reported to the provincial medical administrator in Gweru and was paid by the government, even though nominally he worked for the Lutheran church. Even more than the others, Zshiri thought it was almost too good to be true that they had managed to recruit an American doctor to a place like Mnene.

Zshiri and Swango soon became friends. Zshiri couldn't get over how talkative Swango was, always eager for conversation and filled with curiosity. After his arrival, Swango had garnered glowing reports from patients and staff members. He was soon known to everyone as "Dr. Mike." It was true that he lacked experience in general surgery and obstetrics, two areas most in demand at Mnene. After a month at Mnene, Zshiri sent him to Mpilo Hospital in Bulawayo, where Swango spent the next five months gaining additional clinical experience. The doctors at Mpilo wrote glowing recommendations, and Swango was far more confident and proficient when he returned to Mnene in late May. He was seen as a nearly tireless worker, able to complete forty-eight-hour stints without sleep. He even worked extra shifts, giving up his free time. Of course, at Mnene, there was little else to do. Even the indefatigably cheerful Swango finally complained about the isolation, asking Zshiri if the church could possibly provide him with use of a car, since he couldn't afford one. Fearful that Swango might decide to leave, Zshiri wrote church officials a letter asking whether there wasn't some way they could accommodate him.

Swango often made extra rounds to check on his patients, sometimes at night or during afternoons when he was otherwise off-duty. So when Dr. Swango arrived in the surgery recovery room one May afternoon in 1995 to check on Keneas Mzezewa, the only patient there, no one thought it unusual, even though Swango had already completed his rounds that morning, and technically Mzezewa wasn't his patient.

Mzezewa had recently had his foot amputated by Dr. Larsson. A farmer in the Mberengwa area who was also a part-time laborer at the nearby Sandawana emerald mine, Mzezewa had come to the hospital the previous week complaining about severe pains in his leg. A tall, slender man with a wide smile, Mzezewa had reacted calmly to the news that his infected foot would be amputated. The doctor reassured him that he would be fitted with a prosthesis and should be able to lead a normal life once he returned to his farmstead. The operation had been uneventful, but Mzezewa had been kept in the recovery ward for close monitoring, which was routine in amputation cases. Dr. Larsson had been pleased with his progress, and mentioned to Zshiri how well Mzezewa was doing.

That afternoon Mzezewa was awakened from his nap by the new doctor, Dr. Mike. Before the doctor gave him the injection, Mzezewa noticed, he neglected to swab the skin with disinfectant. Mzezewa also noticed that when Dr. Mike put the used syringe in his jacket pocket, the needle's cover fell to the floor near his bed.

Still, it seemed a routine visit. Despite the large size of the needle, Mzezewa didn't mind the pain. He relaxed and lay back on his bed, prepared to resume his nap. But as the drug given him by the doctor spread through his body, he began to feel a strange loss of sensation in all his muscles. With mounting alarm, he realized that he couldn't turn over and couldn't move his arms or legs. He wanted to speak or cry out, but his jaws, tongue, and throat wouldn't respond. Then the room, brightly lit by the afternoon sun, grew dim. Soon all was darkness.

Mzezewa didn't know how much time passed while he lay there, alive and conscious but paralyzed and terrified. But then the darkness began to lift; he could see, though he still couldn't move his head. A nurse's aide entered the recovery ward and came over to his bedside. She held a thermometer and told him it was time to take his temperature. Mzezewa's mind was racing. His heart beat furiously. He wanted to cry out, but he couldn't make a sound. He could hear the aide, but he couldn't move; his muscles wouldn't respond. She asked him to move his arm so she could put the thermometer in his armpit. He lay motionless. She asked him again. Suddenly the aide looked alarmed, and ran from the ward.

Moments later, Mzezewa regained his voice. He screamed and began shouting to attract attention, though he still could not produce recognizable words. A nurse came rushing into the ward, followed by the aide. She came and stroked his hand, trying to calm him, asking him what had happened. But he was still unable to speak. Two more nurses arrived.

Slowly Mzezewa regained his voice. "Dr. Mike gave me an injection," he finally gasped. The nurses were puzzled, for while Mzezewa was taking oral painkilling medication, he was not scheduled for any injections. In any event, injections were administered by the nursing staff, not by the doctors.

Then Swango himself came into the ward, coolly appraising the commotion. Mzezewa looked terrified. The nurses fell silent.

"Did you give him an injection?" a nurse finally asked. "What was it?"

Swango seemed mystified. "He must be delirious," he said. "I didn't give him any injection."

CHAPTER ONE

SOUTHERN ILLINOIS, the triangle of land north of the junction of the Mississippi and Ohio Rivers, 350 miles from Chicago, feels more like the Deep South than like the industrial Midwest. Summers are hot and steamy, and in June 1979, most of the students and faculty members at Southern Illinois University in Carbondale who could get away after graduation had fled, leaving the campus feeling sleepy and underpopulated. An exception was the medical school, whose year-round schedule enabled students to complete the standard four-year medical school curriculum in three years. They began during the summer, spent the first year at SIU's main campus in Carbondale, then moved to SIU's campus in Springfield, the state capital, to complete their degree.

Late one June night, James Rosenthal, a newly admitted member of the SIU medical school class of '82, was sitting in a college dorm room, sweating from a combination of the heat and his anxiety over an enormous stack of introductory medical texts: anatomy, physiology, biochemistry. . . . The topics seemed endless, the books huge. He should have been asleep. He turned out the lights and noticed that another window in the adjacent dorm was still brightly lit.

It was Rosenthal's classmate Michael Swango, wearing military fatigue pants and doing jumping jacks. Swango was lean and muscled at a time when fitness was far from most students' minds. He'd been in the Marines, and his name was stenciled on the military garb he usually wore to class. It was weird, Rosenthal thought. Many of his classmates had been antiwar protesters. Swango was the only member of the class he knew who had been in the military.

Swango's military garb and fanatical devotion to fitness were noticed by just about everyone in his class at SIU. Besides the military fatigues, he wore combat boots to class. When Rosenthal and other classmates struggled out of bed in the morning after a late night of studying, they would often see Swango outdoors doing early-morning calisthenics, chanting Marine cadences. Sometimes, at breakfast in the cafeteria, they teased him about his uniforms and military bearing. Swango bridled at their ribbing and increasingly kept to himself.

Everyone in the class was soon nearly overwhelmed by the workload and the battery of tests administered to first-year med students. As a relatively new medical school, SIU had been able to build a curriculum from the ground up, unfettered by traditional approaches. It was the first medical school in the country to create a written set of criteria for the medical degree, criteria derived from an extensive survey of medical educators. The goal was to graduate students prepared for careers in primary care—family practice, internal medicine, pediatrics, and obstetrics/gynecology—as opposed to research or the subspecialties, such as ophthalmology and cardiology. Every first-year medical student was required to take and pass 476 written tests during the first year. Each test covered a curricular "module," such as heart murmurs, within one of the core topics, such as the heart. Ten to fifteen closed-book tests were given every Saturday morning on the modules that had been covered in classes that week. Notes and textbooks weren't allowed in the exam room.

That didn't deter Swango, however, from using his notes during the exam. He would choose one of the tests, take it, then choose his next test topic and sprint from the room back into the hallway. There he would frantically page through his notes and books, cramming for the second test. Then he would return, take that test, and repeat the process. His fellow students were dumbfounded, and some were disgruntled. Dashing into the hallway between tests seemed perilously close to cheating, though it wasn't expressly forbidden. As the weeks went by and Swango continued the pattern, several students mentioned to him that they thought it wasn't fair, but Swango was defiant, and continued his cramming. Inevitably, other students began to do likewise, which led to considerable faculty concern. Finally Chandra Banerjee, the first-year professor of pulmonary medicine, admonished his students: "Goddammit, no Swangoing." A new word was coined. "Swangoing," the noun, or "to Swango," the verb, described the practice of racing into the hall and cramming between tests.

Swango was notorious not only for his test-taking regimen. During their first year, medical students dissect a cadaver. A ritual familiar to every medical student, the process bonds students and they usually remember it for the rest of their careers. At SIU, the first-year students were divided into groups and each student was assigned one part of the cadaver to dissect and present to the rest of the group. Swango's assignment was the hip and buttock region, including the gluteus muscles.

Students had keys to the anatomy lab and could come and go on their own time. Many worked late into the night, though the lab was busiest in the afternoons, when faculty members were on hand to offer advice and suggestions. But Swango never came in during the day or evening, preferring to work on his dissection after midnight, when the lab was usually deserted. Indeed, some members of his group, who never saw him in the anatomy lab at all, wondered how he was going to make his presentation.

What Swango gained in privacy from his unorthodox hours he lost in guidance from faculty and other students. For when his presentation finally came, and he unveiled his dissection, his fellow students gasped. He had transformed the hip region of his cadaver into an unrecognizable mess of tangled flesh and bone. As some classmates described it, it was as though he had done his dissection using a chain saw rather than a scalpel. Even Swango finally recognized that he couldn't adequately describe the region's anatomical characteristics using his own handiwork. He abandoned the cadaver and completed his presentation by showing his group pictures from an anatomy text.

Swango had few, if any, friends at SIU; his fellow students later realized they knew almost nothing about his past, his family, his education, or his military service. Yet the combination of his weird garb, chiseled physique, odd nocturnal habits, "Swangoing," and now the cadaver mishap, made him one of the best-known of the seventy-two members of the class, much talked about and derided at the many class parties and gatherings, from which he was usually absent. The cadavers remained on display in the anatomy lab, and members of Swango's group made a point of showing their friends Swango's mangled handiwork, generally with a comment like, "Can you believe this?" One classmate, Kevin Sweeney, paraded nearly half the class through the anatomy lab to see it.

The experience must have been humiliating for Swango, who had received almost nothing but praise and perfect grades before enrolling in med school. Michael was the second of Muriel and John Virgil Swango's three sons. (Richard Kerkering, Muriel's son from a previous marriage, lived with his father.) Michael had excelled at the private Catholic boys' high school he attended in Quincy, Illinois, beginning in 1968. Bob and John were educated at public schools, but—largely at the insistence of his mother, who recognized that he was academically gifted—Michael was enrolled in Christian Brothers High School. The family wasn't Catholic (his father once described his religion as "the brotherhood of man"), but Christian Brothers was perceived as academically superior to the public schools. John Virgil Swango also liked the strict ethical and moral foundation of the Catholic curriculum. He didn't want Michael to become an antiwar activist like his older brother, Bob.

Virgil needn't have worried; Michael seemed oblivious to the social and political upheavals sweeping the country. While Bob listened to Bob Dylan and the Rolling Stones, Michael's favorite popular music group was the brother-sister duo the Carpenters. He was a model student, named to the honor roll every year. He took the usual precollege course load, but the only topic in which he seemed to show unusual interest was the Holocaust, which was covered in world history. He ranked in the ninety-seventh percentile on his college aptitude tests. Though he ran on the track team during his freshman and sophomore years, he wasn't very athletic. He participated in a whirlwind of extracurricular activities: he was a class officer, and served on the student council, yearbook, and newspaper staffs.

His main interest mirrored his mother's love of music. He was a talented pianist and spent many evenings playing classical music for his mother. He was the band's first-chair clarinet, as well as its president, and he sang in the glee club. As a senior, he performed the demanding Mozart clarinet concerto in the band's spring concert, the only student featured as a soloist. Mrs. Swango had bought him a Buffet clarinet, an expensive brand manufactured in Paris and used by many leading players. He was so precocious that his clarinet teacher, who played in the Quincy Symphony and taught at Quincy College, recruited Michael for the Quincy College Wind Ensemble, which toured Illinois during Swango's senior year in high school.

When Michael graduated from Christian Brothers in 1972, he was showered with honors: the "Outstanding Musician" and John Philip Sousa band awards (followed by a party for band members and their parents hosted by his mother); a citation as a National Merit Scholarship finalist; and the place of class valedictorian. A flurry of articles in *The Quincy Herald-Whig*, the local newspaper, memorialized his achievements. His mother clipped the articles and circulated them among relatives. A 1972 yearbook picture shows Michael in his band uniform, smiling, with tousled blond hair. Curiously, in the same yearbook he described his "ambition" as "to be an Illinois State Trooper."

As his class valedictorian and a National Merit finalist with high test scores, Swango would have been highly sought after by top colleges and universities all over the country. But minimal college counseling was available in Quincy, his parents were relatively unsophisticated about higher education outside the military, and almost all his classmates stayed close to home; consequently, Swango's horizons seem to have been limited. He decided to attend Millikin University, a small, private liberal arts school in Decatur, Illinois, about a three-hour drive from Quincy, where he received a full-tuition scholarship in music. Millikin's music department was highly regarded in Illinois, and was considered the school's strongest department.

As he had in high school, Swango excelled academically at Millikin, earning nearly perfect grades during his first two years. But during his first year, a girlfriend broke off their relationship. Though he had typically worn a sports jacket to class, which was unusual in the early seventies, after the breakup he began to dress in military garb. He painted his old Ford Fairlane in camouflage olive green. When a friend asked him about this, he said he planned to join the military and was fascinated by guns. About this time, too, he first mentioned an interest in pre-med courses. And he showed

an intense interest in photos in the local paper of car crashes, which
his classmates found peculiar. By the end of his sophomore year, he
was spending more time alone, and his friends and roommate had
less and less contact with him. That summer, he enlisted in the
Marines, and didn't return for his junior year. No one ever heard
him play the clarinet or the piano again.

Michael completed basic training at the Marines' boot camp
at San Diego, where he was trained as a rifleman, earning the
designation of sharpshooter. His personnel record states that he
entered the service at St. Louis, attended administrative procedures courses at Camp Lejeune, North Carolina, and Washington, D.C., and was working at Camp Lejeune in 1976, when
he received an honorable discharge. He received a National
Defense Service Medal and a "Meritorious Mast," a minor commen-
dation.

When he returned to Quincy after his discharge, Swango was
lean and fit and carried himself with military bearing. He announced
to his family that he wanted to become a physician, something that
especially pleased his mother, who had once worked as a medical
secretary. He enrolled in pre-med courses at the local community
college and had no difficulty gaining admission to Quincy College
for the following fall. A small, private college founded by the Fran-
ciscan Brothers in 1860, and still affiliated with the Catholic church,
the school had long drawn applicants from students at private
Catholic high schools, mostly in Illinois. But the population of such
students had been dwindling. With his near-perfect grades at the
more competitive Millikin and his outstanding high school record,
Swango must have been one of the college's top applicants. Still,
after he was admitted he decided to embroider his record. On a
form he submitted to the college's public information office, he
falsely claimed that he had received both a Bronze Star for heroism
in combat, and a Purple Heart for combat wounds during his relatively brief tenure as a Marine.

Swango was an outstanding student at Quincy College. Having
abandoned music, he plunged into the sciences, earning a 3.89
grade-point average with a double major in chemistry and biology.
He studied prodigiously, working late into the night at the college
library or in the science labs. In contrast to high school, he pursued

few outside activities. He didn't participate in any sports; and in the yearbook he listed the biology club and the college radio station as his only extracurricular activities. In a further reflection of his newfound interest in medicine, he worked part-time as an orderly at Blessing Hospital in Quincy and became a certified emergency medical technician.

During his senior year, Swango wrote a paper, evidently his senior thesis in chemistry, on the poisoning murder of a prize-winning Bulgarian writer living in exile in London. It isn't hard to fathom why the death of Georgi Markov might have drawn Swango's attention. As the Bulgarian crossed the busy Waterloo Bridge in central London in September 1978, he felt a faint pricking on his thigh. A heavyset man mumbled, "Sorry," to Markov as the man stooped to pick up an umbrella he had dropped. That night, Markov developed a high fever and then violent nausea. He died four days later.

An autopsy discovered a tiny capsule, about the size of a head of a pin, embedded in Markov's thigh. The capsule, which could have been carried on the tip of an umbrella, contained a poison called ricin, a castor-bean derivative that causes fever, vomiting, and finally massive blood clots throughout the body. In sufficient doses it is invariably fatal; "there is no specific treatment . . . other than making the person comfortable," according to the U.S. Navy's Bureau of Medicine and Surgery. There was also no pathological test for the presence of ricin, which left no identifiable trace in the bloodstream or body. Though the Bulgarian secret police were suspected in Markov's death, the murder remains unsolved.

DURING his senior year, Swango took the Medical College Admission Test (MCAT) and applied to a number of medical schools. He graduated summa cum laude in 1979 and won the American Chemical Society's award for academic excellence.

Competition for admission to any accredited American medical school in the spring of 1979 was intense, as it had been ever since the baby boom generation began graduating from college in the late sixties and applying in droves to professional schools. This was the case not just at the country's most prestigious institutions, but also at newer, less well-known medical schools such as Southern

Illinois University. Demand for doctors was so strong that lucrative careers awaited med school graduates. Huge numbers of applicants with good records were rejected from every medical school to which they applied, and many migrated to medical schools in foreign countries, Mexico being a common destination. Swango's classmate Rosenthal, despite good grades in his science classes at highly regarded Knox College and decent scores on the MCAT, had been rejected outright by sixteen schools before securing a place on SIU's waiting list. Another of Swango's classmates had applied for seven years in a row before she was accepted.

Applications to U.S. medical schools were funneled through a centralized office in Washington, D.C., which sent preliminary applications to the medical schools named by the applicant. If a medical school thought it might be interested, then, and only then, would it send a candidate its own application. Besides needing outstanding grades in a pre-med curriculum and high MCAT scores, applicants had to sit for a personal interview in which their maturity, commitment, and aptitude for medicine were evaluated.

Because it was founded in part to improve medical services in southern Illinois, SIU accepted only Illinois residents and looked for a commitment to family practice in small-town or rural Illinois. After a committee evaluated all the information candidates submitted, SIU (like other medical schools) placed them into one of three categories: "Reject," "Accept," or "Accept When Place Available."

Muriel proudly reported to family members that Michael had been accepted at several medical schools. Given his excellent academic record and test-taking ability, Swango would have been a strong candidate. His work in a hospital as an orderly would also have worked in his favor. And SIU would have been especially interested in someone like Swango, who was from Quincy, part of the area the medical school was meant to serve.

Yet his classmates speculated that Swango had been admitted from the waiting list, because he moved into the dorms late, along with students who, like Rosenthal, had been admitted at the last minute. They surmised that Michael hadn't performed well in the admissions interview and wondered what he had answered when asked why had wanted to become a doctor. Among his classmates, the decision to become a doctor formed a large part of their getting-acquainted conversations. Swango never participated in these conversations; he seemed blank when the topic surfaced. Swango never expressed any interest in patients.

Still, apart from the cadaver incident, nearly everyone conceded that Swango seemed hardworking and disciplined. Some classmates were astounded to learn that he was working as a paramedic for America Ambulance in Springfield while a first-year student. Not only was outside employment during the first year frowned upon (Rosenthal had to get permission from the dean to teach a Sunday school class in Carbondale), but Swango was commuting to a city one hundred miles away. And his violation of the antimoonlighting policy was particularly brazen, for the Springfield hospitals the ambulances served were affiliated with SIU and staffed with many SIU residents and professors. These staffers soon realized what Swango was doing, but no one on the faculty complained. He passed all 476 tests, however unorthodox his methods, and all of his courses, including anatomy. One member of the class had to repeat the first year, and one person flunked out, but when the rest of the class moved on to the second year in Springfield, Swango was among them.

THE central Illinois city of Springfield, with a population just over 100,000, seems a metropolis compared with Carbondale. It boasts the state capitol building and is steeped in the lore of its most famous resident, Abraham Lincoln, whose restored home is a major tourist attraction. The city is attractive to SIU because its two hospitals, St. John's and Memorial, are much larger than any in Carbondale, and it is there that SIU medical students gain their first clinical experience. Beginning with the second year, the medical school's curriculum turns away from basic science and anatomy to disease-oriented courses, including pharmacology, radiology, and pathology. Pathology, which includes toxicology, the study of poisons, seemed particularly to fascinate Swango. It was taught by a popular professor, Dr. John Murphy, who was favorably impressed by him.

During their third year of SIU's medical school, students undergo a series of rotations, including pediatrics, obstetrics and gynecology, internal medicine, and surgery. In the surgery rotation, students were assigned in pairs to give oral presentations. Rosenthal and Swango were partners, and at Rosenthal's suggestion, they chose to discuss the repair of certain defects through open-heart surgery. A relative of Rosenthal's was a heart surgeon and volunteered some original papers the students could use. But Rosenthal ended up having very little contact with his partner. This may have been because Swango was still working for the ambulance corps and frequently was either unavailable or fidgeting because he was going to be late for ambulance duty. But it was also because Rosenthal didn't like being around Swango. He was jumpy, nervous, and seemed unable to relax. He wore a beeper and would rush off whenever the ambulance service called. The pair ended up giving their presentation in two discrete sections, which might as well have been separate reports. Swango had assembled several slides and gave a creditable, if unmemorable, performance.

But given that the topic was heart surgery, his subsequent performance in class was baffling. Swango's class assembled at the start of each day for what's called morning conference; one day Dr. Roland Folce, the chairman of surgery, led a discussion of X rays. He put a chest X ray on a screen and pointed to a shadowy area in the middle of the image. He looked around at the class, then focused on Swango. "Mike, tell us what's in this picture," he said. Swango was silent. Finally he said, "I don't know." There were some titters from other students. "That's the heart, Mike," Folce said, sarcastically emphasizing the word "heart." It was almost as big a debacle as the cadaver incident, for any medical student this close to getting his degree should have been able to recognize the heart on an X ray. It was so obvious that his classmates concluded that Swango must simply have panicked and frozen.

Yet the episode was one of many that led some of his classmates to conclude that Swango was taking a surprisingly cavalier approach not only to medical school, but to the well-being of his patients. One of the first clinical assignments medical students receive is to take histories and perform physicals—"H & P's"—on hospital patients. Students interview patients, record their medical histories, undertake routine physical examinations, and post the results on the patients' charts. Depending on the patient, the procedure can take anywhere from a half-hour to ninety minutes. His classmates observed that Swango was completing his entire rounds in less than an hour, sometimes spending what seemed like as little as five minutes with a patient. Yet he filed complete H & P's. In at least one instance, another student charged that Swango had plagiarized or fabricated his entire write-up. The claim triggered renewed talk and concern about Swango among his classmates; Rosenthal and several others even wondered whether Swango should be reported to the Student Progress Committee, a group of twelve faculty and two students that heard complaints of student misconduct. But no one did so.

Within their third-year rotations, students can choose areas of specialization. There was a standing joke at SIU that the dumb and the lazy chose anesthesia; the smart and the lazy went into radiology; the dumb hard workers chose pediatrics; and the smart hard workers went into neurosurgery. Thus, it came as a surprise to many when Swango concentrated his courses in neurosurgery, especially considering the cadaver incident. Neurosurgery, involving delicate operations on the brain and other parts of the nervous system, is one of medicine's most demanding (and highly paid) specialties. It is emotionally taxing, because patients needing neurosurgery are often in dire straits, and because deaths and catastrophic incidents on the operating table are probably more common than in any other area of practice. Still, competition for internships and residencies is intense. But Swango was no more forthcoming to his classmates about his choice of a specialty than he had been about why he had chosen medicine as a career.

Swango's decision came as a particular shock to his classmate Sweeney, who had been so dismayed by the cadaver incident and thought Swango was ill-equipped to practice medicine at all, much less neurosurgery. Furthermore, neurosurgery happened to be Sweeney's area of concentration as well, so he and Swango would share patients and work closely together.

The two were jointly assigned to a resident, Mark Zawodniak, who would oversee their work and act as a mentor. Though that meant Sweeney and Swango had to see each other virtually every day, they avoided each other as much as possible. Though most students sharing a neurosurgery specialty would observe each other's surgeries, Sweeney stayed away from Swango's—he was horrified by the prospect of what he might see—and Swango never showed up at Sweeney's, either.

Zawodniak, though he was genial and friendly, also developed an aversion to Swango. When Swango was out of earshot after one particularly frustrating encounter, Zawodniak turned to Sweeney and lamented, "What did I fucking do to deserve him?"

But finally, in the person of a faculty neurosurgeon, Dr. Lyle Wacaser, Swango seemed to find a kindred spirit. Wacaser raved about Swango. He would brook no criticism of Swango's alleged haste, sloppy habits, or indifference to patient care. The two seemed all but inseparable, Swango eagerly accompanying the neurosurgeon on his rounds and into his surgeries. Indeed, Swango had persuaded the nursing staff to beep him on his ambulance pager whenever they learned that one of Wacaser's patients was about to be admitted. That way Swango was usually on the scene even before Wacaser, and sometimes before the patients themselves. This naturally froze Sweeney out of numerous opportunities for clinical experience, and it hardly endeared Swango to fellow students. (The first-come, first-served system for assigning medical students to patients was subsequently changed.) But naturally, Swango's eagerness made a favorable impression on Wacaser, who found him remarkably pleasant and industrious. He thought Swango's patient write-ups were close to perfect.

Wacaser was one of several Springfield doctors in private practice who also served as clinical instructors. He was popular among students and highly respected in his field, and the fact that he championed Swango went a long way to ease student concerns about Swango's competence. He was also eccentric. Wacaser drove around town in a truck that had emblazoned on it in bold letters, "Lyle Wacaser, M.D., Neurosurgery and Light Hauling." Recently divorced and in his early fifties, Wacaser would often invite students for post-surgery beers at his spacious office in a house across the street from the hospital, where he displayed the brain of a former patient in a jar of formaldehyde on the fireplace mantel. He also threw numerous parties. His office phone could be connected to the hospital's public address system; Wacaser would get on the system and announce, "Fluid and electrolyte rounds in progress." The signal sent medical students flocking to the parties, which were often rowdy affairs where they could blow off steam. But Swango didn't drink alcohol and, despite his close relationship to Wacaser, never attended the parties. Indeed, after Swango's surgery rotation ended, Wacaser hardly ever saw him, and later realized that he knew nothing about Swango's background or personal life, even who his parents were or whether they were alive.

During their third year at SIU medical school, students have significantly more contact with patients and are responsible for hundreds of H & P's in the course of the year. Swango's classmate Rosenthal noticed that Swango seemed unusually interested in, even preoccupied with, the sickest patients. The hospital maintained a large blackboard on which were written patient names and treatment remarks. When a patient Swango had seen died, he scrawled "DIED" in large capital letters across the person's name. Rosenthal and other students found this distasteful, almost as though Swango were celebrating the demise and wanted to call attention to it. When Effie Walls, a kindly patient whom Rosenthal had met, and whom Swango had been treating for an injury, died suddenly after a visit from Swango, he scrawled "DIED" over her name as well. Rosenthal went up to Swango and asked him why he did such a thing. "Don't you feel bad that she died?"

Swango gave Rosenthal a blank look. "No," he replied. "That's just what happens."

It happened often with Swango. A standing joke among the students was that if they wanted to get rid of a patient, they should assign Swango to do an H & P.

One day Zawodniak mused to Sweeney that unusually often, it seemed, when he assigned Swango to do an H & P, the patient would suddenly "code," meaning suffer a life-threatening emergency. "Do you think it was just coincidence?" But even as Zawodniak spoke, he dismissed the thought, and the two laughed it off. Swango was correct, after all, that death is a regular occurrence in a hospital.

Zawodniak, Sweeney, and many of their classmates were developing a black sense of humor under the twin pressures of medical school and hospital life. After about five deaths in patients who seemed to be recovering satisfactorily, all of them soon after an

H & P by Swango, Zawodniak coined a nickname for his seemingly disaster-prone protégé: Double-O Swango.

Other medical students thought the nickname was hilarious, and soon it was in widespread use. "Double-O Swango" meant License to Kill.

CHAPTER TWO

D URING SWANGO'S last year of medical school, in January 1982, his mother called him and his brothers, Richard, Bob, and John, with the news that their father was dying and that they should return home to Quincy as soon as possible. Michael drove from Springfield. Richard, Virgil's stepson, made the trip from Florida, where he was working as a certified public accountant, and Bob flew back from Eugene, Oregon, where he was an orderly at a nursing home. John, the youngest, stayed at his Air Force base in Italy. But Muriel's call to her sons had come too late. Virgil died on January 29 at Quincy's Blessing Hospital before the family had converged.

Colonel Swango was given a twenty-one-gun salute and was buried with full military honors in a brief graveside service attended by a handful of family members and friends. At his request, there had been no visitation or memorial service at the funeral home, either. Michael was the center of attention—clean-cut, neatly dressed in blazer and tie, easily the most handsome of the colonel's sons. Along with his girlfriend, an attractive brunette, he was at his mother's side through the ceremony. None of the sons spoke. Muriel sat rigidly, saying nothing and showing no emotion at her husband's death. But she seemed to glow with pride afterward as relatives congratulated Michael on his progress in medical school, his work as a paramedic, and his seemingly bright future as a doctor.

Muriel had always favored Michael over the other boys, and she did so now, too. The attention galled Bob, who had long, unkempt hair, had never graduated from college, and still looked like a hippie. At the funeral, people kept referring to him as "Mike's

brother." He hadn't spoken to Michael in years, but he thought his
brother's poise, his charm, and his earnest-young-professional demeanor were an elaborate charade.

The military hero's farewell accorded Virgil glossed over the
reality that the Swango family had for all practical purposes disinte-
grated. Virgil had died from cirrhosis of the liver, lonely, living in a
mobile home, his Vietnam exploits long forgotten. He and Muriel,
though never divorced, had legally separated. She had had no contact with him since he left the family home in 1976, following a prolonged bout of heavy drinking and an altercation in which he struck
her. Muriel had said that she wouldn't tolerate physical abuse, and
she insisted that he move out. Though she was in touch with his
doctors, she did not visit or speak to her husband during his final
days in the hospital.

Like many Vietnam veterans, Virgil Swango had had a difficult
time adapting to civilian life. He went to work in Quincy as a real
estate agent for Richard "Hap" Northern, an old family friend, but
his sales and commissions were meager. His father, John Harvey
Swango, had been a prominent Democrat and served as Adams
County recorder of deeds for twenty-eight years, a remarkably long
tenure for an elected position. Confident that he would have high
name recognition and would be greeted by voters as a war hero, Virgil tried to pursue a political career, running as a Democrat for a
post as county supervisor. The campaign was his first indication
that Vietnam veterans were viewed not as heroes, but as "losers," as
he later put it. He was painfully disappointed when he came in last
in a four-man race.

With his political hopes dashed, Virgil immersed himself in pa-
triotic and veterans' organizations—the American Legion, the Veterans of Foreign Wars, and the Reserve Officers Association—and
made the rounds of Quincy's many neighborhood taverns. When
he was cited for valor by the State Department in 1976, he commented bitterly to *The Quincy Herald-Whig* that "Vietnam is old hat
now. Everybody's forgotten about it." The same article mentioned
Virgil's "pride" in his son "Michael, at 21 following in his father's
footsteps with the military as a sergeant with the Marine Corps."

It is ironic that in his last years, Virgil looked to Michael as a
source of paternal pride. For he had almost no contact with him or

his other sons, and had had only sporadic involvement with them as children. The family moved sixteen times in the course of Virgil's military career, from Washington State, to Fort Benning, Georgia, to Fort Worth, Texas, to San Francisco. From 1968 to 1975, the stretch when Virgil served in Vietnam, the family lived in Quincy, where Michael entered junior high school. Virgil visited once every six months, and then seemed only too eager to return to Southeast Asia. A photo from his time in Vietnam shows him relaxed and smiling, sunbathing on a webbed lounge chair outside his trailer with a drink in hand.

When he did spend time with the family, he ruled with military precision. When the boys were young and the family was living at Fort Benning, he trained them to march in formation, salute, and execute military commands. Whenever visitors came to the spacious house reserved for the family because of John Virgil's rank as an officer, he put the boys through their paces, then dismissed them. He also enforced a disciplinary code derived from the military principle that an officer is responsible for the conduct of those he commands. In the Swango household, this meant that the oldest child was responsible for his younger brothers, so Bob was punished whenever Michael or John misbehaved. (Dick, Muriel's oldest son from her prior marriage, had left to live with his father, in part to escape the rigors of life with Virgil.) But the actual punishment was usually delegated to Muriel, except on a few occasions—such as the time Bob stole $10 from his father, or when he referred to an officer named Maloney as Baloney—when Virgil whipped Bob with a belt. Michael, on the other hand, was never subject to corporal punishment, nor was John. Still, all the boys were afraid of their father.

Muriel herself had little stomach for discipline, which tended to flag whenever Virgil was away. One day at Fort Benning the boys returned home to find her sobbing, slumped over the kitchen table. It was the first time any of them had seen her cry. When they asked what was wrong, she explained that a colonel who lived next door had berated her for "letting your children run wild." The boys rode their bikes and roamed the neighborhood unsupervised, and while watching professional wrestling on TV, Bob and Mike often wrestled, too, which sometimes threatened to get out of hand.

But the boys were no more unruly than most children their

age, and despite the neighbor's criticism, Muriel seemed determined to be a good mother. She read to the children, helped with their homework, created math problems for them. She belonged to the Book-of-the-Month Club and was always giving them books. (She especially loved mysteries and true-crime thrillers.) Muriel did her best to maintain a routine of family meals. Thanks to Virgil's military salary and the low cost of living, the family was well provided for, and the boys were clean and neatly dressed.

At the same time, Muriel was oddly distant emotionally. Virgil's sister, Louise Scharf, and her husband lived with the Swangos for a while in Quincy, and later visited them at Fort Benning. They rarely saw Muriel kiss or hug any of the boys or display any other affection toward them. Nor did they ever see her cry. When Virgil's handsome, popular, much younger brother Robert died suddenly of kidney failure at age twenty-four, emotionally devastating the Swango family, Muriel shed no tears at the funeral, even though she had been close to her brother-in-law. (She named Michael's older brother Bob after him.) Louise had worked in Quincy as a waitress at the Dug-Out, a popular restaurant where Muriel and her first husband, Richard Kerkering, often went out for dinner. Muriel struck Louise as very reserved and formal in her demeanor.

At Christmas, none of the boys' presents were ever wrapped. Muriel simply put them in paper bags, which she stapled shut. When the boys clamored for a pet, Muriel said no, citing their father's allergic reaction to animal hair. But the children never saw any evidence of such allergies. When Michael was in first grade, the boys were given a rabbit for Easter. It lived in a chicken-wire cage behind the house for two weeks, until a neighbor's dog got into the cage and ate it.

The Swango clan, most of them gregarious and affectionate by nature, generally found Muriel and Virgil's home cold and inhospitable, but they chalked it up to Muriel's upbringing. Muriel's father, John Strubhart, was a barber in tiny Breese, Illinois, due east of St. Louis. Of German background, he was a strict disciplinarian who maintained a stereotypically Teutonic distance from Muriel and her sister. And Muriel's failed first marriage to Richard Kerkering, who turned out to be a heavy drinker, had done nothing to bolster any inclination toward warmth or intimacy.

Virgil met Muriel near the end of World War II, when he was

home on leave. She was recently divorced and working as the office manager for the Swango family physician. A slender, attractive brunette, she had been raised a Catholic, but never attended church or said much about religion. Virgil was tall, handsome, solidly built, sociable, and had worked for his father in the recorder of deeds' office before joining the Army.

At the end of the war, Virgil, who held the rank of captain and was serving in Korea, was among the American signatories to the Japanese surrender. He had been married twice before, both times briefly, and had a daughter from his first marriage. He wrote his second wife from Korea to tell her he wanted a divorce; she was devastated by the unexpected news. He had another girlfriend at the time, but after meeting Muriel, he courted her assiduously; they were married in 1947. A few years later, he returned to Korea. Virgil was away when Bob was born, in 1950, and Muriel moved back to Breese to live with her parents until her husband returned in 1953. The family moved to Fort Lewis in Tacoma, Washington, where Michael was born in 1954, and then to Fort Richardson near Anchorage, Alaska, where John was born. Snapshots from Alaska show an apparently happy, laughing young family in a snowy landscape, with Bob and Michael on miniature skis. After three years there, Virgil was transferred to Fort Benning.

In later years, Muriel and Virgil never said anything about their romance and courtship or early years together. Bob sometimes compared his parents to the prim Ward and June Cleaver on *Leave It to Beaver*, a television show the family watched. Muriel and Virgil slept in twin beds and there were no signs of physical affection between them. Not even the boys ever saw them kiss or trade affectionate hugs. Still, they always assumed their parents were happily married. The only mention of sex came when Bob was in the eighth grade. Virgil took him aside and in serious tones told him it was time "to teach you the blood lines." Though Bob waited expectantly, that was all his father ever had to say on the subject.

Despite living in far-flung military outposts, the Swangos stayed in touch with their families in Breese and Quincy. Although the boys pleaded for trips to Disneyland or a national park, visits to relatives constituted the family's only vacations. Until Virgil left for Vietnam, every summer he loaded the family and their luggage into a station wagon and they set out for visits to the grandparents. The boys were lodged in the rear of the unair-conditioned car for what seemed like unending treks across the sweltering Southern or Plains states. Their parents sat in the front seat, chain-smoking. Virgil ran the expeditions like military maneuvers, barking orders at the boys, rejecting pleas to visit tourist attractions along the route or to make brief stops, even to use a rest room. They stopped only when he deemed it appropriate. On these trips, he referred to Muriel as "the navigator."

When Virgil returned from Vietnam in 1963, after his first tour there, he was assigned to teach military science in the ROTC program at Texas Christian University in Fort Worth, and the family moved to Texas. But Virgil, plainly chafing at his classroom assignment, eagerly volunteered to return to Vietnam less than a year later. The family moved back to Quincy. Then, in 1966, Virgil was transferred from Vietnam to San Francisco, where the family lived at the Presidio. After nearly twenty-six years, his Army career was winding down, and it was clear he would soon be retiring with a generous pension. But he made little pretense of any interest in the family. Even though he was now back in the United States, with a routine desk job, he was out late almost every night, and Muriel and the boys rarely saw him.

One evening Bob, Michael, and John were watching TV and doing their homework when their father returned. They heard their mother confront him. "Why are you never home?" she angrily demanded. Some kind of argument ensued, with shouting, that left Muriel in tears. Virgil stormed out of the house. The boys were shocked. This was only the second time they had ever heard their mother weep, and they had never seen her openly angry at their father. They thought maybe their parents would divorce. But nothing more was ever said, and in September 1967, after Virgil was promoted to full colonel and almost immediately announced his retirement, the family returned to Quincy. They moved into a spacious new ranch-style brick house on Maple Street. Michael entered the seventh grade at Quincy Junior High School.

Virgil talked vaguely about entering politics, but he had barely settled in when he joined the U.S. Agency for International Development (AID) and studied briefly at the Foreign Service Institute in Washington, D.C. He flew to Vietnam, arriving in Saigon on December 30, 1967, just in time for the Tet offensive, beginning January 30, 1968. On February 1, 1968, Nguyen Ngoc Loan, a Vietnamese national police commander, executed a Viet Cong insurgent in downtown Saigon in full view of an NBC crew, an AP photographer, and some American officials. The resulting photograph, which won a Pulitzer Prize and became one of the most enduring images of the war, shows Nguyen holding a pistol inches from the head of the prisoner, who stands with his hands tied behind his back. Virgil Swango kept a copy of the photograph for the rest of his life, and made a point of showing it to Michael. He may have witnessed the execution, since he was in Saigon at the time.

After a few weeks in Saigon, Swango was assigned to Go Cong province as a senior adviser to CORDS, or Civil Operations and Revolutionary Development Support. Go Cong province, located in the Mekong Delta south of Saigon, is often cited as one of the few successful U.S. efforts at "pacification" of the Vietnamese countryside. The fertile rice-growing area experienced relatively few combat operations.

A photograph from the period shows Colonel Swango escorting visiting American defense secretary Melvin Laird; in another snapshot, he is with South Vietnamese president Nguyen Van Thieu. Swango was also close to the American military adviser John Paul Vann, the subject of Neil Sheehan's Pulitzer Prize–winning book *A Bright Shining Lie.* The two had fought together at the pivotal battle of Ap Bac in 1963, a significant early defeat for the American and South Vietnamese forces. In 1970, Vann shifted Swango to Chau Doc province, noting that since Go Cong had been successfully pacified, Swango "must be bored."

While the full history of AID's involvement in Vietnam remains murky, the CORDS operation embraced both military and civilian operations. During Swango's tenure, CORDS was staffed in part by CIA agents, many with military backgrounds. The CIA also ran the Phoenix Program, a "pacification" project that overlapped and sometimes merged with CORDS operations until 1969, when responsibility for Phoenix was transferred to the military. The Phoenix Program gained notoriety for torturing and executing suspected Viet Cong agents operating in the South. Bob and Michael later told others that their father was in the CIA and served in the Phoenix Program—"murdering people and burning villages," as antiwar Bob described it—but while he surely would have known the extent of CIA activity and counterinsurgency operations in his region, there's nothing to suggest that Virgil was directly involved. On the contrary, his colleagues and friends in Vietnam at the time say that Swango was a bona fide AID official who oversaw agriculture and civilian development projects and believed passionately in the American cause.

In 1972, Virgil Swango prepared a lengthy report on his activities in Vietnam, which is relentlessly optimistic and, with benefit of hindsight, almost touchingly naive. "While Free World Military forces battle the enemy with guns and grenades," he wrote, "there is an equally vital, if less publicized, battle underway. No less than 40 nations of the Free World are involved in this battle—the struggle against hunger, poverty, ignorance and fear. Each success in this field makes the enemy's appeal weaker, and makes the job of the fighting man easier."

To his colleagues in Vietnam, Virgil made no mention of a family in Quincy. He lived in a mobile home decorated with knick-knacks he'd picked up during vacations in Southeast Asia. One plaque quoted the chronically inebriated W. C. Fields: "Water? Who drinks water? Fish fuck in it!" There were no family photographs. Virgil drank heavily and liked to socialize with colleagues. They knew he had been married more than once, but not that he still had a wife or children.

Perhaps the reason for his silence was that he was living with a Vietnamese woman. According to a family member in Quincy in whom he confided, he had fallen in love. He made brief, sporadic visits to Muriel and the boys only out of a sense of duty. After he was featured on the *NBC Nightly News* in 1972, the *Herald-Whig* ran a brief article about his being on TV. Interviewed by the paper, Muriel said she hadn't known he was going to be on television and hadn't seen the program.

Back in Quincy, there was almost a sense of relief among his sons that Virgil had returned to Vietnam for what seemed an indefinite stay. Since the incident at the Presidio, relations between husband and wife had been even cooler than usual. On his visits home he seemed restless and eager to return. He told his wife and sons little about his life or activities in Vietnam. He maintained that disclosing details of his work, even to his family, would be a breach of security, but his reticence may have fostered the boys' speculation that he was engaged in violent CIA-directed exploits. As the boys grew older and more independent, they increasingly resented their father's military strictures.

Once they moved back to Quincy, the semblance of a family life steadily eroded. Muriel gave up on the family meal, preferring to spend her evening hours bowling or playing bridge with friends—two activities she pursued avidly. She left a supply of TV dinners in the freezer, and the boys simply heated their own meals whenever they wanted, almost never sitting down together. One Thanksgiving she baked a turkey and made rolls, but then seemed to give up, for there was nothing else on the table.

When Muriel was home, she spent her time with Michael, listening to him play the piano or clarinet, typing his homework, or discussing the mysteries and thrillers that she loved and that he had begun to read almost as avidly. As early as the sixth grade, Michael had been a reader of true-crime magazines and comic books, as had Bob. But Bob soon moved on to science fiction, whereas Michael began buying copies of the *National Enquirer,* scanning its pages for sensational crime stories. He clipped some of the articles, and Muriel helped him assemble them into a scrapbook.

Bob and John began to feel left out. Whatever love their mother could muster for her children seemed to be allocated disproportionately to Michael. Only he received the music lessons, the expensive clarinet, the private-school education. But not even Michael received motherly hugs or kisses. Muriel seemed incapable of expressing any physical affection. Bob and John increasingly sought emotional contact and a family life outside their home, and were all but adopted as surrogate sons by their friends' parents. Bob dressed in tie-dyed overalls, let his hair grow, and hung out with hippies. Though Michael seemed to have a few close friends in high school, he seemed content, even eager, to stay at home with their mother whenever she was there.

Michael's aunts, Louise Scharf and Ruth Miller, and other relatives were concerned about Muriel's blatant favoritism toward

Michael. But she always defended it, saying Michael was much smarter than the other boys, was gifted, and needed special attention. Louise and Ruth disagreed. Michael was undeniably smart and talented, but so were Bob and John. Virgil's sisters thought Michael was arrogant and rude, in part because he was spoiled by his mother. Once when relatives were visiting the Swango home, some from out of town, Michael entered the living room, looked them over briefly, then went to his room without so much as saying hello.

On another occasion, Muriel mentioned to Ruth and Louise that Michael had wrecked his car. "What happened?" they asked.

Muriel said, "I don't know."

"What do you mean you don't know?"

"He didn't tell me, and I didn't ask," she replied.

After Bob left home, Muriel complained to Ruth that she'd had to hire a yardman because Michael didn't want to mow the lawn. "If I had a strapping young man like you do at home, I certainly wouldn't hire someone" was Ruth's indignant reaction. Yet Muriel seemed indifferent to their concerns. As the family members said on many occasions, for Muriel "the sun rose and set" in Michael.

Given Virgil's work in Vietnam and devotion to the American cause, Bob's dress, friends, and increasingly antiwar politics were bound to cause trouble. Muriel expressed no views of her own on the Vietnam conflict, saying only, "Your dad's there so you should support him." But Bob and Virgil argued violently on his rare visits home and grew increasingly estranged. Muriel worried that Bob's views would influence Michael and John, and that further conflict might erupt in the already fractured family.

Bob graduated early from high school and enrolled for his freshman year at Quincy College. In the spring of 1970, he wrote his father a letter reiterating his opposition to the war and concluding, "How can you call yourself a Christian, doing what you're doing to these people?" He showed the letter to his mother. "You can't send that," she protested. "It will really upset him." Despite the warning, Bob posted the letter.

Several days later, Muriel told Bob that his father was flying home to see him. When Virgil arrived after the twenty-two-hour flight, he met with Bob alone, grim-faced and determined. Virgil said his son was nothing but a "Commie fag," gave him $20, and ordered him out of the house. He had paid for one night at a downtown hotel, after which Bob would receive no financial support and would be on his own.

Bob vacated the house as ordered. His brothers seemed stunned into silence. Michael didn't even say good-bye. Muriel showed no emotion at his departure, saying only that it had been his father's decision, and it was his duty to accept it. The next morning, less than twenty-four hours after arriving, Virgil left for Vietnam.

Bob lived with friends in Quincy and then with his half-brother Richard in Florida for the summer. The following fall, Muriel relented and, without telling Virgil, let Bob live at home temporarily while he continued his studies at Quincy College. She also paid his tuition. But after his sophomore year he dropped out and hitchhiked to Oregon, leaving home this time for good. Bob never saw his father again, nor did he see Michael until Virgil's funeral.

In the tumultuous waning days of America's involvement in Vietnam, Virgil was placed in charge of evacuating the cities of Nha Trang and Qui Nhon. North Vietnamese troops had cut off the road from Nha Trang to the airport, so Americans, anticommunist Vietnamese, and foreign nationals had to be moved by military helicopters, which were mobbed by panicking refugees. In his nomination for an Award for Valor, Swango was cited for "courage, coolness and discipline . . . that brought the crowd under control and prevented deaths, injuries, and damage to the helicopters." He was nonetheless unable to evacuate the woman with whom he had been living; she stayed behind in the Delta. "I left Vietnam in 1975 with only my boots, pants, shirt, and glasses," he later said.

After the evacuation, Virgil retired from the State Department and returned home to an America bitter about the war and indifferent to its veterans. Despite the nomination, no medal ever materialized. Virgil confided in his sisters, Ruth and Louise, that he was bored with being a husband and father. Relations with Muriel remained strained, and the tensions culminated in the fight that caused Muriel to order him out of the house. Within a year of Virgil's return from Vietnam, she was granted a formal separation, though divorce proceedings were later suspended. Michael made some attempts at getting his parents to reconcile, but to no avail. Virgil moved into a mobile home that oddly replicated his quarters in Vietnam. One of his close friends from the war called him there from his bachelor party in Washington, D.C., to include Swango in the festivities. Virgil seemed touched by the gesture but wrapped in loneliness.

Swango spent his last years drinking Jack Daniel's whiskey, chain-smoking cigarettes, and reading books about Vietnam. He was mugged at gunpoint one night outside the Plaza, a popular Quincy restaurant and bar. Increasingly infirm from cirrhosis of the liver, he moved into the Illinois Veterans Home the year before he died. He was bitter over the American defeat and his reception as a Vietnam veteran. When the *Herald-Whig* interviewed him for a 1979 retrospective on the conflict, he maintained that "the war was lost in Washington . . . the enemy was aided and abetted by the anti-war attitude and knew it would eventually lead to victory. . . . We came home the losers when we could have been the winners.

"In World War II," he continued, "the GIs came home to open arms. Their jobs and sweethearts were waiting. They were heroes. In Vietnam, nothing like that happened. They came home to people who somehow blamed them for the war."

AFTER Virgil's funeral, Muriel discovered a box of books and papers that had belonged to her husband, and in it she found a scrapbook of articles and photographs of car crashes, disasters, and other incidents of violent death. Knowing he would be interested, Muriel later gave the scrapbook to Michael. "I guess my dad wasn't such a bad guy after all," he said.

Michael had had a fascination for articles about violent death since childhood, when he began clipping *National Enquirer* articles. He dutifully clipped articles and photographs and entered them into an ever-expanding library of scrapbooks, which probably explains why his classmates at Millikin noticed an interest in car crashes. Sometimes, when he was busy, his mother clipped and pasted the articles into the books for him. Ruth Miller thought this peculiar; she once asked Muriel why she kept articles on such grisly subjects for Michael. Muriel just shrugged and said that Michael had asked her to clip and save anything about violent death. "Mike likes to keep up on these things," she explained, presumably in connection with his work in emergency medicine.

Working with America Ambulance in Springfield brought Swango into regular contact with victims of car crashes, heart attacks, and violent crime. His fellow paramedics, many of whom thought highly of his work, nonetheless noted his unusual fascination with violent death, and were familiar with the scrapbooks. They often saw him cutting out the articles while waiting for an ambulance call. Once, a coworker asked him why he clipped and saved the articles. "If I'm ever accused of murder," he replied, the scrapbooks "will prove I'm not mentally competent. This will be my defense." No one took this seriously.

Absent his fixation on violent death, it is hard to understand why he commuted to Springfield during his first year of medical school, and worked up to twenty-four-hour shifts during his second and third years, crowded with clinical and academic demands, for a job that paid ten cents above the minimum wage. Swango told fellow paramedics that he could maintain such a schedule because he subsisted on only two to three hours of sleep a night. Indeed, colleagues in the ambulance service were amazed that Swango would sleep only thirty minutes, then jump up and work for twelve hours straight, almost manic with energy. They'd never seen anything like it.

Even so, his work on the ambulance crew increasingly took a toll. He became so angry one day that he kicked in a cabinet door in the kitchen area of the ambulance headquarters. (He had to pay for it.) His long hours also affected his performance as a medical student. Whereas he had prepared feverishly during his first year, some of his fellow students now found him ill-prepared, careless, and hasty to the point of negligence, always rushing from one class or task to another, interrupting his work whenever his pager indicated he was needed for an ambulance run. Still, when it came time to apply for internships and residencies, Swango secured a glowing letter of recommendation from Dr. Wacaser, the neurosurgeon who had been his mentor, which he sent to about ten teaching hospitals. Wacaser inscribed a handwritten addendum to each copy of the letter—"He'll really do a good job for you"—the only time Wacaser had gone to such lengths for one of his students.

Much as they do in applying to medical school, graduating medical students apply for internships and residencies through the

Association of American Medical Colleges in Washington, D.C., which forwards applications to teaching hospitals with openings. After the initial screening of applications, hospitals winnow the field and conduct personal interviews with candidates who seem attractive. Then they rank the candidates, returning the list to the national match program, which then compares the applicant's preferences with the hospital rankings.

Every year, the third Wednesday in March is known in medical schools nationwide as Match Day.* At noon, Eastern Standard Time, students and hospitals all over the country learn whether they have gotten their first-choice internships and candidates. It's possible for a student to receive no match at all. Though pleased, even Wacaser was surprised when Swango told him that he had been accepted for an especially prestigious internship in neurosurgery at the University of Iowa Hospitals and Clinics in Iowa City. Given that SIU's medical school was not especially well known, had no recognized neurosurgery program of its own and no nationally known surgeons to serve as mentors, and awarded only pass-fail grades, Swango's success was hard to fathom even apart from the fact that most of his classmates thought he was weird and incompetent. It was especially galling to Sweeney, the other classmate specializing in neurosurgery, and to Rosenthal, who remained the most vocal of Swango's student critics.

With his postgraduate career seemingly secure, Swango all but gave up any pretense of interest in his medical studies and indulged his growing fascination with the car crashes and emergencies he encountered on the ambulance crew. All that remained at SIU was his eight-week rotation in obstetrics and gynecology, a requirement that most students completed before their last year and that they had to pass (as they did all mandatory rotations) in order to graduate. Rather than take OB/GYN early, Swango had opted for the more difficult surgery and medicine rotations, and was already concentrating on neurosurgery.

In the OB/GYN rotation, students were assigned to spend one week observing an OB/GYN doctor in the community—in Swango's case, Dr. Robert Prentice. This was the doctor's first ex-

* The day of the week was changed to Thursday in 1998.

perience with an SIU student, and the school was eager for Swango to make a favorable impression. But he didn't show up.

Students were also required to attend OB/GYN surgeries, such as cesarean deliveries and hysterectomies. Swango was again absent. All examinations in the rotation were conducted orally. Swango missed most of them.

Dr. Kathleen O'Connor was the chief resident in OB/GYN at the SIU hospitals, in charge of overseeing Swango's work. An SIU graduate herself, in her fourth and last year of residency at Springfield, she became increasingly dismayed by Swango's disregard of the school's requirements. When she tried to locate him, she was told he was working as an emergency medical technician. She also heard that he had been restricted in his activities at the ambulance corps: He'd been banned from any direct patient contact, though she wasn't told why.

O'Connor found this odd, but she was less concerned about Swango's performance as an EMT than she was about his absence from the rotation. When she finally caught up with him, she asked him to perform a history and physical on a patient who was scheduled to undergo a cesarean delivery. She saw him enter the patient's room, and leave ten minutes later. Thus she was somewhat surprised when he promptly turned in an impressively thorough three-page write-up.

Given that he had spent a mere ten minutes with the patient, the carefully written report was perhaps too complete and polished, and it raised doubts in O'Connor's mind. She visited the patient to inquire about Swango's visit, and learned that the woman had barely talked to Swango. He hadn't conducted any physical examination; he'd never even touched her.

Stunned, O'Connor concluded that the entire three-page report was either a fabrication, a plagiarism from an earlier H & P by a resident, or a combination of the two. She had never encountered such behavior by a student.

O'Connor took her findings to the full OB/GYN faculty, which hastily convened a departmental meeting to consider Swango's status. The faculty members were appalled and angry at Swango's brazen misconduct and dishonesty, which very well might have posed a threat to a patient's health. They determined to fail Swango,

which meant he wouldn't graduate and wouldn't be with his classmates at the June graduation ceremony, now less than a month
away. The department's determination also automatically triggered
a hearing on Swango before the Student Progress Committee, one
of whose members, William Roddick, happened to be chairman of
the OB/GYN department.

WHEN Swango learned that he was going to fail OB/GYN and
wouldn't graduate, he was enraged, though outwardly he remained
calm and confident. He hired a lawyer; administrators worried he
would sue the school.

   While the details were confidential, word that Swango had
failed his OB/GYN rotation and was going to be brought before the
Student Progress Committee coursed through the school, causing
passionate divisions among students and faculty. Wacaser rallied to
Swango's defense, saying that he had been an "outstanding" student
and that charges he was lazy or hadn't done his assignments were
not believable. To fail him in the OB/GYN clerkship would be "dis-
graceful," he maintained. Dr. Murphy, Swango's professor of
pathology and toxicology, became so worked up in a conversation
with the dean over the injustice of Swango's plight that he burst into
tears. At least a few students also argued that to bar Swango from
graduating was too severe a punishment. It is a paradox of the medical profession that while medical schools reject hundreds and thousands of applicants, thereby dashing long-held hopes of a medical
career, they almost never expel them once they've been admitted.

   But the turn of events also precipitated action on the part of
Rosenthal and five of his classmates, now more outraged over
Swango than ever. Rosenthal drafted a letter to the Student Progress
Committee, urging the extreme measure that Swango be expelled.
The shared experience of the rigors of medical school ordinarily
creates a strong bond among classmates, one that can last a lifetime.
Thus, the letter was an extraordinary step for a group of students to
take against a classmate. The students' letter wasn't so much triggered by the OB/GYN situation, or even the mysterious deaths
that seemed to follow Swango, as by a more general sense that he
was incompetent. He hadn't progressed at all during their years together; he showed no interest in any patients; his attitude toward

medical education seemed to border on contempt. None of the group felt they would ever want Swango to be their doctor. He was not, in their view, capable of functioning as an intern. Time was running out, and Rosenthal and the others felt that he had to be stopped.

It was in this highly charged atmosphere that the Student Progress Committee convened in May 1982. Ten committee members were present, two students and eight faculty. Besides Roddick, they included Dr. Murphy and a member of Swango's class, David Chapman, who knew Rosenthal and was familiar with the letter. The immediate mandate of the committee was to review Swango's failing grade in the OB/GYN clerkship, but because of the nature of the evidence, the letter from Rosenthal, and Chapman's urging, the committee decided to consider expelling Swango.

In preparation for the hearing, Kathleen O'Connor had gone to the patient files to retrieve Swango's report on the cesarean delivery patient. It had vanished. It suddenly occurred to her that other reports by Swango had been suspiciously thorough as well. She quickly looked for some of them in the files. They, too, were missing.

O'Connor reported this to the committee. She also testified about Swango's performance in the OB/GYN rotation, detailing his frequent absences and presenting the evidence suggesting he had fabricated at least one patient's history and physical, and perhaps others.

Other allegations, some contained in the Rosenthal letter and others contributed by student members of the committee, also surfaced: the "Swangoing," other incidents of cursory or fabricated H & P's, his dubious performance in several classes, his work as an emergency medical technician, and his fascination with violence. But there was no reference to any suspicious patient deaths or to the "Double-O Swango" nickname. That still seemed a joke, too far-fetched to be true.

Swango appeared on his own behalf. He was at his most earnest and charming. He denied that he had failed to examine any patients or had removed any files. He denied plagiarizing or fabricating the cesarean patient's H & P. Almost tearfully, he explained that he had no choice but to moonlight as an emergency medical

technician because his father had died earlier that year, and he was
virtually the sole support of his mother and two brothers. And he
argued that not allowing him to graduate with the class would be a
terrible hardship, since he would lose his coveted internship at the
University of Iowa.

Most members of the committee, especially the two student
members, were unmoved. Roddick flatly called Swango a "bald-
faced liar" and said that alone was sufficient grounds to expel him.

But Dr. Murphy rallied to Swango's defense. Murphy had
grown up in a large family, and he felt that competing with his siblings had given him an instinctive sympathy for the underdog. His
father had also died recently. He understood and sympathized with
Swango's need to support his family, and he felt other students in
the class were unfairly picking on him simply because he was different. Swango had been his student, and while his performance had
not been exceptional, Murphy found it entirely adequate, better
than that of some other students who were going to graduate. At
one point in the debate Murphy turned to Chapman, who was arguing strenuously for Swango's dismissal, and said, "Your whole class
is full of goof-offs and jerks. Why pick on him?"

Murphy had done some investigation of his own. From the
records department of the maternity ward, he told the committee,
he'd learned that at about the time Swango was supposedly examin-
ing the cesarean patient, another doctor had asked that student
comments be expunged from patient records. That, he argued,
might explain the absence of any entry by Swango on the patient's
chart and the disappearance of the files.

But no one investigated Swango's emotional claim that he was
supporting his widowed mother and family. In fact, Muriel had a
well-paid job as business manager at the Casino Lanes bowling alley
and received a pension as the widow of a military and Foreign Service officer; she was helping to pay for Michael's medical school education.

When the deliberations ended, the committee took its vote, on
which all Swango's hopes to become a medical doctor rested. Any
decision to dismiss a student required unanimity. Eight members
voted to expel Swango. One abstained. And one—Dr. Murphy—
voted to give him another chance.

• •

DESPITE the outcome of the committee vote, serious concerns had
been raised about Swango's character and fitness to practice medicine. Even Dr. Murphy agreed that some form of punishment was
warranted, and that Swango's record should reflect what had happened. The dean and several faculty members went so far as to consult several psychiatrists, who advised them that if Swango really
suffered from a significant character disorder, as some testimony
suggested, or was a habitual liar, as most committee members had
concluded, he would not be able to conceal these traits if he was
placed under close scrutiny.

It was one thing to fail Swango on the basis of certain objective
criteria for a course, but the school worried that it would be difficult to defend any action taken on the basis of relatively vague concerns about his character—especially in light of the fact that
Swango had a lawyer. A series of negotiations ensued between SIU's
lawyers and Swango's lawyer, and a compromise was reached that
averted litigation. Swango would not be allowed to graduate with
his class. But neither would he be expelled or asked to withdraw. He
would be required to repeat his OB/GYN rotation. He would also
be given assignments from some of the faculty's strictest professors
in other specialties, all of them aware of the allegations against him.
If he passed these assignments, he would be allowed to graduate. If
not, he would be dismissed.

IN Quincy, Muriel Swango had been looking forward to her son's
graduation for weeks, mentioning it to friends and relatives. Though
she was careful about expenses, she bought a new dress for the occasion. To Louise Scharf and Ruth Miller, Mike's graduation seemed to
fulfill all Muriel's hopes and to validate the attention she had lavished
on him throughout the often lonely and painful years of her marriage.

Muriel was nervous about making the two-hour highway drive
to Springfield alone, so she asked Ruth to accompany her. Ruth was
thrilled. No member of the family had ever received a medical degree. After the graduation ceremony, Muriel planned to host a dinner in Mike's honor, and had invited Ruth, Louise, and Louise's
grandson, who was living in Springfield, to join them at the motel
where Muriel and Ruth would be spending the night.

Louise, too, was excited about the occasion, though more for Muriel than for Mike. Her nephew had been studying and working in Springfield for two years, but he hadn't visited or even called, and she'd seen him only once. She had been visiting a friend in the hospital, and saw Mike in the corridor, wearing his paramedic jacket. She called out, but he didn't respond, instead quickly walking in the other direction. She was sure he had seen her.

The day before the graduation, the Springfield *State Journal-Register* ran a list of all the graduates, and Louise eagerly scanned it for Mike's name. There was no Swango. She looked over the entire list again, just to make sure. Mike's name was missing.

Louise called Ruth in Quincy. Ruth in turn spoke to Muriel. Michael had said nothing to his mother about the troubles of the preceding weeks, and certainly nothing to indicate that he might not graduate. Ruth called Louise back, saying the newspaper must have made a typographical error. "Well, I'm not so sure," Louise told her. "Maybe you should double-check." But Muriel and Ruth were determined to be there to see Michael graduate. Because of Muriel's concerns about highway driving, they rose at dawn so they could drive at a leisurely pace and still arrive in plenty of time.

The SIU medical school class of 1982 graduated on June 5, 1982. Michael Swango was absent. Because he failed to graduate, the University of Iowa withdrew its offer of an internship. Some of his classmates, especially Rosenthal, were jubilant—mostly because they were graduating, but also because they felt their campaign to block Swango had at least partly succeeded.

After the ceremony, Dr. Murphy, whom Rosenthal had especially admired, followed him off the stage and into the hallway. Rosenthal greeted him, expecting a slap on the back and some congratulations. Instead, Murphy lambasted him for his campaign against Swango. "If you'd spend half as much time worrying about your own performance as you do others," Murphy told him, "you might be the doctor you think you are."

When Louise arrived at the motel that evening for the celebratory graduation dinner, she knew immediately that something had gone wrong. Muriel looked ashen. Ruth was tight-lipped, but seemed to be fighting back tears. Louise sat down and they all ordered a drink. Then Muriel announced that Mike hadn't graduated with his class and that she and Ruth hadn't attended the ceremony. Just before leaving the motel, about an hour before the graduation, Michael had told her that because of a computer mix-up, he had inadvertently been dropped from the list of graduates. Whatever emotions she must have felt were held firmly in control. Muriel didn't express any shock or disappointment.

Louise found the explanation hard to believe, but Muriel said firmly that if Michael said so, then that was what had happened.

They waited, but Michael never showed up for dinner.

CHAPTER THREE

AFTER HIS BRUSH with expulsion, Swango was a model medical student. He dutifully repeated the OB/GYN rotation, attending all the required surgeries and oral examinations, and he acquitted himself satisfactorily in his other supervised assignments.

Dean Richard Moy had taken an additional step that he believed might put others on notice that SIU had experienced problems with Swango's performance. Every graduating medical student receives a "dean's letter," which reviews his or her strengths and weaknesses and is used in applications for internships, residencies, and other employment. Though another administrator usually drafted such letters, Dean Moy took a personal interest in Swango's. It was carefully written to call attention to the fact that he had not graduated with his class, that he had failed a rotation and been required to repeat it, and that there had been concern about his professional behavior. Given the school's anxiety about possible legal liability, this was as far as Moy felt the letter could go. He was confident that, at the least, it would cause a teaching hospital to call SIU for more explanation before admitting Swango for further training.

Yet on Match Day, March 16, 1983, Dr. William Hunt, director of the department of neurosurgery at Ohio State University in Columbus, offered Swango a residency in neurosurgery after the successful completion of a year's internship in general surgery to begin on July 1. That year, Ohio State, one of the most prestigious residency programs in the country, had received about sixty applicants for its neurosurgery residence program and had invited twelve for personal interviews, Swango among them. He was the only student finally offered a position. Swango's success seemed even more astounding than his offer from the University of Iowa had been the year before.

Michael Swango was graduated from SIU on April 12, 1983. Though there was no ceremony, he received his diploma in the mail, and Muriel spread the good news of his graduation and acceptance at Ohio State to family members. These developments lent credence to Michael's explanation that a computer glitch had postponed his graduation. No one questioned why it would have taken nearly a year to correct such an error. Nor did Michael mention to anyone in Quincy, let alone at Ohio State, that shortly after his graduation from SIU he was fired by America Ambulance.

Already on probation there because of his violent outbursts, Swango had responded to an emergency call in Rochester, Illinois, a small town close to Springfield. The patient, gasping for air and in acute pain, was suffering a heart attack. Swango's instructions were to administer any emergency treatment called for and then transport him in the ambulance to the nearest hospital. Instead, he made the patient walk to his own car and told the family to drive him to the hospital themselves. The patient survived, but the family called America Ambulance to complain about Swango. No one could explain his cavalier behavior. It was both medically unsound and a clear violation of the ambulance corps' rules. Swango offered no adequate explanation and was fired.

But Michael was no doubt indifferent to his dismissal now that he had graduated from SIU. He returned to Quincy and was promptly hired as a paramedic by the Adams County Ambulance Corps. He worked there for just three months, since he had to be in Columbus, Ohio, by July 1 to begin his internship.

ANNE Ritchie first met the new blond intern on the ninth floor of Rhodes Hall, one of the largest buildings in the Ohio State medical complex. She did a double-take. She thought he was handsome, with an athletic build and angular face, a very all-American look. But what struck her most was that he looked remarkably like her cousin's husband in Minnesota. The similarity was so pronounced that she checked the I.D. tag on his surgical jacket to see if there might be some family relation. That was why she remembered his name: Michael Swango.

Attractive, popular, and vivacious, Ritchie was the daughter of a physician, and had always wanted a career in health care. She loved working in the Ohio State Hospitals, even though as a "casual" or supplemental nurse, working two to four shifts a week whenever she was needed, she ranked fairly low. Swango didn't seem the least bit interested in his resemblance to her cousin, but Ritchie was accustomed to indifference on the part of doctors. At the Ohio State Hospitals, which maintained a rigid hierarchy among doctors, nurses, and other staff, nurses didn't speak to attending physicians unless specifically questioned by them. The physicians gave their instructions to residents and interns, who in turn passed them on to the nursing staff. Any questions or statements by the nurses were supposed to be directed either to the interns and residents for transmittal to attending physicians, or to their nurse supervisors.*

With over 50,000 students at the time Swango arrived, Ohio State is virtually a city unto itself; it even has its own police force and governance. The Ohio State University Medical Center is located just a few blocks from "the oval," the grassy center of the sprawling campus. After the Ohio State Buckeye football team, the medical center is the crown jewel of the giant state university. It has 1,123 beds and 4,278 employees, and university officials describe it as the second-largest teaching hospital program in the country (after the University of Iowa's). The hospitals sometimes vie for supremacy in Ohio with the prestigious Cleveland Clinic, the highly regarded Case Western Reserve University, also in Cleveland, and the University of Cincinnati. But its size and political clout—the university trustees are appointed by the governor, and the hospitals' board is a Who's Who of prominent Ohio business and civic leaders—usually ensure Ohio State's preeminence. Graduates of the medical school dominate Ohio's medical establishment and institutions.

So Swango joined an elite group of medical school graduates

---

* Ohio State denies that there is any rule or policy preventing nurses from initiating a conversation with attending physicians, but every nurse I interviewed insisted that such a practice prevailed.

for his first assignment as a surgical intern, which was in the emergency room. Given such competition, it didn't take long for some of his shortcomings to surface. Each doctor in charge of a surgical rotation evaluates the interns at the conclusion of the rotation, and Dr. Ronald Ferguson, the doctor in charge of transplant surgery, who oversaw Swango's work from mid-October until mid-November, told Dr. Hunt that he was going to fail Swango, and that he didn't believe he was competent to practice medicine.

While the details of Swango's performance have been shrouded in secrecy by Ohio State (the school has said only that nothing of a criminal nature was contained in Swango's evaluations), Ferguson complained specifically about Swango's brusque and indifferent manner with patients, his cursory H & P's—charges that echo the criticisms of his performance at SIU—and a general sense that Swango lacked the temperament and dedication necessary to be a doctor. Swango also alarmed at least one other of his supervising physicians with remarks suggesting a fascination with the Nazis and the Holocaust. (This fascination was noted in his student record.)

Some of the residents, who spent more time with Swango than the attending physicians did, also complained to doctors on the faculty that Swango was "weird." While making rounds, residents often give interns tasks and then critique their performance. Whenever they criticized Swango—as they often did, because of his incompetence—Swango would immediately drop to the floor and begin a strenuous set of push-ups. He could do hundreds of them. It was almost as if he were still in the Marines, and this was his self-imposed punishment. Of course, the residents thought his reaction not only peculiar but highly inappropriate for a doctor making rounds. Despite their admonitions, he persisted.

At the time Swango was hired, no one from Ohio State called anyone at SIU. Indeed, no one appears even to have noticed that he should have graduated from SIU a year earlier than he did. But now, troubled by the negative report from Ferguson and other comments about Swango's odd behavior, Dr. Hunt got on the phone to SIU's Howard Barrows, the associate dean for medical education. Barrows was in charge of student recommendations, including the dean's letters signed by Moy, and had helped draft Swango's. With an edge of annoyance, Hunt asked about Swango. "What kind of guy did you send us?"

Barrows said that Hunt should have seen plenty of warning flags in Swango's dean's letter. "Well," Hunt retorted, "I don't read dean's letters."

Barrows asked him if he'd kept the dean's letter in Swango's file, and Hunt said he'd check. Soon after, Hunt called back: he'd found the letter.

"Oh, my God," Hunt said. "You're right. You did tell me."

Still, no consideration seems to have been given to terminating Swango's internship. On January 14, 1984, Hunt met with Swango and warned him that he had received a failing evaluation from Dr. Ferguson that might threaten his residency. He reminded Swango that the offer of a residency in neurosurgery was contingent on successful completion of the one-year internship. Swango took the news calmly; he seemed suitably concerned and sincere in his desire to improve. He was sufficiently charming and contrite that Hunt helped him plot strategies for overcoming the negative review and continuing with his residency. Hunt recommended that Swango appeal Ferguson's evaluation to the Residency Review Committee, made up of doctors from the surgery department. Swango took him up on the suggestion, and the committee met later that month to reevaluate him.

RITCHIE and Swango didn't have much contact after their initial meeting, when she had examined his name tag, though she did talk fairly often to his new girlfriend: a fellow nurse named Rita Dumas, who also often worked in Rhodes Hall. The relationship surprised many on the nursing staff, because Dumas hardly seemed a catch for a promising and handsome young intern. She was reasonably attractive, but her personality had caused some of the other nurses to keep their distance. Divorced a few years before, with three young children, she was always complaining about something. She worked the night shift, returning home at seven in the morning, just as the children were awakening. She said she was never able to get enough sleep, which might have accounted for her often surly mood.

But she seemed transformed by the romance with Swango. Though she still kept mostly to herself, she acquired a new glow of confidence, and her attitude toward life seemed to improve. A few of the other nurses noted the changes with a touch of envy. Dumas had been going through a difficult period. Swango had been tender and supportive. He was wonderful with her children, and they loved it when he performed feats of juggling for them. She later said, "I do not think that I would have survived had Swango not been there for me."

On February 6, Anne Ritchie reported to Rhodes Hall for the morning shift, and was assigned to a neurosurgery patient in Room 968, named Ruth Barrick. Barrick was a pleasant, elderly woman who had been admitted to the hospital on January 17. She had fallen and hit her head at home ten days earlier and suffered a cerebral hematoma. Though her condition was serious, it had never been considered life-threatening until she suffered respiratory arrest and nearly died on January 31—just after Swango's appeal of his negative evaluation was rejected.

No one told Ritchie what had happened. But on January 31, another nurse, Deborah Kennedy, had given Barrick her breakfast and assessed her condition. The patient seemed to be doing well. She was sitting up in bed, talking, and responding to directions. At about 9:45 A.M., Dr. Swango had come into Barrick's room and told Kennedy, "I'm going to check on her." Kennedy thought this was peculiar, since doctors rounded at 6:30 A.M. and rarely returned unless there was a specific problem. In such cases, it was the attending physician, not an intern by himself, who would call on the patient. But Kennedy gave the matter little thought. She left Swango alone in the room with Barrick.

About twenty minutes later, Kennedy returned to check on Barrick. Swango was gone. Barrick was now reclining and seemed to be asleep, but when she drew close to the bedside, Kennedy was alarmed. Barrick was barely breathing. Her skin was taking on a bluish cast, a sign of imminent death from respiratory failure. Kennedy immediately called a code over the intercom, and doctors came rushing to the room. Swango was the first to respond, but others too began working to resuscitate her. After forty-five minutes Barrick's vital signs seemed to stabilize and she was transferred to intensive care. There she recovered without any evident lingering effects, and returned to her room.

At about eight A.M. on February 6, Ritchie gave Barrick a bath. The patient was alert, talking, cheerful, and seemed to be recovering. But Ritchie noticed that the central venous pressure (CVP) was low in the central line, an intravenous tube supplying medication to the major blood vessels. She called to ask that a doctor check the line, and then left the room to check other patients. A few minutes later, she saw Swango enter Barrick's room, remembered him as the new doctor who looked like her cousin, and felt relieved that an M.D. had responded to her call. Ritchie might have given the matter no further thought, but some time passed and she didn't see Swango emerge, which made her think that there might be a problem with the central line. This wasn't unusual, because the central line, connected as it is to the major blood vessels, often requires some delicate work if a blockage occurs, and there is a particular risk of air getting into the tube, which can be fatal. So Ritchie went back into Barrick's room to see if Swango needed help.

Swango had drawn the curtains entirely around Barrick's bed, which meant that neither Barrick's roommate nor anyone passing the room's open door could see what was happening. Ritchie found this odd. She stuck her head through the curtains. Swango was hovering over Barrick's chest area and seemed startled. "Do you need any help?" she asked cheerfully. "No," Swango replied. Ritchie left.

Ten minutes later, concerned that Swango still hadn't finished, Ritchie entered the room, saw the closed curtains, and again asked if Swango needed any help. He said he didn't. Three minutes later, Ritchie returned, opened the curtain, and looked in. This time she saw that Swango was using two or three syringes. One was stuck directly into the central line. Another was resting on Swango's shoulder, as if he was waiting to insert it whenever the other syringe had emptied. Had Swango simply been using the syringes to clear the line, there should have been blood in them. But there was no blood. Swango again said he needed no assistance and Ritchie left the room.

Just a few minutes later, Ritchie saw Swango finally leave. "Good," she thought to herself. "That's finally over." Whatever was wrong with Barrick's line had evidently been corrected. Almost immediately—no more than ten seconds had elapsed— she went back into the room to check Barrick's dressing where the central line entered the body.

Ritchie was stunned. Barrick had turned blue. She gave one terrifying shudder and gasp, then stopped breathing. Ritchie screamed "Code Blue! Code Blue!" then began mouth-to-mouth resuscitation, desperately trying to get breath into Barrick's lungs. She looked up and saw Dr. Swango coolly watching her from the back of the room, doing nothing to assist her or the patient. "That is so disgusting," Swango said of her efforts at mouth-to-mouth resuscitation, his voice tinged with contempt.

Still in shock, Ritchie stared at him in disbelief. "You jerk!" she shouted, before returning frantically to the patient. Other nurses and doctors rushed in and began chest compression, to no avail.

Ruth Barrick was dead.

The last entry in Barrick's "physician progress notes" was made by Swango and dated February 6 at eleven A.M.:

PT [patient] suffered apparent respiratory arrest witnessed by R.N. No pulse present, Code Blue called at 10:25 hrs. PT did not respond to resuscitative measures . . . pronounced dead at 10:49. Dr. Joseph Goodman and family notified per Dr. Arlo Brakel.

Swango.

The death certificate cited the cause of death as "a. Cardiopulmonary arrest, due to, b. Cerebrovascular accident," a stroke in lay terms.

Ritchie was astounded and appalled when Swango insisted he wanted personally to convey the news of Barrick's death to her family members. (She later saw him leading relatives into a private room.) And she could hardly believe what she had witnessed. She was almost certain that something Swango had done had killed Barrick. Still, it never crossed her mind that he might have killed her deliberately. She assumed that he had accidentally allowed an air pocket to enter the central line, causing a fatal embolism in the bloodstream. Such accidents did sometimes happen, which was one of the reasons only doctors were allowed to adjust central lines. But why hadn't Swango acknowledged the error? Why had he acted as he did? And what was he doing with those syringes?

These troubling questions were still swirling in Ritchie's mind

that afternoon when she responded to an urgent call in another
room. The head nurse, Amy Moore, was with a patient who was
having serious trouble breathing. Ritchie was alarmed to see that
Swango was also in the room. With the patient gasping for breath,
he ordered Ritchie to fetch a heart monitor.

Moore seemed incredulous: Using a heart monitor would take
valuable time. "We don't need a heart monitor to check her lungs!"
she exclaimed. It was rare for a nurse to defy a doctor, but the
patient's condition plainly suggested blood clots in the lungs. She
needed to be rushed to another floor for testing.

Swango was insistent. "She has to have a heart monitor."

"No she doesn't!" Ritchie interjected, fearing that the patient
would die while they delayed dealing with an obvious condition.

But Swango was adamant. Moore said she could handle the situation, and told the visibly upset Ritchie she could leave. Moore got
the patient to the other floor in time to save her life.

After her shift ended that day, Ritchie was driving home on
Route 315 to the northwest suburbs where she lived. She couldn't
get the day's disturbing events out of her mind. Barrick's death,
Swango's unfeeling reaction to it, and his jeopardizing another patient made her consider the possibility that his actions had been
deliberate. Her heart started racing; her head felt light; and she
feared she would faint. She pulled over to the side of the busy
highway to collect herself, but she still felt waves of anxiety. As
soon as she could, she got off the highway and drove to her sister's
house, where she broke down in tears. She told her sister about
Ruth Barrick, and then about the other patient. Her sister called
their father, the doctor, who said he'd check on Anne as soon as he
could. Meanwhile, she did deep breathing exercises in an effort to
stem the anxiety and calm herself. Surely she was wrong about
Swango; Barrick's death was an accident. Eventually her pulse returned to normal, she regained her strength, and she was able to
drive home.

The next day, in line with the hospital protocol that any irregu-
lar incidents should be reported to one's immediate superior,
Ritchie told Amy Moore her suspicions that Swango had caused
Barrick's death. She also talked with several other nurses about what
had happened. Given hospital practice, she didn't dare say anything

to any doctors. And in any event, she was afraid to mention the real cause of her anxiety attack: her suspicion that Swango's actions had been premeditated and deliberate.

THAT same evening, February 7, Swango and several other doctors made their evening rounds, stopping to see Rena Cooper, a sixty-nine-year-old widow who had had an operation that morning for a lower back problem, and Iwonia Utz, age fifty-nine, who was scheduled for, but had not yet received, treatment for a brain tumor. For twelve days the two had shared Room 900 in Rhodes Hall; over that time, they had become friendly. Cooper, a former seamstress and, for nineteen years, a practical nurse, and Utz, also a widow, and the mother of nine children, had discovered that they shared a strong Christian faith. (Cooper described herself as "born again.") On the evening of February 7, they had dinner, watched some television, and were avidly discussing the Bible when the doctors arrived. The doctors noted nothing unusual and continued their rounds. When they left, Cooper was lying comfortably on her side, with an intravenous tube for antibiotics connected to her left arm.

About an hour later, between nine and 9:15 P.M., an Ohio State nursing student, Karolyn Tyrrell Beery, came in to Room 900 for a routine hourly check and was surprised to see Swango there. Cooper had requested more pain medication, asking Utz to hold the call button down for her because she couldn't reach it, and Swango had apparently responded to the call. He was standing at Cooper's bedside, only about three feet from Beery, and the student noticed that he was adding something to Cooper's intravenous tube by inserting a syringe. "Her line must have clotted off" was her only thought; she assumed Swango was clearing a blockage. Beery stepped outside to enter data on Utz's chart. She was running late, and ready to move on to her next patient when, no more than two minutes later, she heard Utz call out, "Are you all right, Mrs. Cooper?" Then Beery heard a violent rattling of bed rails, followed by Utz's screams.

She rushed into the room. Utz cried out, "There's something wrong!" Cooper was turning blue and had stopped breathing.

Panicked, Beery rushed to the nurses' station for help, and returned to the room with a regular nurse, John Sigg. Sigg took one look at Cooper, then called a code. Two doctors, Rees Freeman, the chief resident in neurosurgery, and Arlo Brakel, another resident, were among the first to arrive, along with several nurses.

The genial, easygoing Freeman was referred to by nurses as "California Boy," since he'd grown up there. He was also a vitamin and mineral enthusiast, frequently handing out zinc tablets to patients, which the nurses also thought was a very West Coast habit. Brakel was often disheveled and tardy; as a joke, the nurses gave him an alarm clock with two large bells on top.

Swango, though he had just been in the room, didn't immediately respond to the code. As the senior resident, Freeman took charge of the emergency. He asked Beery what had happened. "Doctor," she said, "you know, Dr. Swango was in here and he left."

"Dr. Swango was in here?" Freeman asked, somewhat incredulous, since the doctors' rounds had been concluded some time earlier and Cooper wasn't scheduled for any follow-up visits. "What was he doing here?"

"I don't know," Beery said, adding: "This doctor's a real jerk."

Freeman asked what medication Cooper had taken, and another nurse said it was only codeine, a mild pain remedy. Beery then remarked that she had seen Swango giving Cooper something through the intravenous tube, but the doctors seemed skeptical, and she was convinced that neither of them believed her, probably because she was just a student nurse. Their skepticism may also have been rooted in the hospital custom that nurses, not doctors, adjust IV tubes (as opposed to the more complicated central lines). While doctors may inject drugs directly into IV lines, Cooper hadn't been scheduled for any such medication.

With the code and all the commotion in her room, Utz had become hysterical—by her own account, she was "screaming like mad"—and Freeman ordered her removed. As nurses converged on Utz, she called out that "a doctor with blond hair did something to Mrs. Cooper." Between sobs, she elaborated to the nurses: the "blond-haired doctor" had come into the room with a syringe and "something yellow that you wrap on your arm when you draw blood." She had heard him tell Cooper that "he was going to give her something to make her feel better." Utz said she had watched as the doctor wrapped the yellow tube around Cooper's arm, injected her with the syringe, and then "ran" from the room. Then Cooper's bed rails began to shake. Utz tried to press her emergency call button, but couldn't reach it, so she began screaming for attention. By the time Utz had finished her story, she had been moved to a private room down the hall, so only nurses heard the full account.

In any event, the doctors at this point were more concerned about saving Cooper than they were about determining the cause of her mysterious paralysis. Brakel later noted that Cooper "was not breathing. She was unconscious. She had no movements to any stimulus, even deep pain." But she wasn't dead—she had a good pulse and heartbeat. The doctors checked her pupils and noticed that there was faint, sluggish reaction to stimuli. But the doctors were surprised by what they called her "total flaccidity"—"she didn't even have any reflexes," as Brakel put it. The doctors inserted a tube down her throat to facilitate breathing. This is normally a painful procedure, but Cooper showed no reaction, and the doctors concluded she was essentially paralyzed.

Joe Risley, a nurse's aide, had responded to the code, and was standing outside Cooper's room when he heard Beery, who was a friend of his, tell Freeman that Swango had injected something into Cooper's IV. He moved west down the corridor and rounded a corner, checking to make sure there were no other patient emergencies while the medical staff was preoccupied with Cooper. As he neared Room 966, Risley saw Swango, wearing his white medical coat, come out the door. Risley knew Swango had just been in Cooper's room, and knew of no reason he would be in 966. But what really struck him was a peculiar look of satisfaction on Swango's face when he looked Risley directly in the eye. As Risley later put it, "He had a goofy look on his face. . . . It's an old cliché, like a kid with his fingers in the cookie jar. I mean, it was basically just a shit-eating grin."

The two said nothing to each other as they passed, but Risley, his suspicions aroused, immediately went into the room. On the bathroom sink, located just inside the door, were an 18-gauge needle and a 10cc syringe with the plunger depressed. An 18-gauge needle is large, used on patients only in unusual circumstances when a large dosage needs to be injected at high speed. Lily Jordan, the charge nurse, who supervised other nurses on the floor, was walking by, and

Risley asked her if anyone had been assigned to give an injection in Room 966. No, she replied, not that she knew of. Risley asked her to look in the bathroom, and pointed out the huge needle and syringe. "Did you leave that there?"

"No," she said emphatically.

"I just found it," Risley said.

The two thought the location of the abandoned syringe was peculiar, since a sharps container—a box for disposing of used needles and syringes—was located just behind the sink.

Risley told Jordan that he'd just seen Swango coming out of the room with a strange look on his face, and the significance of their discovery immediately sank in. Jordan took a paper towel, wrapped it around the syringe and needle, and carefully placed them in a cabinet under the sink.

"You are my witness," she told Risley, who nodded gravely.

BACK in Room 900, Cooper was responding to resuscitation efforts. Within fifteen minutes she was breathing on her own, and the paralysis throughout the rest of her body quickly eased. Though the tube down her throat prevented her from speaking, she indicated with gestures that she wanted to write a note. The supervising nurse on the floor that evening, Sharon Black, fetched a notebook and pencil and handed them to her. Cooper scrawled, "He put something in my IV." Black took the note, dated it "February 7, 1984," and wrote Cooper's name and patient number on it. Cooper was immediately removed to the intensive care unit, where she again asked for pencil and paper. This time she wrote, "Someone gave me some med in my IV and paralyzed all of me, lungs, heart, speech" and "someone gave me an injection in my IV and it paralyzed my lungs and heart."

As soon as the tube was removed and Cooper could speak, Dr. Freeman asked her what had happened. She reiterated that a blond-haired person had injected something into her IV; she had seen a syringe in the person's hand. She had never gotten a clear look at this person's face. As soon as he gave her the injection, she felt a "blackness" spread through her body, beginning in the left arm attached to the IV, then spreading from the left to the right side of her body. She became frightened when she tried to speak and couldn't, and with her dwindling strength began shaking the bed rails to attract attention. Then, she said, she saw a "white angel of death" at her bedside and stopped breathing.

Though Beery had the impression that none of the doctors believed her, Dr. Freeman pursued her declaration that Swango had been in the room. He described Swango to Cooper as a "tall, blond doctor" and asked if he might have been the person Cooper saw inject something in her IV. Cooper replied, "Yes, it was that person." Freeman ordered a blood test on Cooper to see if the cause of the paralysis could be determined.

Freeman returned to the ninth floor, where Swango was still on duty, and confronted him with the allegation that he had given Cooper an injection. Swango denied that he had even been in Cooper's room after the doctors finished their rounds. Later, after hearing more reports from nurses, Freeman again asked Swango if he was sure he had never been in the room. Swango repeated that he had had no contact with Cooper. As Freeman later put it, "I confronted him and did question him and he said he was not in the room. Nor did he see her just previous to the incident."

WITH Cooper seemingly safe in intensive care and the immediate crisis over, a sense of shock descended on the nurses. Though none of them had ever confronted anything like this in their careers, they felt that something had to be done. Black, the supervising nurse, told Nurses Beery and Jordan to write down everything they could remember, and she did the same. Beery wrote that Swango was in the room and "it appeared" that he injected something into Cooper's IV tube. Black collected their statements and placed them in a sealed envelope, which she left for the director of surgical nursing, who would be in the next day. Just after eleven P.M., Black also took the unusual step of calling Amy Moore, the head nurse, at home, and told her what had happened. Then Jordan, too, called Moore to tell her about the syringe Risley had found in Room 966. Moore was alarmed, especially since she had heard about Swango that same day from Ritchie, who had told her about his involvement in Barrick's death. She told Jordan to retrieve the syringe and place it in her, Moore's, briefcase, which was in her office.

Moore was already concerned about the startling increase in the number of codes and deaths on the ninth floor of Rhodes Hall in the prior few weeks, though only now did she begin to link them specifically with Swango. On January 14—just after Swango's meeting with Dr. Hunt—Cynthia Ann McGee, an attractive young gymnast from the University of Illinois, had been found dead in Room 901. Six days later, twenty-one-year-old Richard DeLong was found dead in Room 964. A nurse had said Dr. Freeman, who responded to a code on DeLong, "was definitely stunned" by the sudden and mysterious death. Another patient on the ninth floor, forty-three-year-old Rein Walter, died unexpectedly on January 24 after a nurse found him gasping for air and turning blue. Swango had been working on the floor at the time of all of these deaths, and the coincidence was hard to miss. As one nurse, Lynnette Brinkman, had put it, there had been more codes on the ninth floor since Swango began his neurosurgery rotation than there had been in the entire prior year.

The next morning, Moore went to Jan Dickson, the associate executive director for nursing, the highest-ranking nurse at Ohio State. Dickson had earned high praise for restoring morale and building up the staff after a bitter and debilitating nurses' strike that had preceded her arrival. She loved working at large teaching hospitals, and had been in charge of nursing at the University of Kentucky before moving to Columbus. Dickson, forty-two, had grown up on a farm in northeast Missouri, not far from Swango's hometown of Quincy, where she had relatives. An attractive blonde, she had a warm, down-to-earth manner and the ability to bridge the often large gulf between nurses, doctors, and hospital administrators. She was dating Donald Boyanowski, an associate executive director of the hospital, so she also had unusual access to the hospital's inner workings and politics.

Dickson had never encountered a head nurse so shaken and upset. Moore related the previous night's incidents, told how she'd been called at home by both Black and Jordan, and mentioned her fears about the sudden increase in mysterious deaths on the floor where Swango was working. The story was so incredible that had Dickson not known Moore so well and trusted her judgment and maturity, she wouldn't have believed it. It was obvious to Dickson that something was terribly wrong in Rhodes Hall—so wrong, in fact, that she thought the police would have to be notified.

That, however, was not a decision she could make alone. Dickson dispatched Moore to talk to Dr. Joseph Goodman, a professor of neurosurgery and the attending physician who had operated on Cooper's spine. Dickson also called to arrange a meeting with Donald Cramp, the hospital's executive director and top administrator. Cramp was alarmed and upset, and readily agreed with Dickson that there was an emergency. He immediately called Dr. Manuel Tzagournis, the university vice president for health services and dean of the College of Medicine, who scheduled a meeting for six that evening.

In Columbus, few figures are viewed with more reverence than Tzagournis, the quintessential Ohio boy made good. Though he reported directly to Ohio State's president, Edward H. Jennings, Tzagournis was close to members of the hospital's powerful board, some of whom were also university trustees. The board included such local luminaries as Charles Lazarus, chairman of the department store chain; John Wolfe, owner and chairman of *The Columbus Dispatch;* and Dean Jeffers, chairman of Nationwide Insurance. Tzagournis, a native of Youngstown, earned both his bachelor's and medical degrees from Ohio State and was a specialist in endocrinology, the study of the glands and hormones. He had cemented his ties to the hospital board by treating some of its members, not to mention prominent state legislators. Tzagournis's cousin, Harry Meshel, was the Ohio state Senate minority leader, and Vernal G. Riffe, Jr., the speaker of the Ohio House of Representatives, was one of Tzagournis's patients. (Ohio State received $229.4 million in state aid in fiscal 1984.) Tzagournis had become dean in 1981, transforming the office into a highly visible fundraising position. Charming, sociable, and urbane, Tzagournis cultivated not only state legislators, but the local business and professional elite.

At the time, Tzagournis had been overseeing what was arguably the hospital's most important campaign—the Arthur G. James Cancer Hospital, named after an oncologist at Ohio State and initially financed with $40 million from the state government. Ground was about to be broken on the new hospital when the Swango matter surfaced. The new hospital's prestige, success, and future operations depended on Ohio State's ability to attract additional donations, major research grants, and $12 million in additional funding from the state. This potential scandal could not have come at a worse time.

Before the scheduled meeting, Dickson summoned Beery and Jordan and asked them to read and sign typed versions of their handwritten statements from the previous night. Jordan took the opportunity to tell Dickson in greater detail about the McGee, De-Long, and Walter deaths and the nursing staff's suspicions of Swango—a topic that was dominating conversation among the nurses that day. Like Moore, Jordan was extremely upset, and Dickson grew even more alarmed.

But the nurses were receiving a very different reaction from Dr. Goodman. Though relatively young, Goodman was perceived by some nurses as the epitome of the cold, detached, aloof, even arrogant surgeon. He was especially disdainful of questions from patients. Some complained they couldn't get answers from him, and nurses assigned to work with Goodman were warned that, as one put it, "he doesn't have much of a bedside manner."

Though nurses tended to be especially circumspect in Goodman's presence, Moore related the story she'd told Dickson. She told him about Risley's discovery of the syringe, and said she had the syringe in her briefcase. And she mentioned the other mysterious deaths, and the fact that Swango had been present for all of them. Goodman thanked her, then dismissed her without asking any questions or offering further instructions. He said nothing about what to do with the syringe.

Goodman's major concern was that the nurses' "grapevine," as he later put it, was overreacting and recklessly spreading virulent and unfounded gossip about a fellow doctor. He was annoyed that Swango was being arbitrarily linked to every death or unusual event in the hospital for the past year, and felt the situation was getting "out of hand." He didn't find anything unusual or suspicious about finding a used syringe on a hospital sink.*

---

* Dr. Goodman later explained that he didn't know the syringe had been found in a room from which Swango had just emerged. He said he was also under the impression that it had been found the next morning, not the night of Cooper's respiratory arrest.

After conferring with Dr. Larry Carey, the chief of surgery, who had been notified by Cramp, Goodman asked Swango to come to his office. He told Swango that questions had been raised about his treatment of Rena Cooper, and said he thought he should take some time off from the hospital until the matter was cleared up. Goodman later observed that Swango appeared calm, even placid. He seemed entirely unaware that there had been any problem the previous night, and didn't show any undue concern or anxiety, a reaction that only reinforced Goodman's suspicion that nurses' gossip was the root of the problem. Goodman didn't ask Swango for any explanation or account of his activities.

Dr. Carey, too, spoke to Swango, mentioning that there had been an "incident report" concerning him that would need to be investigated. Unlike Goodman, Carey did ask Swango specifically whether he had "done anything" to Cooper or "injected anything in her IV." Swango said no, but then volunteered a detailed account that differed sharply from his answers to Dr. Freeman the night before. He said that he had gone into Cooper's room because either Cooper or Utz—Carey couldn't remember which—had told him her feet were cold, and asked him to fetch her slippers. He did so and left immediately, without doing anything to an IV line.

Carey told Swango that a committee would be meeting that evening to consider his status, and suggested he wait outside for the results.

Dr. Carey also spoke to Dr. Hunt, the head of neurosurgery, who had admitted Swango to the residency program. Goodman was widely viewed as Hunt's protégé, though Hunt was more personable and outgoing. Hunt, too, was a graduate of Ohio State's medical school, and was a Columbus native. Hunt had been married for years to Charlotte Curtis, long the highest-ranking woman at *The New York Times*, a member of the paper's editorial board. After her death he married Carole Miller, a former resident of his who had joined the neurosurgery staff at Ohio State. Hunt had long taken a professional interest in the residents' program; as a member of the American Board of Neurological Surgery, he was in charge of graduate medical education. Hunt was urbane and nationally known, spending time in New York and at his summer home on the coast of Maine.

Both Hunt and Carey were aware of some cases at other hospitals in which residents sued after being fired and the hospitals were ordered to reinstate them. They didn't want to be sued by Swango as a result of unfounded charges and nurses' gossip, and then be ordered to reinstate him.

Hunt immediately called Cramp, the hospital's executive director, and said a lawyer should attend that evening's meeting. Hunt thus appears to have been the first person involved in the matter who recognized that the situation might threaten Ohio State with possible legal liability. Besides fears of a lawsuit by Swango, there were also possible suits by patients to consider.

The questions about Swango coincided with what is generally referred to as the second malpractice insurance "crisis." The first of these occurred in the mid-1970s, when doctors' insurance premiums shot up, on average, 500 percent. During the second "crisis," in the mid-1980s, the U.S. General Accounting Office reported that malpractice insurance costs for physicians nearly doubled between 1983 and 1985, rising from $2.5 billion to $4.7 billion. The St. Paul Fire and Marine Insurance Company, the largest underwriter of medical malpractice insurance, reported a 55 percent increase in claims from 1980 to 1984. And the GAO reported that damage awards increased over 100 percent in some states in the same period. This "crisis" received enormous publicity, especially in the medical press, and fueled intense concern and resentment on the part of many doctors.

The issue of potential legal liability was especially sensitive at Ohio State, because, as a large state-financed and taxpayer-supported institution, the university was largely self-insured. Though individual doctors carried malpractice insurance and were subject to the explosion in premium costs, judgments against the hospitals, the medical school, or the university itself were paid by the university, which meant the money ultimately came out of taxpayers' pockets. Because of Ohio State's unusual status, the office of the Ohio attorney general, an elected official, served as the university's lawyer. One assistant attorney general, Robert Holder, maintained an office on the Ohio State campus and worked full-time on university matters, including issues at the medical college. Indeed, Holder and Tzagournis had worked closely together and had become friends. Cramp called Holder, who was out that day. He then called Richard Jackson, vice president of the university for business and finance. Jackson in turn asked Alphonse Cincione, a probate lawyer with a downtown Columbus law firm, to represent the university at the meeting.

The group convened at 6:30 that evening in a large conference room at the university hospital. Tzagournis did not attend, nor did Michael Whitcomb, the hospital's medical director, whom no one had been able to reach. Dickson was there as head of nursing, as were hospital administrators Cramp and Boyanowski. Cincione functioned as legal counsel. The only doctors present were Goodman, Carey, and Hunt. Goodman and Hunt had already expressed their skepticism of the nurses' claims.

Just a few years earlier, Carey had hired and brought to Ohio State a surgeon with a criminal record. The surgeon, an old friend of Carey's, had been fined and sentenced to six months' hard labor after pleading guilty to eleven counts of attempted sodomy, indecent assault, committing lewd and indecent acts, and using his position to solicit sexual favors from women subordinates while he was chief of surgery at a Philadelphia hospital. Though the prosecutor had characterized the offenses as "crimes of violence, crimes that shock the conscience," in 1982 Carey recommended to the Ohio Medical Board that the doctor be licensed to practice medicine, saying that the sex crimes were "misbehavior at worst. From my point of view, they are not the kind of charges that ought to permanently damage a man's career." Tzagournis had approved hiring the surgeon even after Carey informed him of the doctor's criminal record.*

Knowing this history, Dickson considered the possibility that the doctors' first instinct might be to rally around Swango, a fellow doctor. She had seen how protective of one another doctors were, both at Ohio State and in other hospitals where she had worked. Yet these circumstances were extraordinary, with the lives of patients possibly at stake. She took the lead, presenting the evidence she had been able to collect during the course of the day. She reviewed the

* The doctor received psychiatric treatment, and there have been no further incidents reported at Ohio State. The doctor remains on the medical faculty.

Cooper incident, described Utz's observations, mentioned the syringe found by Risley, and briefly reviewed the McGee, DeLong,
Walter, and Barrick cases. Then she listened with mounting dismay
as the doctors undercut the gravity of her disclosures. She thought
the doctors seemed more concerned about Swango's rights than
they did the patients' lives.

Hunt immediately cast doubt on anything Utz might have
said, noting that she was awaiting treatment for a brain tumor. The
group discussed what might have caused Cooper's respiratory arrest, and while conceding that a toxic drug might be one explanation, the doctors noted that there might also be many others.

Dickson and Boyanowski thought the evidence was sufficiently serious and compelling that the police should be notified.
Cincione, the lawyer, disagreed and said there was no evidence any
crime had been committed, nor was there enough evidence to know
how to proceed. Cincione recommended that the hospital's medical
staff—the doctors—conduct a discreet internal investigation.

Dickson, Boyanowski, and Cramp all thought it was a mistake
for the hospital to try to investigate itself, but they deferred to Cincione's legal judgment. Dickson was expressly ordered not to question any nurses further—this because of the fear, first expressed by
Dr. Goodman, that to do so would only fuel the nurses' "tensions
and concerns," which might in turn alarm patients. Instead, Goodman himself, who from the outset had been highly skeptical of the
nurses' claims, took charge of the investigation. He agreed to report his findings to the group at a meeting the following Saturday
morning.

The meeting ended at about eight P.M. Swango had been sitting
on a bench in the lobby. Dr. Carey suggested he "go home for a few
days" because of the incident report. Swango took the news calmly.

Dickson was upset by the meeting, but felt if she could only
get her message across to Tzagournis, whom she knew and respected, he would surely recognize how serious the situation was.
She couldn't reach the dean, so she called Holder, the assistant attorney general, who had been briefed on the meeting by Cincione,
to try the same tack. She asked him to meet with her in her office,
which he did the next day. Holder insisted on deferring to Cincione's judgment that there wasn't any credible evidence of a crime

and they should await the results of Goodman's investigation, but
he did agree to pass on Dickson's request to meet with Tzagournis.
The next day, Dickson narrated the alarming events to the dean; she
thought he at least listened carefully. Tzagournis seemed to recognize the gravity of the matter, and though he made no commit-
ments, she felt she was making headway.

On February 9, the day after the meeting, Goodman began
what would prove to be a pivotal investigation of Swango's activities. His investigation had three components. At 3:30 P.M., he interviewed Cooper; next, he reviewed the files of seven patients who
had died since Swango began his neurosurgery rotation; last, he
considered the results of a blood test on Cooper. He did not interview either of the residents, Freeman and Brakel, who responded to
the code on Cooper. Had he interviewed Brakel, he would have
learned more about Swango's involvement in Ruth Barrick's death
the same day, since Brakel had responded to Barrick's code as well.

Nor did Goodman interview any of the nurses who witnessed
the events, or the orderly who discovered the syringe, or Utz,
Cooper's roommate. He did not ask to see the syringe, still in
Nurse Moore's custody. He didn't speak to any witnesses to any of
the patient deaths, such as Nurse Ritchie. No autopsies or physical
tests were ordered for any of the possible victims, nor were any experts in toxicology or anesthesia consulted for possible explanations of the deaths and of Cooper's apparent paralysis. While
Goodman did not purport to be a trained investigator, the extremely limited scope of his inquiry is hard to comprehend unless
he had already largely concluded that Swango was innocent and that
the nurses' "grapevine," as he had put it, was largely to blame for the
rumors sweeping the hospital. These were sentiments he had expressed from the outset.

The following statements appear in a memorandum Goodman
wrote the next day, summarizing the interview with Cooper:
"Someone was standing by the bed and injected something into the
I.V."; "Blonde, short, unable to see face"; "Yellow pharmacy jacket."

Goodman's principal reaction to the interview seems to have
been distress that Cooper was spreading stories that were agitating
other patients. He called Cramp, the hospital chief, at 4:30 P.M. to
complain that rumors about Swango were "rampant" on the floor

and to say he was moving Cooper to a private room to stop them. Although Cramp objected, Goodman did so. He also ordered that only Amy Moore, the head nurse, would be allowed contact with Cooper; this move, too, was intended to contain her inflammatory allegations.

That Saturday morning, the initial group involved in the matter met to hear Goodman's report and conclusions. Three important people joined this meeting: Holder, Tzagournis, and Michael Whitcomb, the hospital medical director, a close friend and protégé of Tzagournis. Although Dickson and others had urged that the university president, Edward Jennings, and Richard Jackson, the vice president, attend, Tzagournis had decided that there was no need.

To Dickson's amazement, Goodman was even more dismissive of the allegations against Swango than he had been at the first meeting. His interview with Cooper, he assured the group, had gone a long way toward eliminating the possibility that Swango had been involved in foul play of any kind. Goodman reported that Cooper had identified the alleged assailant as a "female" and "neither a nurse nor physician on the hospital staff." Since his notes also indicated the person was wearing a "yellow pharmacy jacket," he concluded the suspect was probably a woman pharmacy technician, and he had already determined that there was no one who fit that description.

Virtually everything about Goodman's conclusions and interview with Cooper is puzzling. Cooper insisted she never described her assailant as a "female." Indeed, in her numerous other accounts of the incident, Cooper said consistently that she couldn't see the person's face, and whenever she identified her attacker's sex she said he was male. In her first handwritten note she referred to the assailant as "he." Nor, she maintained, did she ever mention anything about a yellow pharmacy jacket; her roommate *did* refer to a yellow tourniquet. Goodman said that Nurse Moore was a witness to the interview and, by implication, would support his account. However, Cooper herself said she remembered that only Goodman was present.* In any event, at the time participants in the meeting had only Goodman's version.

* Moore declined my requests for comment.

Goodman also reported on his review of the files of patients who died. While he conceded that seven deaths in a little more than two weeks was abnormally high (he said the norm was two or three), he said that all the patients had been "extremely ill" and that the deaths were "clearly explainable medically." As another doctor put it, sometimes the "grim reaper of death" just sweeps through a hospital. While Goodman also conceded that Swango had been present when at least half the patients died, this was only to be expected given that he was an intern assigned to the floor, working long hours. The only death that caused Goodman any concern at all, he said, was that of Cynthia Ann McGee, the young gymnast. Goodman noted that she had been improving and that the sudden death had come as a surprise. But an autopsy had been performed, and Goodman said he'd been told the cause of death was a pulmonary embolism. Such embolisms aren't uncommon in cases where patients have been transported, as McGee had been from Illinois, he explained. Goodman's colleague and mentor Dr. Hunt said he, too, had reviewed the patient files and seconded Goodman's conclusions.

McGee's autopsy results in fact cite "cardiopulmonary arrest due to incipient pneumonia" as the cause of death. There is no mention of a pulmonary embolism.

Finally, the group discussed the results of the blood test on Cooper. But no such blood test results were ever found in Cooper's medical file. It is at least possible that the blood test ordered by Freeman was never administered, or that the results were lost. The notes of the meeting don't make clear whether Goodman reviewed the results himself, or relied on a hearsay report that they were normal. In either case, the results may have come from a blood test given Cooper when she entered the hospital; they were in her file and, not surprisingly, showed nothing suspicious.

That was the end of the investigation as far as Goodman was concerned.

The group did consider some troublesome evidence that seemed to call Goodman's conclusions into question. Dickson, for example, circulated the written eyewitness accounts of the Cooper incident she'd collected from the nurses, including Karolyn Beery, who had been only several feet from Swango when she saw him inject something into Cooper's IV line. She also showed the meeting participants Cooper's handwritten notes. Dr. Carey reported on his conversation with Swango, in which he denied injecting anything into Cooper's IV, a statement also in conflict with Beery's observations. But the doctors, especially Goodman and Whitcomb, dismissed their significance, noting disdainfully that Beery was a student nurse. "What does a student nurse know?" one of the doctors asked, to knowing snickers around the table. The comment left Dickson quietly seething.

Swango's file was reviewed, and the group discussed the evidence suggesting that he had "attitudinal problems." Carey mentioned the residents' reports that Swango had "weird ideas about death," that he was fascinated by the Nazis, and that his work was "sub-standard." But Cincione's sketchy notes of the meeting conclude only that "this discussion shed no light on the situation at hand." Nor could any support for the proposition that a pharmaceutical technician was the culprit be produced. Boyanowski, the administrator, had investigated that possibility, and there were no "blonde, female" technicians. Cooper hadn't been scheduled to receive any medication during the relevant time period.

The group also discussed at some length what might have caused Cooper's respiratory failure, a fact which could hardly be ascribed to nurses' paranoia. Potassium was mentioned as a chemical that, when injected, can easily cause cardiac arrest, but the doctors pointed out that Cooper didn't suffer a heart attack; she experienced a respiratory failure. Her IV line had been discarded, so no tests on it were possible. Curiously, the mention of possible tests on the IV line triggered no mention of the syringe by Goodman, although he had been told of its existence by Nurse Moore. The group concluded that the cause of Cooper's seizure was probably unknowable.

Then the lawyers weighed in. Without knowing the cause of Cooper's code, Cincione told the group, they had no legal basis for accusing Swango of a criminal act or, for that matter, even removing him from the intern program. But while the lawyers seemed to have been focusing on Swango's rights and the potential liability of Ohio State, they seem to have given no consideration to an Ohio statute that requires any "physician" to report "any serious physical harm to persons that he knows or has reasonable cause to believe resulted from an offense of violence." In any event, these requirements were never mentioned at any of the group's meetings, despite the presence of two lawyers, Holder and Cincione.*

The meeting lasted about three hours. At its conclusion, Tzagournis ordered that Swango be returned to the hospital, but watched closely. He asked Dr. Whitcomb to conduct a "quiet inquiry" into the matter, and report his findings at another meeting in three days. At least some participants understood that the report was to be in writing. Both Dickson and Boyanowski objected, again arguing that the hospital couldn't effectively investigate itself, and that there was enough evidence to justify notification of the campus police. But Tzagournis disagreed, no doubt in part because he was steeped in the medical profession's tradition of "peer review," in which only other doctors are deemed competent to evaluate a fellow physician. Dickson, increasingly troubled by the direction of the inquiry, asked if she could assist Whitcomb by at least being present at interviews with the nurses. Tzagournis said no.

As Ohio State's medical director, Whitcomb held the number two medical position in the hospital, just under Tzagournis. Like his boss, Whitcomb was an Ohio native and graduate of Ohio State, though he attended medical school at the University of Cincinnati. He worked at Walter Reed Army Hospital before returning to Ohio State in 1974. He was largely given responsibility for the investigation by virtue of his position as medical director, and because he was a pulmonologist, or lung specialist, it made some sense to assign him to investigate what appeared to be a respiratory failure.

But Whitcomb looked terrible, as if he hadn't had much sleep. It hadn't surprised anyone that he couldn't be located in time for the first meeting. It was much discussed in the hospital that he had been having an affair with his secretary, and was involved in a messy divorce. At the meeting Whitcomb's hands were visibly trembling, so much so that Dickson later asked if he was suffering from some neurological condition. (He later publicly acknowledged a drinking problem.)

Some who felt Swango should be vigorously investigated were

---

* The Ohio statute is R.C. 2921.22(B). A later investigation by Ohio State concluded that there was no need to report the incident.

dismayed that Whitcomb was put in charge, and their concerns were soon borne out, for Whitcomb's investigation was even more cursory than Goodman's. He spoke to Goodman and reviewed his notes; interviewed Beery, the student nurse; and, significantly, interviewed Swango. He did little else. Incredibly, he may not even have interviewed Rena Cooper, relying instead on Goodman's notes. (Cooper later insisted that Whitcomb never interviewed her.) Whitcomb kept no notes of his investigation and prepared no written conclusions. He delivered his report orally on February 14, 1984, to the same audience, which included Tzagournis and Holder.

Whitcomb concluded that no one in the hospital fit the description of a blond female wearing a yellow pharmacy jacket. For all practical purposes, that description ruled out Swango as a suspect. In any event, Cooper's observations weren't reliable. She was no doubt "confused," he said, which wasn't surprising since she had been given an anesthetic for her surgery earlier that day. Utz, the roommate, was also unreliable, as Hunt had earlier noted, because she had a brain tumor. Whitcomb hadn't interviewed her, either, but he did go over her patient file.

During Whitcomb's interview, Beery, the student nurse, had softened her earlier account. Under what must have felt like cross-examination by Whitcomb, Beery acknowledged that she was "not certain" she actually saw a syringe in Swango's hand. This, Whitcomb maintained, was inconsistent with her earlier statement that it "appeared" that Swango had injected something into Cooper's IV. Because of this, Whitcomb told the group that Beery's "identification testimony" was "shaky," noting that she had been in the room only a short time. As he had suspected, she was an unreliable witness and her statement should be discounted accordingly. Thus, Beery's statement in every interview that she had seen Swango in Cooper's room and had been only a few feet away was also discarded as unreliable.

In diagnosing the cause of Cooper's respiratory arrest, Whitcomb identified the fact that she shook the bed rails as all but incontrovertible evidence of a seizure followed by paralysis. (The possibility that Cooper could have rattled the rails before a paralyzing drug took full effect does not appear to have been considered.) Whitcomb had spoken briefly to Dr. George Paulson, a neurologist at Ohio State, who said that it was "possible" for a seizure to be followed by paralysis. By contrast, drugs such as muscle relaxants might cause paralysis, but not a seizure. On that basis, and without speaking to any other specialists, such as anesthesiologists, Whitcomb diagnosed Cooper's problem as "grand mal," a severe form of epilepsy characterized by seizures and loss of consciousness—but not paralysis.

Whitcomb told the group he'd interviewed Swango, and that Swango had given him a version of the "slippers" story, in which Cooper had complained that her feet were cold. However, Whitcomb later told police an entirely different story: that Swango told him he was in the room to draw blood.

Nonetheless, Swango's account appears to have been accepted as credible, even as Beery's and Cooper's versions were dismissed as unreliable and confused.

That was the end of Whitcomb's report. As Hunt later summed up the evidence, "All we have is a crazy patient who had an unusual episode and a nurse who saw something. Is that enough to prove anything?" Tzagournis ordered that Swango, who had already returned to his work in the hospital, should resume his internship. The residents who worked with him in Rhodes Hall should be told that there wasn't any evidence against him, but that he should nonetheless be "closely observed."

The nurses, on the other hand, should be told only that Swango had been exonerated. And other doctors, including those on Swango's future rotations, would be told nothing. On Tzagournis's orders, there would be no further inquiry or investigation into the matter, and the police would be told nothing of the incident or the sudden increase in deaths.

Dickson had by now fallen into stunned silence. Swango's accusers were all female nurses; his defenders, male doctors. She was convinced that the entire point of the so-called investigation had been to exonerate Swango and thereby avoid any liability or embarrassment to the university. She had tried to see the patient files herself; she was denied access. She felt it would now be impossible to observe Swango closely in the hospital. There was too much to do, and too few doctors who had been alerted to Swango's suspicious activities, to keep him under close surveillance, especially if the

nurses and most of the doctors were kept in the dark. Still, she felt
she had done what she could, at considerable personal risk. Now
that Swango was back at work, and she had emerged as the
strongest advocate for his dismissal, she thought it likely that someone on the medical staff would tell Swango. She was afraid to walk
her dog at night alone, even in the safe neighborhood where she
lived. She was afraid Swango would kill her.

Karolyn Beery, the discredited student nurse, was also frightened, and tried to avoid Swango. She and other nurses usually
brought bag lunches to work, which they labeled with their names
and kept in a refrigerator. "Who's been messing with my lunch?"
Beery asked a group of nurses one day, explaining that for several
days, it had been obvious that her food had been rearranged in the
bag. Then she started to feel nauseated, and developed headaches.
She thought she might be pregnant, but three separate pregnancy
tests were negative. After several weeks, when Swango left the neurosurgery rotation, her symptoms eased. She wondered if she was
just being paranoid.

Dr. Carey met with all the residents on the rotations remaining
on Swango's schedule. He told them he was "worried" about
Swango, that he wanted them to watch him closely and "report to
me any untoward events, any patients that had complications or difficulties that weren't expected." As he later put it, "Our intent was
to do everything possible to protect people from harm and get him
out the door at the end of the year without risk that a court would
order us to reappoint him."

ON the same day as the meeting in which Swango was exonerated,
Charlotte Warner, a seventy-two-year-old leukemia patient, had a
routine splenectomy performed by Dr. Marc Cooperman. The operation went well and she recovered sufficiently to be transferred
out of intensive care to Room 968 in Doan Hall.

Swango began working in Doan Hall on February 18 as part of
his general surgery rotation. The next day, Cooperman met with
Warner, found his patient to be doing very well, and talked with her
about when she wished to be released from the hospital. That night,
a nurse found her slumped on the floor by her bed. She was dead.
An autopsy concluded she had suffered massive and unexplained

blood clots all over her body, including the liver, lungs, kidneys, and left coronary artery.

Dr. Cooperman was mystified and upset. As he later put it, "Basically what happened is she had developed clots in the arteries in her heart, in the vessels to the intestine, in the vessels to her kidneys, to her liver, and to her lungs. And I could never understand why this thing would have happened to somebody who had undergone a straightforward surgical procedure five days earlier and was walking around having no problems."

That same month while Swango was in general surgery, he examined another surgical patient, Evelyn Pereny, with her attending physician, Dr. Carey. Later, the chief surgical resident, Gary Birken, was urgently summoned to Pereny's bedside. She was bleeding all over her body—even from her eyes. As Dr. Birken noted, her coagulation was "off the wall," as if she had been bitten by a poisonous snake, such as a "cobra."

On the afternoon of February 20, Mary Popko came to visit her twenty-two-year-old daughter, Anna Mae, who had undergone intestinal surgery for a deformed bowel. She was sitting with her daughter when Swango asked her to leave the room so he could give Anna Mae an injection to raise her blood pressure. Popko asked to remain so she could hold her daughter's hand. Swango refused, and she reluctantly left the room. Later that afternoon, Swango summoned Popko to a small conference room. He leaned back and put his feet on the table. "She's dead now," Swango said of Popko's daughter. "You can go look at her."

Popko later complained about what she considered Swango's inappropriate comments and demeanor. "It seemed like it lifted his ego or something," she said of her daughter's death. "He just seemed so happy."

Despite Dr. Carey's warning, none of the residents who had been alerted about Swango reported anything unusual.

SWANGO completed his general surgery rotation and in April moved to Children's Hospital for his pediatrics rotation. Swango had often mentioned to his fellow interns and residents how much he loved fried chicken, and one night he offered to get Kentucky Fried Chicken for the residents on duty with him. Thomas Vara, the senior resident, said that would be fine, but suggested, "Instead of getting separate boxes, why don't you get a big bucket for all of us to eat?"

"No, no," Swango said. "Let's keep it separate." He insisted on taking everyone's chicken and drink order. He returned with the orders about five P.M.

"It's extra spicy chicken," Swango told Ed Hashimoto, one of the residents, as he gave him his food. That was news to Hashimoto. He knew that Kentucky Fried offered "extra crispy" chicken, but he'd never heard of "extra spicy."

Vara, Hashimoto, and a third resident, Douglas Hess, ate the chicken. About three hours later, all three fell violently ill, with fever, nausea, and vomiting that lasted over a week.

As Vara later described it, "It's as sick as I've ever been. We were sick there at the hospital. The other guys were, Jesus . . . like in the operating room vomiting in their masks and stuff. That's how bad it was."

When the doctors later discussed the episode, they thought maybe they'd suffered a violent reaction to something in the chicken. But then they tended to discount their own theory. After all, Swango, too, had eaten Kentucky Fried Chicken. He hadn't been sick at all.

COOPER, the elderly born-again Christian whose brush with death had triggered the investigation of Swango, recovered from her back surgery and mysterious respiratory arrest without further incident. Before she was released, the hospital prepared a written "discharge summary," which became a part of her permanent hospital record, something that would be produced in the event of any lawsuit. The summary contains a description of the Swango incident:

> Post operatively during the evening of surgery, the patient had a witnessed pulmonary arrest. She was noted to have seizure-like activity just prior to this arrest . . . when the patient received adequate oxygenation via endotracheal intubation. She was awakened and was intact neurologically. However, her sensorium was noted to be unusual in that she had apparent paranoid ideation as to the cause of her respiratory arrest. The patient gave indi-

cation that she entertained some paranoid ideation regarding the cause of her respiratory arrest and felt that it may be due to unnamed person or persons. The patient was carefully observed for further psychologic parameters of this nature. . . .

In other words, in the official opinion of the hospital that had treated her, and where she nearly died, Cooper was mentally unstable—"paranoid."

CHAPTER FOUR

THE RESIDENCY REVIEW COMMITTEE at Ohio State met in late February 1984 to consider Swango's status. At the end of his neurosurgery rotation earlier that month, Dr. Carole Miller—who, despite supervising Swango's work, claims she was never told of the Cooper incident and investigation—had written a letter to Dr. Hunt (her future husband) concluding that Swango "didn't demonstrate the qualities required of a neurosurgeon." She based her assessment on Swango's failure to inspire confidence in patients and other staff members rather than on any specific incident. Dr. Ferguson, who had given Swango such a negative evaluation in the transplant rotation, went so far as to write a letter urging Swango's firing after he heard reports about the Cooper affair. As a result, the committee voted not to continue Swango's residency when he completed his internship at the end of June. But in keeping with Tzagournis's orders, and out of fear that Swango might sue Ohio State, he was allowed to complete his internship and continue his work in the university hospitals. Dr. Hunt notified Swango of the committee's decision by letter dated March 2.

But just five days after the letter rescinding Swango's residency appointment, three doctors on the university's medical faculty submitted recommendations on his behalf to the Ohio State Medical Board, to which Swango had applied for a permanent license to practice medicine. Two of these "certificates of recommendation" were made on a standard form supplied by the medical board. One was from Dr. Whitcomb, who had been in charge of the hospital investigation of Swango. He rated Swango's "medical knowledge and technique," his "ability to work well with peers and medical staff," and "his relationship with patients" all as "good." Whitcomb left blank the space for "personal comments, evaluation and recommendation." The other recommendation was submitted by Dr. Gary Birken, who had treated the patient with the mysterious bleeding. In the same categories, he rated Swango as "excellent," "excellent," and "exemplary."

The third recommendation was submitted by Dr. Carey, the head of surgery, who was also involved in the hospital's investigation. The form he used differed slightly from the other two. He rated Swango as "good" in the three areas mentioned. But in the space for comments, he said he was recommending Swango with "reservations." This triggered an inquiry from the medical board in May, and Carey elaborated briefly on his recommendation in a letter dated June 5. He wrote that while Swango had completed his internship at Ohio State, he had not been appointed to a second-year residency. Carey also wrote: "There was a suggestion concerning a patient's demise with regard to Dr. Swango having been in attendance proximate to the demise. This was investigated rather thoroughly and Dr. Swango was exonerated." Though he didn't mention the patient by name, Carey must have been referring to Cooper, even though she didn't die, since none of the *deaths* linked to Swango had been investigated at all, let alone thoroughly. Carey's letter went on to say that Swango's performance had been "substandard," that he had "difficulty relating to paramedical personnel," and that he did not relate well to nurses and other hospital employees.

Carey's letter thus reduced Swango's troubles at Ohio State largely to an issue of personality differences with paramedics and nurses—hardly sufficient grounds to deny an otherwise qualified doctor a medical license. Virtually all of Carey's major assertions are, at the least, open to question: Cooper didn't die, but survived as an eyewitness; Swango was more than a bystander who was "proximate" to the incident—he was alleged to have caused it; the investigation wasn't thorough; and Swango was hardly "exonerated." Even Tzagournis had ordered that Swango be watched closely; Carey himself had told the residents he was worried about Swango.*

---

* When I asked him about this, Carey said he had no recollection of the letter, but said that "the people who read these [would] know" that he was trying to warn

Despite Carey's "reservations," the letter did nothing to deter the Ohio State Medical Board. In September 1984, it granted Swango's application and licensed him to practice medicine in Ohio.

AT the Ohio State Hospitals that summer, head nurse Amy Moore was going through her desk when she came across the syringe, still wrapped in a paper towel, that Joe Risley had found in Room 966 the night of Cooper's respiratory arrest. Several months had passed since those terrifying events, but the discovery brought back bad memories of the whole affair. Moore couldn't understand why no one had seemed interested in the syringe, which she and the other nurses had been so careful to preserve. She'd told Dr. Goodman about it in their meeting, but he never mentioned it to her again. She'd never been asked for it in the course of any investigation. Then she heard that Swango had been cleared.

Moore was about to dispose of the thing, but for some reason she hesitated. She turned to another nurse and said she was going to throw the syringe away. "Do you think it's okay?"

"Well, sure," the nurse replied. "It's gone now. It's over with."

Moore dropped the syringe into a waste container.

IN July Swango moved back to his hometown of Quincy, as he had during other intervals in his career. He told his mother and relatives that he hadn't liked the doctors he worked with at Ohio State, and as a result had left his residency there. He planned to apply for a medical license in Illinois and in the meantime, work as a paramedic for a few months before resuming his medical career. He was immediately hired by the Adams County Ambulance Corps, where he had worked the previous spring and part-time while he was at Quincy College. Though his hours were unpredictable and he often worked weekends, he frequently made the eight-hour drive to Columbus so he could see his girlfriend, Rita Dumas, and her children. As in the past, he managed to function on amazingly little sleep; he once mentioned that he'd made the long drive to Colum-

---

them about Swango. The later Ohio State investigation concluded that Dr. Carey "cannot be faulted for his handling of the recommendation to the State Medical Board."

bus, visited Dumas for just an hour, and then driven back and reported for work, all without any sleep.

Quincy had changed little since Swango's childhood—or, for
that matter, since its heyday as a Mississippi River port in the mid-
nineteenth century. Maine Street, its central thoroughfare, runs
through a national historic district lined with stately mansions built
by riverboat captains and early industrialists. Swango rented an
apartment on Eighteenth Street, just north of Maine, at the upstairs
rear of an attractive older brick house. It had one bedroom and a
screened porch. It was within walking distance of Quincy's two
hospitals, Blessing and St. Mary's. Though Quincy had a population
of just over 40,000, its distance from any major city (Springfield was
two hours away) had made it a regional medical center, serving a
large rural area.

The ambulance corps was headquartered at Blessing Hospital,
in a suite adjacent to the hospital's emergency room. The paramedics shared a central room with a large round table, comfortable
chairs, and a television; a kitchen and bathroom; and several sleeping rooms. Paramedics worked twenty-four-hour shifts, responding
to ambulance calls whenever they came in, and often ate and slept at
the hospital. Since they spent so much time together, they were a
close-knit group, drawn together by a shared temperament that
thrived on the crisis, violence, mayhem, and serious accidents that
trigger ambulance calls. The work required a strong stomach. The
paramedics' demeanor could at times seem vulgar and coarse to outsiders, and they often indulged in black humor to relieve the pressure of their work. Lonnie Long, who was in charge of the
paramedics, and who hired Swango, was a guns and weapons enthusiast. Copies of *Soldier of Fortune* and the National Rifle Association magazine were often lying about the paramedics' quarters.

Still, even by the standards of paramedics, Swango was considered bizarre. Nearly everyone knew him from his previous stint
with the corps. An exception was Mark Krzystofczyk. Somewhat
soft-spoken, dark-haired, and nice-looking, Krzystofczyk was
twenty-seven and had graduated from SIU before moving to
Quincy in 1982. He wondered why a resident at a big hospital like
Ohio State would be coming to work as a paramedic in Quincy.
"Wait till you meet Swango," his coworkers told him when they

learned their former colleague would be returning in July. "He's different." But when Krzystofczyk asked why, they just grinned and shook their heads. "You'll see."

If anything, the qualities that had made Swango "different" were now even more pronounced. The paramedics who had worked with him before noticed that he was restless, on edge, constantly pacing around the room. He rarely sat down and relaxed with the other paramedics. He kept saying he wished something would happen so he could get on the ambulance. Still, they felt he was an effective paramedic and admired his medical degree and hospital experience, which put him on a different plane educationally from his colleagues. Long, in particular, told Swango that he envied him his education and internship, and warned Swango not to forget the paramedics when he resumed his career as a doctor. Long believed that most doctors had swelled heads and egos.

Soon after Swango started work, he ran into Jim Daniels, a fellow graduate of the SIU medical school and Quincy College, who'd been a year behind him at SIU. Daniels was now doing his internship at Blessing Hospital, and was assigned to the emergency room for his first rotation, just as Swango had been at Ohio State. "I thought you were a neurosurgeon," Daniels said.

"No," Swango answered. "It didn't work out."

Daniels thought Swango might elaborate, but he said nothing further. Swango was similarly vague with Krzystofczyk, who was often his partner on ambulance runs. Krzystofczyk also wondered what his fellow paramedics had been talking about when they warned him about Swango. All that struck Krzystofczyk about him in the first weeks they worked together were Swango's "Beaver Cleaver" all-American looks, and how hard he was willing to work. He always volunteered for extra shifts. As if their long hours weren't enough, even when he was off-duty Swango monitored ambulance calls with a shortwave radio and then would show up at the scenes of emergencies, sometimes even before the ambulance arrived. When he wasn't on an emergency run or visiting his girlfriend, he seemed to be exercising. Krzystofczyk often saw him jogging in one of his old Marine sweatshirts.

Gradually, however, Krzystofczyk began to understand what his coworkers had meant when they said Swango was "different."

Perhaps in the nearly all-male, gun- and violence-oriented atmosphere of the ambulance corps, Swango simply felt freer to express the kinds of interests that had surfaced only intermittently in college, at SIU, and at Ohio State. In any event, he now revealed far more about his fantasy life and fascination with violence than he ever had before. Krzystofczyk noticed that his colleague seemed extremely excited when they reached an accident and discovered a fatality. The normally talkative Swango grew even more animated than usual, often exclaiming "Wasn't that great?" after they removed a body. Krzystofczyk thought maybe he was just testing him, trying to get a reaction. But then Swango started phoning him when he missed out on a gruesome call. "What did it look like?" he would ask. "What did you see?" Swango wanted even the goriest details repeated.

Another paramedic, Brent Unmisig, relayed a comment by Swango that seemed odd coming from someone who was trying to save lives. Unmisig had been driving with Swango down a busy Quincy street one day when a motorcyclist passed them. "That's my friend," Swango said.

"Why is that your friend, Mike?" Unmisig asked.

"He doesn't have a helmet on," Swango replied.

Swango was so interested in death that he mentioned to several of his fellow paramedics that he'd like to get the job of deputy coroner. Indeed, he approached the coroner, Wayne Johnson, asking for the job.

Swango's interest in articles about violent death, first manifested when he was a child, now became an obsession, as he himself described it. Krzystofczyk and the other paramedics noticed that when Swango was on duty and waiting for an ambulance call, he spent much of his time working on four or five large scrapbooks. He'd spread out articles on the table and carefully paste them into one of the books. One day Krzystofczyk went over to the table and looked at some of the articles. Many were about fatal car crashes, and quite a few about poison. He could tell Swango didn't like him sifting through the clippings. Swango told him that while he was living in Columbus, a cleaning woman had "messed up" the order of the clippings, and he said he'd "blown up" at her. Krzystofczyk took that as a warning.

Just to be friendly, Krzystofczyk mentioned that media mag-
nate Rupert Murdoch had very recently purchased the *Chicago Sun-
Times,* published in Krzystofczyk's hometown, and he told Swango
he might want to subscribe, given Murdoch's reputation as a tabloid
publisher. "It's going to have all kinds of lurid articles," he said.
Swango thanked him for the suggestion.

"How'd you get started on this?" Krzystofczyk continued.

Swango explained that he'd been on an ambulance call in which
someone was killed, and the next day he'd seen an article about the
accident in the paper. He'd gotten a charge out of it, so he cut out
and saved the article. Since then, he said, clipping articles about accident fatalities had developed into an "obsession."

Krzystofczyk also asked Swango specifically about why he had
so many articles on poison. "It's a good way to kill people," Swango
replied matter-of-factly. Krzystofczyk shrugged. Was that a joke?
He never knew when to take Swango seriously.

Few things distracted Swango from work on the scrapbooks,
but on July 18, not long after his arrival, the paramedics were
watching TV in their quarters when a news bulletin announced that
an out-of-work security guard armed with a rifle and shotgun had
killed twenty-one people at a busy McDonald's restaurant in San
Ysidro, California, before being gunned down by a police sharpshooter. Television crews had rushed to the scene, filming the gruesome spectacle of the dead and wounded, many of them children.
Swango was relaxing in a recliner, but at the first mention of the
massacre, he leaped to his feet, rushed to the television set, and
turned up the volume as far as it would go. "Don't do that," shouted
one of his colleagues, Greg Myers, annoyed at the earsplitting
sound. Swango turned it down slightly, but then, still standing in
front of the TV as he absorbed the news, he shouted gleefully,
"That's just great! I love it!" When the segment ended, he continued, "I wish I could have been there!" He talked about the killings
the rest of the afternoon, jumping up every time CNN repeated the
news and footage.

"Man, you're crazy," Myers thought, but he didn't say anything.

"Did you hear about the McDonald's massacre?" he asked
Lonnie Long when he came in. "Every time I think of a good idea,
somebody beats me to it."

The next day, Swango mentioned the killings to another paramedic. "Wasn't that something about that McDonald's massacre?"
he said. "I'd give anything in the world to have been there and
seen it."

Sexual banter wasn't uncommon among the mostly male staff,
but there, too, Swango set new standards. He loved to tease the one
woman paramedic, Sandy Ivers, who also happened to be dating his
boss, Lonnie Long (and later married him). "Sandy, do you know
what I'd like to do to you?" he asked her. He then described in lurid
detail what he called a "sexual fantasy" that culminated in his plung-
ing a hatchet into the back of her head. After the first recounting of
this "fantasy," Ivers would say, "Get away from me, Swango," but he
nonetheless repeated it in her presence on several occasions, within
earshot of other paramedics.

In addition to his visits to Rita Dumas in Columbus, Swango
was now dating a nurse at St. Mary's Hospital. While he never confided any details of his actual sex life, he often spoke of fantasies in
which violence and sex were closely linked. His fellow paramedics
detected a sexual element in his excitement over the McDonald's
massacre. He once told Krzystofczyk that "the best thing about
being a doctor" was "to come out of the emergency room with a
hard-on to tell some parents that their kid has just died from head
trauma."

"Mike, you are very weird," Krzystofczyk told him.

To another paramedic, Swango said he'd love to take a gun into
the emergency room "and start blowing people away."

And then there was what he described as the "ultimate call."
Nearly all the paramedics, at one time or another, heard Swango re-
count, with only minor variations, his fantasy of this "ultimate"
emergency. In this scenario, Swango is called to the site of an accident in which a busload of children has been hit head-on by a trac-
tor trailer filled with gasoline. As Swango arrives on the scene,
another bus plows into the wreckage, causing a massive explosion
of the gas-filled truck. The force of the explosion throws the children's bodies onto nearby barbed-wire fences. Swango "would see
kids hurled into barbed-wire fences, onto the telephone polls, on
the street, burning," as Unmisig put it, describing what Swango had
told him. Again, the paramedics sensed a sexual undercurrent to

Swango's excitement as he narrated the ghastly details of burning children thrown onto barbed wire.

Later that summer, Krzystofczyk and Swango were drinking coffee together, waiting for a call, while they watched a public television special on Henry Lee Lucas, who at the time was believed to be the nation's most prolific serial killer. Lucas had just been convicted of the murder of an unidentified woman known only as Orange Socks, the first of more than twenty victims he confessed to killing along Interstate 35 in Texas. In a widely watched televised interview, Lucas claimed to have crisscrossed the country with a partner, wantonly raping, robbing, and murdering. As he said on television, "We killed 'em every way there is except one. I haven't poisoned anyone. We cut 'em up. We ran 'em down in cars. We stabbed 'em. We beat 'em. We drowned 'em. There's crucification [sic]. There's people we filleted like fish. There's people we burnt. We strangled 'em. We even stabbed 'em when we strangled them. We even tied 'em so they would strangle themselves."

Krzystofczyk was amazed at how excited Swango was by the program. "Wouldn't that be great?" Swango exclaimed after the interview. "To travel around the country killing people! Just moving on, killing some more—a great lifestyle!"

EARLY on the morning of September 14, Swango showed up at the paramedics' quarters in the hospital with a box of Honey Maid doughnuts and put them on the table. Krzystofczyk was mildly surprised. It wasn't unusual for the paramedics to bring food to work, but he couldn't remember Swango ever showing much generosity. Usually it was Lonnie Long who brought in doughnuts or sweet rolls. Krzystofczyk had gone along with Swango recently when he stopped by to see his mother. Muriel gave Michael a chocolate cream pie she had baked. Krzystofczyk had expected Swango to offer him a piece when they returned to the hospital. Instead, Swango had devoured the entire pie himself.

"I got you guys a bunch of doughnuts," Swango said as he put the box on the table. Krzystofczyk took a doughnut, as did the three other paramedics in the room that morning. But Swango didn't take one; he sat down near the TV. This in itself was somewhat unusual, because Swango usually had so much energy that he stood up or paced in front of the TV while watching CNN. Krzystofczyk took a bite. He thought the doughnut tasted okay, though the icing on it looked as if it had melted slightly, maybe from exposure to heat. It was a warm day for September.

One of Swango's colleagues chided him: "What did you do, buy day-old doughnuts?"

"They're fresh, just bought them this morning," Swango replied cheerfully.

About a half-hour later, one of the paramedics began to feel nauseated, flushed, dizzy, and had to rush to the bathroom to vomit. Within another fifteen minutes all four who had eaten the doughnuts were ill with similar symptoms.

"What did you do, Mike, poison us?" joked Unmisig. Swango looked incredulous, sitting forward in his chair and shaking his head earnestly.

"No, I didn't," he replied, staring down at the floor as he said it. "You know I wouldn't do anything like that." He picked up the box with the remaining doughnuts, saying he was going to take them down to the nurses' station.

As their condition worsened, the paramedics reported to the emergency room, where they told the doctor on duty that they'd all just eaten doughnuts and become violently ill. The doctor suspected food poisoning and gave them a drug to retard vomiting. But if anything, the drug seemed to make matters worse. All four had to leave work.

The incident was reported to the Adams County Health Department as a case of suspected food poisoning, and two investigators for the department interviewed the paramedics and personnel at the Honey Maid doughnut shop. The shop owner was indignant at the suggestion that there was something unhygienic about his operation, and personally ate six doughnuts on the spot. The investigators inspected storage conditions and packaging materials, but nothing suggested food poisoning. With nothing more to go on, they concluded that an unidentified virus was to blame, and the matter was closed.

Krzystofczyk's symptoms hadn't been as bad as the others'— he wasn't sure he'd even finished the doughnut—and he later returned to the hospital. As he got out of his car in the parking lot, Swango materialized.

"How are you feeling?" he asked, seemingly genuinely concerned. Krzystofczyk said he'd been sick, but was feeling a little
better. "How are the others?" Swango asked, eagerly pressing him
for details.

Swango also called the homes of the other victims, asking relatives or roommates how they were feeling and how their illnesses
were developing.

THE next evening, a Friday, Swango was assigned to work at the
Quincy Notre Dame High School football game, where two ambulances are always on duty in case of injuries to players. Swango was
assigned to the backup ambulance rather than (as he preferred) to
the primary emergency vehicle. Swango's alma mater, Christian
Brothers, had merged with the private Catholic girls' school in
Quincy, and the combined schools used the name Notre Dame.
With marching bands, cheerleaders, and enthusiastic students,
the football games were festive occasions that attracted large
crowds. Swango had once marched with his clarinet in the half-
time shows.

Swango's partner on the ambulance that evening was Brent
Unmisig, who was in his twenties, easygoing, and popular, especially with nurses. With a twinge of envy, the other paramedics
sometimes teased him about his good looks. Unmisig was still feeling sick from the doughnuts and had barely been able to make it to
the game after his violent illness. The game was proceeding un-
eventfully when, just before half-time, Swango offered to get Unmisig a soda. Unmisig said he'd like a Coke.

Swango returned with a cola in a paper cup and gave it to his
partner, who took a sip. He'd drunk about half the cup by the time
half-time began and the players left the field. Soon after, Unmisig
felt a renewed wave of nausea. He sat the cup on the spare tire of the
ambulance, ran behind the vehicle, and vomited. When he returned,
he noticed the cup was gone, though he was too ill to care. By the
end of the third quarter, he was again vomiting behind the ambulance and suffering severe stomach cramps. He had to go home.

Unmisig lived with his aunt, Connie Meyer, who worked as a
secretary in the emergency room. The next day, Swango called her
to see how Unmisig was doing, asking whether he'd have to miss his

next shift and probing for details of his symptoms. Suffering from an intense headache, continued nausea, and dehydration, Unmisig couldn't get out of bed for three days.

Gradually the others, too, recovered and returned to work. Twelve days later, on September 27, several of the paramedics teased Swango over the fact that he'd again been assigned to the backup ambulance rather than the primary emergency vehicle. This seemed to infuriate Swango, which only encouraged them to keep up the banter. Swango, in turn, had been complaining that the other paramedics weren't keeping up with reading the latest literature on emergency medicine and weren't working hard enough.

A little after noon, after responding to an ambulance call, Swango said, "I'm going after some sodas. Does anybody want one?"

"Yeah, I'd like a 7-Up," replied Greg Myers, who hadn't eaten any of Swango's doughnuts. After a few minutes, Myers saw Swango coming down the corridor with four sodas. But then Swango turned suddenly into the men's bathroom. When Swango handed him his 7-Up, Myers noticed that it had already been opened.

"Hey, what the heck did you do?" Myers asked jokingly. "Go in the bathroom and take a whiz in mine?"

"What do you mean?" Swango asked.

"I saw you go into the bathroom," Myers said.

"No, no," Swango said, explaining that he'd opened the 7-Up by mistake.

Though the can seemed full, Myers noticed the residue of some liquid around the opening, and again teased Swango about having urinated in it.

"I wasn't feeling well," Swango said this time, explaining he'd taken a sip of the soda to settle his stomach.

"That's fine, as long as you didn't whiz in it." Myers laughed.

He poured the 7-Up into a cup filled with ice and drank about a fourth of it. Soon after, he started to stand up, then suddenly sat down, overcome by nausea. He rushed to the bathroom, where he was racked by vomiting, the worst he'd ever experienced. While he was in the bathroom, Swango came to the door holding the cup of soda and asked if he wanted more, saying it might settle his stomach. Myers declined. He was so weak he had to lie down. He couldn't even drive home. Someone else had to replace him on the shift.

When Myers's girlfriend, who worked at the hospital, stopped by later that afternoon, he told her, "Something's not right. I never get sick like this." She asked him what had happened, and he told her he'd just drunk some 7-Up that Swango had gotten for him. She mentioned that she'd just passed Swango in the kitchen area, where he was emptying a cup and ice into the sink. Myers suggested she look for the can. She found it in the sink, upside down, drained.

About an hour later, Myers managed to drive himself home, but had to stop three times to vomit en route. That evening, he got a call from Swango, who asked how he was doing and wanted to hear about his symptoms in great detail. Did he have diarrhea? How long had it lasted? Had his headache grown worse? Myers felt that most people would have asked how he was doing and left it at that. Swango was a doctor, but his interest seemed so acute that when he hung up, Myers said to himself, "I think he gave me something."

Several days later, when he had recovered enough to return to work, Myers described the incident involving the 7-Up to Connie Meyer. Her eyes widened as she listened to his story. "Oh my God," she finally said. "That's just what happened to Brent" at the football game. The pattern seemed obvious: Swango had offered both Unmisig and Myers a soda just before they fell ill. But Myers and Meyer were reluctant to share their suspicions. When Myers mentioned them to Lonnie Long, the boss brushed them aside, dismissing as preposterous the notion that someone like Swango might have tampered with their drinks. Nevertheless, the two confided in another paramedic, Fred Bennett, who thought they might be on to something.

About two weeks later, on October 12, while Swango was on duty, two other paramedics brewed some iced tea, then left on a call. They each took a sip of the tea when they returned. Both preferred unsweetened tea, and they hadn't added any sugar. But inexplicably, the tea tasted very sweet. Alarmed by the recent spate of severe illness among their fellow paramedics, they poured out the glasses and began searching for any empty sugar packets that might explain the sweet taste. They found none. Swango, hearing their remarks, dumped out the entire pitcher of tea.

Later that afternoon, after Swango had left on an ambulance run, the two noticed that his duffel was open and a bag stamped "George Keller & Sons" had fallen from it. Keller is a large garden and feed store in Quincy; and when they looked in the bag, the paramedics saw two boxes of Terro brand ant poison. One of the boxes was empty; the other contained a full bottle. The primary active ingredient in Terro ant poison is arsenic, which is concentrated in a sweet sucrose solution. When they shared this discovery with Krzystofczyk, he went into the emergency room and looked up arsenic in the medical encyclopedia. The symptoms of arsenic poisoning—violent vomiting, stomach cramps, and severe headaches—were exactly what they had been experiencing.

Now several of the paramedics baited a trap. They had been careful to keep their suspicions confined to a small group— Krzystofczyk, Unmisig, Myers, Fred Bennett, Connie Meyer, and a few others. They didn't want anyone tipping off Swango. First, they planted some fake ambulance calls that would summon everyone from the paramedics' quarters, leaving them vacant. Swango would hear the calls on his scanner, they assumed; someone in the emergency room would surreptitiously watch the paramedics' room to see what he did. But nothing materialized.

Then, about a week later, on Friday, October 19, Myers brewed a pot of iced tea, adding no sweetener. He and Bennett poured the tea into their glasses, which were marked with their initials. They had taken just a few sips when they received an ambulance call, put the glasses down, and left.

Not long after, Swango drove out of the parking lot and stopped at a busy intersection. Another paramedic pulled up just behind him. Suddenly, as Myers and Bennett approached in their ambulance, Swango pulled over, threw his car into reverse, and backed up at high speed until he could turn into the nearest alleyway.

Curious, the paramedic who'd stopped behind Swango's car at the intersection returned to the hospital, where he told Myers and Bennett about Swango's strange behavior. Unaware of the recent developments, he said laughingly that it seemed Swango didn't want them to see him. Myers and Bennett looked at each other knowingly, then went to their tea. Bennett took a taste.

"Taste this," he said to Myers. Myers took the glass.

"Damn, that's sweet," he said.

Shortly after, Mark Krzystofczyk arrived. "Here," Myers said, handing him the glass of tea. Krzystofczyk tasted it. We've got him, he thought.

But now that the paramedics had the sample of sweetened tea, none of them knew what to do with it. They poured the remaining tea into a plastic container they obtained from the emergency room, then put that inside an empty cottage cheese container and stored it in a brown paper bag in Bennett's locker.

At two A.M., Swango showed up at St. Mary's Hospital, where one of his closest friends among the paramedics, Lamont "Monty" Grover, was on call, sleeping in the paramedics' quarters. Swango woke him up and insisted Grover walk outside with him into the hospital garage. There Swango said, "Sometimes I feel I have an evil purpose in life." Grover didn't know what to say.

The paramedics left the tea in the locker over the weekend. When they told Connie Meyer about it, she called Dr. William Gasser, who in addition to having been one of Swango's chemistry professors at Quincy College also worked part-time helping the pathologists at Blessing Hospital as a laboratory consultant. Meyer told Gasser she had some tea she'd like tested for the presence of arsenic. Gasser said he couldn't test specifically for arsenic, but he could do a relatively simple test that would indicate the presence of heavy metals. Arsenic is a heavy metal, along with cadmium and tin.

Gasser knew only that the liquid was tea. On Monday, he took the sample to his lab at Quincy College. First he tested ordinary tea, which did not show the presence of any heavy metals. Then he tested the sample. It was positive.

Myers took the sample to the Adams County coroner, Wayne Johnson, who forwarded it to the crime lab at the Illinois Bureau of Investigation for further tests. It was positive for arsenic.

Armed with this evidence, the group of paramedics, along with Connie Meyer, met with Gene Mann, the director of the Adams County Health Department, in his office. They shut the door, and laid out their findings. Noticing their absence, Swango asked several secretaries at the emergency room what was going on, but none of them knew.

At the meeting, several paramedics, Krzystofczyk among

them, argued for more time to collect evidence. They knew Swango was smart and cocky, and they were afraid he'd wriggle out of any charges unless they caught him red-handed. But presidential candidate Michael Dukakis was scheduled to arrive in Quincy for a speech at the college later that week. Swango had been talking recently about assassinations, and they worried that such a prominent visitor might be at risk if Swango remained at large.

The paramedics had the feeling that Swango had merely been experimenting with them, though the arsenic dose in the pitcher of tea might have been lethal to anyone who actually consumed it. But they felt that their evidence suggested that Swango, far from the all-American image he projected, was psychologically twisted and fully capable of murder. Mann decided that the police should be notified immediately. He picked up the phone.

SWANGO seemed suspicious that so many of the paramedics had been meeting with Mann, but when he asked what they were doing, Myers claimed it was nothing important. Swango badgered him. "What were you talking about?" he asked. "Nothing I can tell you about," Myers replied.

The next day, Friday, October 26, Swango got a call at work asking if he'd stop by the Adams County Sheriff's Office. He had applied for the deputy coroner job; Sheriff Bob Nall implied that he was about to get the job. When Swango arrived he was instead arrested, read his rights, charged with battery, which under Illinois law includes nonfatal poisonings. Though he said he wouldn't make any statement without his lawyer being present, he gave the police permission to search his apartment.

When police arrived at the neat, two-story house on Eighteenth Street and opened the door to Swango's apartment, they were startled. The place was a mess. Spread out on a table and shelves was a virtual poison lab, with a large book bearing a skull and crossbones on the cover placed prominently amid the vials, needles, and bottles. The book, *The Poor Man's James Bond,* which is said to be popular among paramilitary enthusiasts, is described by its publisher, Paladin Press, as "the undisputed leader in the field of books on improvised weaponry and do-it-yourself mayhem," which tells "how to buy most of the needed chemicals from your grocery and garden store."

As the police report described the scene, "An entire mini-lab set-up was observed. Detectives found numerous chemicals, suspected poisons and poisonous compounds. Underground-type magazines were observed that gave technical information on exotic poisons.... Handwritten recipes for poisons/poisonous compounds were observed." The poisons and recipes included ricin, botulin, nicotine, supersaturated cyanide, and fluoroacetic acid. The report continued, "Detectives also observed numerous newspapers and various scrapbooks etc. The suspect appears to have been collecting information on disasters, car accidents, and even newspaper clippings in regards to the Tylenol murders in the Chicago, Ill. area."

The police seized as possible evidence the *James Bond* book, various pesticides including numerous bottles of Terro ant poison filled to varying levels, chemicals, a large supply of castor beans— the raw material for the poison ricin—syringes, needles, and a gallon jug of sulfuric acid. The police also confiscated a small arsenal: a Mossberg twelve-gauge pump shotgun with a combat stock; a Llama .357 Magnum revolver; a Raven .25 automatic handgun; and two large K-Bar survival knives. But perhaps the most peculiar items dealt with the occult. Among the books confiscated were *The Book of Ceremonial Magic, The Necronomicon,* and *The Modern Witch's Spell Book.* Police also found numerous handwritten spells, incantations, and a bag of stones bearing peculiar markings.

Mostly out of curiosity, the police also checked with the Quincy Public Library. The library's records indicated that Swango had recently checked out two books: *One by One,* a novel by Linda Lee, and *The Healer: A True Story of Medicine and Murder,* by Leonard Levitt. According to its jacket copy, *One by One* describes how a pair of "diabolical psychopaths" injects botulism toxin into food in New York City supermarkets, terrorizing the entire city's population. *The Healer* is a nonfiction account of the 1975 fatal injection of his wife with Demerol by Charles Friedgood, a Long Island surgeon. According to its jacket copy, it is "a fascinating psychological study of a physician-murderer."

NEWS of Michael's arrest stunned the extended Swango family. Muriel Swango was staying in Florida with her son Richard when Michael called Friday afternoon to say he'd been arrested for battery and needed bail money. Muriel called Michael's aunt Ruth Miller in Quincy, and asked her to go to the courthouse and put up the $5,000. Muriel promised to repay her as soon as she returned. Swango was released that evening. Muriel also called Bob in Oregon to tell him about his brother. She was matter-of-fact and unemotional.

When Louise Scharf heard the news in Springfield, she called Ruth for details. "It's all a misunderstanding," Ruth explained. "Michael told his mother it was some kind of fight."

But on the Monday after Swango's arrest, *The Quincy Herald-Whig* ran a brief story that made no mention of any fight or brawl. The headline was "Man Suspected of Poisoning Co-worker":

> Michael W. Swango, 30, 220 N. 18th, was arrested Friday on a charge of aggravated battery in connection with the earlier poisoning of a co-worker.
>
> Police chief Charles A. Gruber said investigators are still trying to learn the exact nature and content of the toxic pesticide. The toxin is being checked at laboratories in Chicago and Atlanta, Gruber said. . . .

Muriel returned to Quincy immediately after hearing the news. Ruth asked her what had really happened.

"He's not guilty at all," Muriel said.

"How can you say that?" Ruth asked.

"Because he told me he wasn't," she replied firmly.

CHAPTER FIVE

THE OHIO STATE UNIVERSITY police department occupies spacious quarters near the football stadium, and with fifty officers, is larger than the police force in many medium-sized cities. Police Chief Peter Herdt, who was forty at the time of Swango's arrest, reported to a university vice president, and though the force often cooperated with the Columbus police, it was autonomous. Indeed, Herdt had been personally assured by President Edward Jennings before he agreed to take the job that he would have unfettered freedom to investigate any crime. So when Quincy authorities called the Columbus police asking for background on Swango, an Ohio State intern, they were referred to the Ohio State force.

OSU police officer Bruce Anderson returned the call; the Quincy police briefed him on Swango's arrest and on the bizarre evidence found in his apartment.

This was hardly the usual fare for a university police officer, even on a campus the size of Ohio State. Anderson, age thirty-four, had a bachelor's degree in microbiology; he had minimal experience in major-crime investigation. He went to the hospital, was told to speak to the chief of surgery, and met with Dr. Carey on the afternoon of October 26, the same day as Swango's arrest. Coroner Wayne Johnson had also phoned Carey earlier that day, but Carey thought he was calling about a job recommendation for Swango and ignored the call. That was why Johnson had turned to the police for help.

Anderson now told Carey that Swango had just been arrested in Illinois, and that he was pursuing a background check for the Illinois authorities. Carey was taken aback. He had largely put Swango out of his mind in the four months since the intern had left Ohio State, and didn't remember much about the internal investigation. He refreshed his memory by looking at Swango's file. Carey told Anderson that Swango's performance as an intern had been substandard, and that he hadn't been reappointed at the end of his first year. He added that Swango had been accused of "tampering" with a patient's IV line. The hospital had conducted an internal investigation, he said, and Swango had been "exonerated," the same language he'd used in recommending Swango to the medical board. Anderson thought Carey cooperative, though he didn't show the officer Swango's file, since it included confidential evaluations of his performance. Carey did tell Anderson that Swango's personnel file should be available in the office of the acting medical director.

The possible import of the news from Quincy wasn't lost on Carey. As soon as Anderson left, he called Tzagournis. (Apparently unrelated to the Swango incident, Whitcomb, the medical director who conducted the internal investigation of Swango, had taken a leave of absence, and Cramp, the hospital's executive director, had resigned.) Tzagournis, in turn, consulted university vice president Richard Jackson and Alphonse Cincione, the outside lawyer brought in for the Swango investigation. This suggests that Tzagournis immediately recognized the potential significance of Swango's arrest.

Tzagournis called a meeting to discuss the latest turn of events; the group included, for the first time in the Swango affair, someone from the hospitals' public relations office. The focus of the meeting seems to have been to limit the legal and public-relations damage to the Ohio State Hospitals. Concern was expressed about the confidentiality of files—Swango's and patients'. Consideration was even given to issuing a press release, since word of Swango's arrest in Illinois was likely to surface publicly in Ohio sooner or later. But that impulse was quickly suppressed. There is no indication that anyone decided to notify the Ohio State Medical Board that Swango had been arrested.*

---

*Later it was concluded that "someone involved, probably Dr. Carey, should have alerted the State Medical Board."

Instead, the upshot of the meeting was that Assistant Attorney General Holder, who had been involved in the earlier investigation and was therefore familiar with the facts, should handle all police inquiries as well as any others. Specifically, no files relating to Swango or patients would be given to the OSU police by anyone at the hospital. In keeping with the hospitals' policy, they were moved to a locked file cabinet to which access was strictly limited. The possibility of cooperating fully with a police investigation—and perhaps finally getting to the bottom of the Cooper incident, not to mention the patient deaths—doesn't seem to have been discussed, even though it was a police officer's request for cooperation that had triggered the meeting.

The decision to position a lawyer between the university police force and the hospital doctors and other personnel—in particular, to use the same lawyer who had already "exonerated" Swango and endorsed the decision to return him to hospital duty the previous February—was surely based on the perceived need to protect patient confidentiality and to limit any potential liability and embarrassing publicity. But it may also have reflected a long-standing deterioration in relations between doctors and the police at Ohio State; similar tensions developed in many American communities during the preceding decades of malpractice litigation and skyrocketing insurance premiums. Many doctors had come to see the police as little more than evidence-seekers for plaintiffs' lawyers. The hospital administrators' defensiveness also reflected doctors' concerns that the police, in their zeal to find and convict criminals, were insensitive to the well-being of patients and the workings of the hospital, which they seemed all too willing to disrupt. But in the case of Ohio State, ill will between doctors and police had reached the boiling point during a recent investigation within the hospitals.

As a result of a spate of reports of gambling and loan-sharking at the university hospitals, the OSU police had mounted a relatively sophisticated undercover operation, using investigators posing as hospital employees. Evidence soon emerged of drug abuse at the hospitals. Fiber-optic cameras were mounted inside, several of them being trained on carts used to store and dispense drugs. The agents obtained footage of doctors, nurses, and nurses' aides taking drugs from the cart. In some cases they injected themselves with narcotics intended for patients who needed relief from pain, then replaced the drugs with a saline solution given to patients. Investigators observed one doctor who was obviously drunk while on duty, and others who appeared to be working while under the influence of marijuana and other drugs.

Chief Herdt took the evidence to Holder, the assistant attorney general now involved in the Swango inquiries, arguing that criminal activity was far more widespread in the hospitals than anyone had suspected and that the investigation should be expanded. Holder sent Herdt to the university's "risk management" committee, which aims to reduce liability. Herdt was later told that hospital personnel suspected of drug and alcohol abuse should be quietly encouraged to seek treatment, but that no other investigative steps should be taken. The surveillance operation was later dismantled. No drug charges were ever filed.

Still, as word of the operation spread within the hospitals, many doctors became angry. They thought the OSU police had been trying to entrap them, and this generated even more distrust of the force. The police, in turn, were angered and made cynical by their perception that the hospitals were more interested in covering up any possible liability or embarrassment than in stopping drug and alcohol abuse in the hospitals.

With these recent tensions still simmering, Holder and Jackson called Charles Gambs, the university administrator who oversaw the police force, and asked him to find out exactly what the police were doing in the hospital. Gambs, in turn, called Chief Herdt.

Herdt, with his rugged good looks, prematurely gray hair, and forceful presence, was viewed by some as overqualified for the university job, not to mention overzealous. He was nationally known in police circles for his work in the seventies on the Oakland, California, police force, where he investigated the Symbionese Liberation Army kidnapping of Patty Hearst. Since then, however, his career had been somewhat less exciting. He had come to Ohio State from comparatively peaceful Springfield, Vermont, where he had been police chief, and the university assignment seemed to make up in job security and benefits what it lacked in drama. For that, Herdt turned to his own imagination, writing crime fiction for *Police* magazine. He had just arrived at OSU and it wasn't yet clear whether he'd be a team player, someone who was equally sensitive to the safety of the community and the reputation of the university.

When Gambs called, asking what Officer Anderson was doing asking questions at the medical school, it came as news to Herdt. The Quincy police request for a background check on a former student had seemed inconsequential—Anderson hadn't bothered mentioning it to Herdt. Herdt spoke to Anderson, then reported back to Gambs that they were simply doing a routine background check at the request of the Quincy police force. But the suddenly expressed interest of an assistant vice president naturally alerted Herdt and Anderson to the possibility that the matter was less routine than Anderson had assumed.

This was confirmed the next day. Anderson returned to the acting medical director's office, expecting to review Swango's files, and was informed that they had been moved to Tzagournis's office. As had been decided at the previous day's strategy meeting, Anderson was told to direct his inquiries to Holder. Instead, Anderson went in person to Tzagournis's office to see the Swango files he thought he'd been promised. He was told to wait. After some time passed, Tzagournis's secretary told him he had a phone call from Holder, which, Anderson assumed, meant that someone in Tzagournis's office had called the assistant attorney general. Once Anderson got on the phone, Holder asked him what he was doing there. Once again, Anderson explained the nature of the inquiry and said he simply wanted to review Swango's personnel file. Holder told him he could not get that information from Tzagournis and suggested that he and Anderson meet to discuss the matter the following week. Anderson returned to headquarters empty-handed.

The Quincy police fared no better in their inquiries at Ohio State. After ignoring the call from Wayne Johnson, Dr. Carey had returned a call from someone who identified himself as a Quincy police officer. But a police secretary said no one by that name worked in the department. Carey leaped to the conclusion that someone might have been impersonating a police officer to gain information about Swango. He apparently didn't consider the possibility that his secretary might simply have gotten the name wrong. He resolved not to respond to any more inquiries over the phone.

The following Monday, November 5, 1984, Gambs met with Herdt in his office. Gambs had now been briefed on Swango by Cincione and Holder, who told him about the Cooper incident and the internal investigation conducted by Dr. Whitcomb under Tzagournis's supervision. Filtered through the eyes of Holder and Cincione, both of whom had been involved in returning Swango to the hospital and allowing him to complete his internship, this account not surprisingly emphasized that the investigation had been thorough and that Swango had been exonerated. Gambs in turn briefed Herdt, who for the first time learned that Swango had been involved in a highly suspicious incident in the Ohio State hospitals.

As a trained investigator, Herdt was less interested in the details of the earlier investigation than in the startling coincidence that someone suspected of tampering with a patient's IV line had now been arrested and charged with poisoning coworkers at another hospital. The events in Quincy had suddenly shed an entirely new light on Swango; rather than a doctor with no known blemish on his record, he was one accused of a bizarre and potentially deadly felony. The situation cried out for a thorough inquiry carried out by trained investigators, not by doctors. Herdt insisted on discussing the need for such an investigation directly with Holder and Cincione, and Gambs arranged a meeting for the next morning.

Herdt believed that he got along well with the mild-mannered Gambs, who had supported him in several other contentious matters, including the controversial undercover investigation in the hospitals. He expected that once Gambs pointed out the need for outside investigators to Holder and Cincione, the group would quickly authorize a thorough inquiry.

But Herdt's expectations proved naive. At the meeting, positions hardened almost immediately. Holder and Cincione argued that the matter had already been thoroughly investigated and there was no point in bringing in the police unless they had specific new evidence relating to the events at Ohio State. Now that the events were several months old, the investigative trail would in any event be "stale," they argued, and unlikely to yield any significant evidence. Gambs agreed. Herdt asked to see Whitcomb's report and notes. The OSU administrators replied that there was no written report, and that Whitcomb kept no notes.

Herdt was shocked. Both he and Anderson, who had accompanied him to the meeting, pointed out that they could hardly produce any new evidence unless they were allowed to investigate. And in any event, Swango's arrest in Illinois was by itself basis enough to reopen the inquiry. But Gambs and the lawyers were adamant. As Herdt wrote in notes to himself immediately after the meeting, Gambs "stated that he sees no basis of a crime happening as was the finding of an already completed investigation. He thought it strange for the police to be investigating matters where there is no crime!" He "sees little point in pursuing this further." In a parenthesis, Herdt continued: "I don't understand his reasoning here; why is he seemingly against our being involved? Why is he saying this?"

All Herdt managed to extract was an agreement that the police could look into any satanic or occult involvement by Swango while he was at Ohio State, a line of inquiry triggered by the books and paraphernalia on the occult found in his Quincy apartment. But even that limited investigation was to be kept out of the hospital. For now, Holder and Cincione specifically barred the OSU police from speaking to any doctors, patients, or former patients, such as Cooper.

Holder and Cincione left. Furious, Herdt stayed behind to vent his anger at Gambs. But Gambs warned him off: "In my view," he said, "the OSU police should not be pursuing this any further."

"You're stonewalling," Herdt angrily accused.

Gambs shrugged. Even if Herdt did investigate, "it will only end in the same result anyway," he said. But if Herdt insisted on pursuing the matter, he should write a memo, which Gambs would pass on to Holder. Herdt took notes as Gambs dictated the questions that he should address:

> What is it that the police intend to investigate in this matter?
> On what basis?
> Specifically, what parts of this investigation by Hospitals staff did the police have doubts or questions about?

Herdt was insulted and angry. He thought such a memo would only waste time, and being made to write it at all was an infringement of the autonomy he thought he'd been promised when he took the job.

Herdt and Anderson left at noon. As Herdt wrote in his notes, "I departed . . . *depressed, shocked, saddened* and visibly *upset.*"

Anderson spoke to Wayne Johnson, who reported that Anderson feared he might be fired. "If I don't cool it" on the Swango investigation, he said, "they'll have my job." *

AFTER the frustrating meeting with Gambs, Holder, and Cincione, the OSU police investigation made scant progress. Herdt wrote a three-page memo responding to Gambs's questions, arguing that the developments in Illinois all but mandated a renewed investigation; that he had learned of other incidents besides the one involving Cooper, including some patient deaths, which ought to be investigated; and finally, that the investigation conducted by Whitcomb was "inadequate."

Herdt's memo—the first *written* criticism of the medical school's own investigation—not only offered a politically charged assertion, given the mutual suspicion between the doctors and the police, but could also be expected to fuel the adverse publicity the university wanted to avoid. It was one thing to investigate Swango, another to investigate the university's handling of the affair. Gambs wrote back that he found the memo unpersuasive, and again expressed doubt that there was any point in further investigation. He also asked for another memo detailing precisely how Herdt proposed to conduct his investigation. But the exchange of memos had already taken a month; Herdt refused to waste any more time on what he considered a stalling tactic.

Anderson had not made any progress with Holder, either. No one in the police force had yet reviewed any of the hospital's files on Swango.

Except for some halfhearted inquiries into satanic practices in and around Columbus, the police inquiry ground to a halt. Anderson, who remained in charge day to day, went on vacation in De-

---

* Later, Anderson denied that his job was ever threatened.

cember. Hospital officials seemed confident that the whole matter would soon blow over, as it had four months earlier.

Then, on December 12, Gambs received an ominous call from Thomas Prunte, the lawyer for the Ohio State Medical Board who had corresponded with Dr. Carey before the board approved Swango's application for a medical license. Prunte also called the OSU police. He had just heard from the Illinois state attorney general, who was looking into Swango's Illinois medical license, and had subsequently spoken to Quincy police. He had thus learned of the Swango matter from Illinois authorities—not from anyone in Ohio, and certainly not from anyone at Ohio State. Now the medical board had assigned its own investigator, Charles Eley, to the matter.

Word of the call from Prunte brought Herdt's frustrations to the boiling point. That same day, he drafted a memo to himself: "If so requested, I will submit my resignation. But first, I will complete this investigation at whatever cost. I'd come to OSU proud of my personal integrity after 15 years as a law enforcement officer and I intended to remain here or leave with it intact. . . . I would never involve myself or department personnel in any type of so-called cover-up. And I believed the 'shit would hit the fan' very soon."

IN Quincy, Swango was formally arraigned on seven counts of aggravated battery on December 20 and entered a plea of not guilty. To defend him, he hired Daniel Cook, who had taught him history in high school before becoming a lawyer and had considered Swango one of his best students. The court continued Swango's bail of $5,000. A condition of his release was that he not leave Adams County without the court's permission, which it granted on one occasion so he could visit his mother and half brother in Florida at Christmas.

Nonetheless, only days after his arrest, at the end of October, Swango had applied for a job as an emergency room physician for the northern Ohio region. Robert Haller II, the regional vice president for National Emergency Service, Inc., in Toledo, had interviewed Swango for the job in November, and was impressed by his credentials, his experience as a paramedic, and his enthusiasm for emergency medicine. Swango remained a licensed physician in both

Ohio and Illinois, and he made no mention of his recent arrest or upcoming trial. Other than *The Quincy Herald-Whig,* no media had carried the story, so Haller knew nothing about it. Haller later said that he introduced Swango to three of the company's medical directors, "all of whom thought Mike was a very personable and professional young man."

There was nothing in Swango's record to suggest otherwise. On the contrary, National Emergency Service verified that Swango had received his medical degree from Southern Illinois and obtained at least two letters of recommendation from Ohio State. Even though Swango was at that very moment once again under investigation, and Ohio State officials now knew he had been charged with poisoning coworkers in Illinois, the university gave National Emergency Service a certificate showing that Swango had satisfactorily completed his internship. The 1984 certificate was signed by both Tzagournis and Carey.

National Emergency Service subcontracts its doctors to area hospitals, and it referred Swango to several of them, including Fisher-Titus Memorial Hospital in Huron County. Dr. Timothy Thomas, who was in charge of emergency services at Fisher-Titus, was impressed by Swango, describing him as "very outgoing . . . he seemed to have interpersonal skills, and he struck me as a pleasant young physician." Thomas described Swango's letters of recommendation from Ohio State as "glowing." Swango told Titus that he had left Ohio State after his internship because he wanted "to take a break" and "pay some bills." He mentioned having worked briefly in Quincy, but said he was now living at the Harvard Square apartments in northwest Columbus, and would be commuting the ninety miles to work. None of this struck Thomas as out of the ordinary, and no one did any further checking on Swango's background.

With what must have seemed extraordinary speed and ease for someone facing felony charges, Swango was again working as a doctor.

HERDT'S prediction that news of Swango's arrest would cause a commotion in Ohio finally materialized. It had taken several months, but an official at the Ohio State Medical Board had tipped off reporters at the Cleveland *Plain Dealer* to Swango's arrest. On

Wednesday, January 30, 1985, Mary Anne Sharkey, a Columbus-based reporter for *The Plain Dealer*, called the university's information office for comment. The information office in turn contacted Tzagournis's office. Sharkey and Gary Webb, an investigative reporter in Cleveland, were asking pointed questions about Swango. *The Plain Dealer* was the most widely circulated and most powerful newspaper in the state; many people at Ohio State felt it harbored a pro-Cleveland bias and was always looking for ways to disparage the rival city of Columbus.

Sharkey's inquiry prompted a flurry of meetings among medical school and university officials and what seemed to be a sudden change in their attitude toward the police. Tzagournis convened a meeting the afternoon of Sharkey's call that included Chief Herdt; Holder and Cincione, the lawyers; Boyanowski, now the hospital's acting executive director; Charles Eley, the medical board investigator; and John Rohal, Eley's supervisor at the medical board. Tzagournis opened the meeting with the statement that Ohio State and the medical school would "do everything necessary to cooperate" in any investigations. Herdt was amazed. Then Cincione seconded the commitment. Tzagournis added that "a newspaper reporter has learned of the incident." Suddenly Herdt understood what had prompted the newly conciliatory approach.

But Rohal, the medical board supervisor, had been talking to authorities in Quincy. The police chief there, Charles Gruber, and Rohal had attended the same police institute in Louisville; Gruber had called Rohal to complain that, as Rohal bluntly told the meeting, "the hospital was blocking the OSU police investigation." Rohal added that, according to the Quincy police, "other deaths might have happened here."

That potentially explosive assertion brought a flurry of denials. Tzagournis emphasized that "there are no other incidents in the files" and reiterated that "we want to give [all] information to the police." In fact, among the files locked in the filing cabinet at the hospital was at least one other "incident"—the one involving Rein Walter, the patient who had turned blue and died unexpectedly.

The seriousness of the latest developments was underscored by the arrival of Richard Jackson, the university vice president, about fifteen minutes into the meeting. Jackson, too, now proclaimed his support for a police investigation: "We ought to get on with this, get to the bottom of this."

Herdt was skeptical, but he nonetheless briefed the group on the limited progress his staff had made, mentioning that Anderson had failed to gain access to Swango's files. Tzagournis turned to Holder. "Can we give them our notes?"

"They've always been available," Holder said, a remark that prompted Herdt to write an exclamation point in his notes.

Ohio State also moved to minimize damage from the fact that Carey, in his June letter to the medical board, had erroneously referred to a patient's "demise," something the *Plain Dealer* reporters were asking about. Without correcting the reporters, Tzagournis ordered Dr. Carey to amend his June 1984 letter about Swango to the medical board. Carey did so, stating that "the patient referred to did not die and ultimately recovered." The correction obviously put the university in a more favorable light, and the urgency of the matter was underscored by the fact that Holder personally hand-delivered it to the medical board that day.

The next morning, January 31, the story the university had so hoped to avoid finally broke. *The Plain Dealer* ran a six-column banner headline, "Medic Probed in OSU Deaths." Written by Webb and Sharkey, the article began, "An Illinois surgeon, charged in the non-fatal poisonings of six paramedics in Quincy, is under investigation in connection with several patient deaths at Ohio State University Hospital, The Plain Dealer has learned."

The article continued, "While at OSU, the medical school investigated Swango in the death of a woman patient, a source familiar with the investigation said. Swango was cleared at the time of any wrongdoing." Like Dr. Carey's letter to the medical board, the passage evidently referred to the Cooper incident, repeating the error that the patient had died.

Despite the previous day's meeting, not to mention the months of meetings, memos, and deliberations that preceded it, an Ohio State spokesman flatly denied the thrust of the article: "OSU spokesman Scott Mueller denied the medical school had been asked for information concerning Swango's activities at OSU by any investigative agency," the paper reported. But the article quoted Quincy authorities contradicting Ohio State's denial.

A Quincy police official said detectives have been in contact with OSU police concerning the patient deaths, but said the detectives were not getting much cooperation.

"We are having a hard time verifying some of our information about what happened at Ohio State," the official said.

Ohio State officials were horrified. When Boyanowski saw the blaring headline, he ran into the hospital's lobby and purchased all of that day's copies of *The Plain Dealer* so patients wouldn't see the article and panic. The article also caused alarm at Fisher-Titus Hospital, where Swango had just completed a twenty-four-hour shift in the emergency room that ended at eight A.M. on Wednesday. As soon as he read the article, Dr. Thomas tried to reach Swango at home, but there wasn't any answer. The hospital immediately suspended Swango's hospital privileges.

(Swango had considered fleeing, but Dumas had persuaded him to return to Quincy, where he was scheduled for a court hearing the next day. Swango and Dumas were en route when Dr. Thomas called.)

The Columbus Dispatch, whose chairman, John W. Wolfe, had been a member of the hospital board until the previous October, had long been perceived as a cheerleader for Ohio State and its hospitals. But the *Dispatch* had to follow the *Plain Dealer* story in its afternoon edition. The relatively brief, unbylined article reported that Swango was under investigation by OSU police and added that "months ago the university launched an investigation into five patient deaths." The article said, accurately, that Swango had been investigated "in connection with a patient's respiratory arrest during his residency, but was later cleared." The *Dispatch*, managing to evade both the Ohio State public relations office and Holder, had interviewed Dr. Carey. He told the paper that Swango had been dropped from the residency program, but said nothing about patient deaths or suspicions that Swango had tampered with anyone's IV. "It was how he got along with people," he explained. "How he responded to calls. The residents thought he was a little funny, but there was nothing specific. They say he had a preoccupation with war; he talked about it a lot."

The promised cooperation with the police that had been stressed at the previous day's meeting quickly evaporated under the pressure of the negative publicity and suspicions of leaks. When Herdt met with Gambs and Jackson that afternoon, he had to leave the room briefly. He didn't take his briefcase, and later, Jackson demanded to know whether he had a tape recorder inside. Furious, Herdt opened the case to prove it contained only papers. Jackson, Gambs, and Boyanowski, who later joined the meeting, were extremely upset by the press coverage, and the discussion soon lapsed into mutual recriminations and accusations of leaking.

Worse was to come, as the Illinois authorities publicly vented their frustrations with Ohio State. The next day, *The Plain Dealer* followed the previous day's scoop with this headline: "OSU Covered Up, Poison Prober Says":

> Wayne L. Johnson, former Adams County (Ill.) coroner, said the medical school tried to cover up an incident last year involving a woman patient who suffered a mysterious seizure after Dr. Michael Swango reportedly injected something into the patient's intravenous tube. Johnson said when he reported the incident to campus police, the medical school refused to give police any records concerning Swango.
>
> "OSU needs to be shaken up on this crud," Johnson said angrily. "This was a very serious situation. They didn't want to tell me anything."

Johnson was also angry that OSU had allowed Swango to return to Quincy and obtain a job in a hospital without alerting anyone. "I have to find fault with OSU for not making his home [Quincy] aware of the circumstances out there," Johnson told *The Plain Dealer*. "They didn't do anything. They just covered it up."

The paper also quoted an unnamed medical school faculty member, who was similarly angry that no one had been warned about Swango after the Cooper incident. "They kept a lid on it," the faculty member told the paper. "You would have thought they would alert us to keep an eye on him, but they did not."

Ohio State also had to retract the denial it had given *The Plain Dealer* the previous day, reporting that the university spokesman,

Mueller, "admitted that [investigative agencies had indeed sought information concerning Swango's time at OSU]. He said the false information was given to him by the office of the medical school dean, Dr. Manuel Tzagournis."*

The next day, Anne Ritchie, the nurse who had been so shaken when Ruth Barrick died just after Swango treated her, called Herdt. The articles about Swango had confirmed her worst fears of the previous February. She told Herdt she felt she must speak out, because no one in the hospital had followed up after she reported the incident the day it happened. She told Herdt how upset she'd been when Swango ordered the heart monitor. Herdt was startled. Although he had heard some talk of mysterious deaths connected to Swango, Tzagournis had denied that there had been any such deaths. Ritchie's account suggested otherwise, and fueled Herdt's mounting concern that the hospital was blocking the investigation.

Jan Dickson, the hospital official in charge of the nurses, who had argued for a more thorough inquiry the previous February, was summoned by Tzagournis and Holder and asked for her recollections of the February 1984 meetings at which Swango was discussed. She described them as well as she could, mentioning that she had circulated the nurses' typed accounts as well as Cooper's handwritten notes, and that she had specifically cited the suspicious deaths linked to Swango.

Dickson could tell Tzagournis and Holder weren't happy with these answers. She felt that they were less interested in establishing what had actually happened than in coordinating a defense that hospital officials had no reason to be concerned about anything beyond the Cooper incident. As she later described her perception of the meeting, "I had a strong feeling they were cross-examining me. It was not subtle. I felt pressure. They wanted me to recall it differently. I kept saying, 'No, no, no. That is not how it happened.' "

---

* The medical school later claimed that Tzagournis hadn't lied, but had responded "no" to the question, "Was there an investigation of Swango by police or highway patrol while he was here?," which was a correct answer, albeit a misleading one, focusing on the phrase "while he was here." The reporter, however, maintained that her question was whether there had been a police investigation of Swango at any time, up to and including the present. Her question was passed through two intermediaries before it reached Tzagournis, which may account for the confusion.

Dickson said she assumed that Whitcomb's written report of his investigation would support her recollection. Tzagournis said there was no written report.

Holder then insisted that Dickson turn over to him all the nurses' typed statements, any handwritten notes by Cooper, and any other evidence in her possession. Dickson complied, but, fearing that the evidence might be lost, she secretly photocopied the original handwritten note from Cooper. She was also instructed not to talk to the press under any circumstances, and to refer any calls to Holder.

Though she remained loyal to the hospital, and wouldn't have spoken to the press in any event, Dickson felt ostracized by Tzagournis, Holder, and other high-ranking administrators after the meeting.

Herdt, too, felt pressure. Top hospital administrators were reeling from the articles in *The Plain Dealer*, especially the comments from authorities in Illinois. They were particularly incensed that Bruce Anderson, the OSU policeman who was reported to have felt threatened with the loss of his job, had declined comment when asked about the matter—even though he was merely complying with instructions not to talk to the press. Gambs told Herdt he should issue a press release saying that Anderson had never been threatened. Herdt refused.

Herdt concluded that, if anything, the defensive, obstructive mentality at the hospital was getting worse. He had never done such a thing before, but at 6:30 P.M. on February 5, he went over the heads of Gambs, Holder, and Jackson and called university president Jennings at his residence using a campus pay phone so the call couldn't be traced. Herdt told Jennings he had to meet with him immediately on a matter of extreme urgency. Jennings told him to come over; Herdt arrived at seven P.M.

Jennings, who served as president during the tenure of then-governor Richard Celeste, had something of a populist bent and loved to tell jokes that made fun of lawyers. Herdt hoped he would be a sympathetic ear. For an hour and a half Herdt briefed him on the Swango affair and the hospital's reaction; he even got into the evidence of physician drug use and drunkenness he'd gathered during the undercover operation into loan-sharking. Jennings said he was "shocked" and had had "no knowledge" of the extent of the problems at the hospital. Jennings promised to protect Herdt by saying that he had initiated the meeting in the wake of all the press coverage.

The next morning, President Jennings met first with Vice President Jackson, then with Jackson and Gambs. Gambs reported to Herdt that Jennings was going to issue a press release announcing that he had asked James E. Meeks, dean of the Ohio State University School of Law, to conduct an investigation into the Swango affair to determine what had happened, how it had been handled by the university, and whether any university policies or procedures had been breached, and to make recommendations. Though Meeks had no experience in criminal investigation, he was widely respected in the community, was trusted by both Jennings and Tzagournis, and, as he later put it, knew where the political "mine fields" were.

That evening, Jackson, chastened by his meeting with Jennings, came to Herdt's office to apologize. Sitting on Herdt's leather sofa, he emphasized that he'd relied on what Cincione and Holder had told him. "There was pressure on me" to go along with the lawyers, he said. He had "no knowledge" of how difficult a time Herdt had been having.

Herdt seized on the occasion to express his frustrations, saying he was unhappy working at Ohio State and felt he was a "figurehead." He told Jackson that Holder was talking with Tzagournis about taking a high-level job at the hospital.

Jackson said he wanted to assure Herdt that he would have his support, and that he felt no personal animosity toward him. "I'm willing to give statements" and "will tell Meeks the truth," Jackson said.

DESPITE the seeming rapprochement, relations between the OSU police and hospital personnel soon broke down again, this time for good.

The following Monday, now armed with what he believed was a mandate to get to the bottom of the Swango matter, Herdt dispatched one of his senior officers, Richard Harp, and the medical board investigator Charles Eley, who was now coordinating his efforts with Herdt's, to the hospital to begin interviewing nurses.

They arrived on the ninth floor of Rhodes Hall, asked a few preliminary questions, and left. While the interviews were uneventful, word quickly coursed through the nursing staff that police had been in the hospital asking about Swango. All the nurses knew officially was that Swango had been cleared of any wrongdoing earlier in the year. But many had never been convinced, and, of course, everyone had now been reading the papers. With Swango free on bail, and for all they knew living in the Columbus area, fear of him had returned with a vengeance. Nurses knew that Dickson and Moore had spoken out and that their concerns had been dismissed; many were now afraid that Swango would seek revenge if they said anything.

In this atmosphere, Officer Bruce Anderson arrived at the hospital the next night. A nurse told him she "was not at liberty" to tell him anything, not even whether the nurse he wanted to interview was still employed at the hospital. Anderson was furious. Despite the rebuff, he went to the ninth floor and tried to talk to some nurses there. When they refused, he accused them of interfering with a police investigation. A state of near-panic ensued, as nurses concluded they were being threatened with arrest and worried that patients would be alarmed. A nurse called Dickson at home; she in turn alerted hospital and university administrators. The matter got all the way to Vice President Jackson, but by then Anderson had left the hospital. Jackson said he'd deal with the problem in the morning.

The next night, a Wednesday, investigators Harp and Eley again showed up at the hospital and went straight to the ninth floor, where Dickson and Boyanowski were still at work. Even though they were the hospital administrators who had pressed most vigorously for an outside investigation, they were also upset over the events of the previous night, the effect on the nursing staff, and the potential harm to patients. Dickson and Boyanowski quickly intercepted the investigators, arguing that they were disrupting patient care. Harp angrily denied it. "Perhaps your definition of disruption is different from mine," Boyanowski responded.

The heated argument proceeded in a conference room on the floor so patients and nurses wouldn't overhear it. Boyanowski refused to let the investigators ask the nurses any questions, though he agreed to arrange future meetings in a conference room located off the floor. Harp and Eley were furious.

"I've been thrown out of better hospitals than this," Harp reported to Herdt when he returned to police headquarters.

MICHAEL Miller, the prosecuting attorney for Franklin County, which includes Columbus, walked into the office of Edward W. Morgan, one of his assistants. Miller said something had come up that he thought Morgan might be interested in: a search warrant at Ohio State. Morgan wasn't excited at the prospect of a routine search warrant, but Miller had something of a twinkle in his eye. "This could turn into something," he told Morgan, adding that Dick Harp would be calling him from the OSU police.

Morgan, forty, tall, good-looking, and a good speaker, liked being in the limelight. He'd joined the prosecutor's office in 1973, after graduating from Ohio State Law School and doing a stint of college teaching in the south. He thought of himself as something of a frustrated actor, and he'd come to love the drama of trials, even though he lost his first one, involving a sixteen-year-old juvenile accused of running a red light. He'd since become one of Miller's most experienced investigators and trial lawyers.

When Harp called Morgan, he explained that the matter involved Michael Swango. Morgan knew immediately why he'd been put on the case. He'd read about Swango in the papers, and given the hospital and university role, he knew, the matter could be explosive politically. Harp explained that the police had identified a storage locker on Kenny Road in Columbus rented by Swango, and needed a search warrant. Morgan helped prepare one, which a judge approved. By the time of the search itself, on February 5, the press had descended, along with the Franklin County sheriff's bomb squad. Because of Swango's fascination with weaponry and violent death, rumors had swirled that the locker might be booby-trapped. As Herdt and other police approached the locker, the crowd surged forward, and Herdt ordered them to back up. "I won't be responsible if anyone gets blown up," he warned.

The result was something of an anticlimax. The locker held some old newspapers, more clippings about accidents and disasters, some used Army clothing.

After the search, Morgan met with Herdt, who asked him to stay involved with the case as the investigation continued. Herdt briefed him on all the problems he'd had with the hospital and how frustrated he'd felt. Morgan, sympathetic, reported back to Miller, who agreed that they should treat the matter as a potential murder case. Together, Miller and Morgan went to the law library to do some reading on poisons and related forensic issues. What they learned was discouraging, especially given the amount of time that had passed since the last suspicious patient death. They read that autopsies typically do not reveal poisons. For some poisons, among them ricin, there was no known test at all. As Morgan remarked to Miller when they finished their research, "Poisoning is the perfect crime."

Of the various investigations now under way, the internal Meeks inquiry was the first to be finished. Meeks had enlisted a criminal-law professor who had been an assistant district attorney to help with the report, and though they did not interview Swango himself, they were the first to interview several critical witnesses. These included Rita Dumas; Rena Cooper; several of the nurses, including Dickson and Beery; and most of the doctors, who were told by Jennings and Tzagournis to cooperate.

Rita Dumas staunchly defended Swango, saying it was impossible for him to have harmed any patients. She tearfully told them how she felt she would not have survived without his support. He had helped her financially when she was nearly destitute, and had helped care for her three children.

The student nurse Karolyn Beery, who had been in the room and had seen Swango inject something into Cooper's IV, "felt very vulnerable," Meeks said. "She was shunted aside. She was upset. She had the most damning eyewitness account."

Meeks questioned Dickson's testimony. She insisted she had told the doctors about the patient deaths and brought the nurses' incriminating observations to their attention at the meetings the previous February, but the doctors involved disputed it, saying they had no memory of Dickson having done so. As Meeks later put it, "Dickson claimed she told the meeting and was ignored. This is possible. But all of the doctors ignored her? That's hard to believe." Like many involved in the investigation, Meeks credited the united front of doctors over the word of a nurse.

Meeks found nearly everyone involved to be cooperative, except for Dr. Whitcomb, who was still on leave of absence in Washington, D.C. Meeks interviewed him by telephone. "He didn't give us very much," the investigator later said. Even if Dickson had presented her suspicions to Whitcomb, Meeks concluded it wouldn't have made much difference. "Whitcomb paid no attention to the nurses," he said. "There was tension between him and the nurses. He ignored them. All he was looking at was the medical record, and there wasn't much there. He was very removed from the reality of the hospital floor."

Meeks also quickly encountered what he described as "open hostility" between the medical personnel and the police force, stemming in part from the abortive undercover operation in the hospital. This tension came as a surprise to him.

The Meeks report was released to the public on April 2, 1985. To say, as Meeks did, that he was operating in a "political mine field" was an understatement. He had the Ohio press, the university president, and even the governor looking over his shoulder. He was charged with investigating some of the most powerful figures in the university community: Tzagournis, the medical dean, with his ties to trustees and legislators; Holder, an assistant attorney general; and Cincione, a prominent outside lawyer. The reputations of the university and its cherished medical school and hospital were at stake.

"We went into the review with completely open minds," Meeks began his report. "We ended the review process with many doubts about what exactly had happened in this very complex episode. Our purpose, of course, was not to determine whether criminal behavior occurred. We leave resolution of criminal issues to the law enforcement officers and the courts. Nor did we enter with any presumption that evil or criminal behavior had necessarily occurred." Indeed, the report concluded that "It is quite possible that there are innocent explanations for the [Cooper] incident, as well as other cases which were never investigated." Meeks also pointed out that "the matter to which our inquiry was directed was a very unusual event in the life of any hospital. For that reason, it was difficult, we think, for anyone to fully grasp its significance or how to deal with it. Medical authorities here and elsewhere have agreed that it was such an aber-

rational episode that it was almost impossible to plan for its handling or to have specific devices in place to try to prevent it."

In several instances, Meeks resolved issues in the university's
favor, concluding that there had been no cover-up and that the hospital did not withhold information from investigators; that the
medical school had cooperated with investigators within the con-
straints imposed by legitimate interests of patients; that the hospital
had not "erred" in the decision as a preliminary step to conduct its
own investigation; and that Dr. Carey, in particular, had been fully
cooperative and had not misled the medical board in recommending
that Swango be licensed to practice medicine.

But even couched in the diplomatic language chosen by Meeks
and his assistants, the report was scathing, especially with respect to
the hospital's initial investigations of the Cooper incident. "Put
simply, [the inquiry] was far too superficial," the report concluded.

> We have been apprised of facts which should have sig-
> naled the need for a more thorough inquiry. . . . The re-
> sults were that there were numerous witnesses who were
> never interviewed; the interviews that were conducted
> were in many instances inadequate; no attempts were
> made to reconcile inconsistencies or clarify ambiguities;
> and the conclusions drawn from some of the key inter-
> views are of questionable validity.

Meeks specifically faulted the treatment of Utz, Cooper's
roommate. "Her basic story has remained unchanged to this day,"
his report noted. "Yet no one in a position to make a medical judgment about what she was saying, not even Dr. Hunt, talked to her
about the incident. . . . The decision to discount her entirely without even a determination of the effect of her disease on her ability
to perceive and recall is highly questionable, particularly in light of
her eyewitness position and the substance of her highly incriminating allegations against Dr. Swango."

The report noted that not one but three eyewitnesses—Beery,
Cooper, and Utz—saw someone do something to Cooper just before her respiratory arrest. Yet all of their testimony was dismissed
as unreliable. "The combined effect of all three statements is quite

powerful and suggests, at the very least, the need to investigate further. Indeed, assuming hypothetically that all three witnesses to an event are psychotic, the fact that they report the same basic facts would preclude rejection of all three versions due to the psychosis of each individual witness."

Nor, the report noted, were various nurse witnesses interviewed; nor was Dr. Freeman, the head resident, who was the first to confront Swango.

"Most disappointing of all," the report continued, was the failure to test the syringe discovered by Joe Risley, which Nurse Moore had brought to Dr. Goodman's attention. "Dr. Goodman never asked to see the syringe and he did not make its existence known during any of the three meetings of the investigative team." While Meeks found Goodman's behavior understandable, "the fact that no one on the investigating team except Dr. Goodman is even aware of its existence to this day is troublesome."

The report harshly criticized the doctors' diagnosis of the cause of Cooper's respiratory arrest as a grand mal seizure and the failure to consult appropriate experts who might have rendered an accurate diagnosis. As Meeks noted,

> We consulted with two anesthesiologists who disputed the view that [Cooper's] symptoms were inconsistent with the use of muscle relaxants such as Anectine [succinylcholine] or curare. Both of these drugs are readily available and frequently used in the hospital, particularly in the emergency room; they are eliminated quickly from the bloodstream and will not usually show up on a routine blood test; and they will cause paralysis and respiratory arrest. . . . Both anesthesiologists we consulted found the use of Anectine or curare quite plausible as explaining what happened here.

The doctors' failure to investigate any of the patient deaths linked to Swango, other than a cursory review of their medical files, even where there were nurse witnesses, seemed inexplicable to Meeks and his assistants. "The failure to follow up on the nurse concerns and suspicions with regard to Dr. Swango's involvement in cases other than the [Cooper] case was, in our judgment, a serious omission." And finally, using what under the circumstances was unusually blunt language, Meeks wrote,

> We still find it astounding that no permanent record was kept detailing the occurrence and what was done about it. We understand the reluctance of those in the health profession to put anything in writing because it could be used in a subsequent civil liability litigation context. Nevertheless, we believe a full formal report of this incident should have been prepared by someone and kept in the hospital records.

"The inadequacy of the investigation . . . undermines the ultimate conclusion not to pursue the matter further, and specifically not to refer the matter to outside authorities," Meeks concluded.

He called for several remedial measures, the most important of which was to establish a new office that would report to the vice president for health services or the hospital's executive director and would be staffed "with persons trained as investigators and capable of handling medically-related investigations." The office "should also monitor deaths and unusual events within the hospital in an attempt to detect illegal or undesired activity."

The report also called for a "statement of principles" to govern police presence in the hospital in an effort to ease tensions between law enforcement and hospital personnel. "To this day," the report noted, "the relationship between the Hospitals administration and the police is quite negative. The police are of the view that they simply get no cooperation from the Hospitals administration at all. The Hospitals administration is of the view that the police conduct themselves with total insensitivity to the special needs and requirements of a health care situation and have no respect for the confidentiality of patient records."

But there was little in the report about accountability, potentially the most sensitive issue. No blame for what had happened was apportioned, nor were any disciplinary measures or personnel moves suggested. Meeks concluded that the "lawyers relied on the doctors" and the "doctors relied on the lawyers," and thus, no one was really at fault. Herdt and Boyanowski, among others, felt that the report papered over what they saw as the real problem: Tzagournis's leadership. They saw the emphasis on police-hospital relations as a red herring.

Dickson, in particular, who had triggered the hospital investigation, was dismayed that the doctors claimed she hadn't brought the patient deaths to their attention, and that Meeks was skeptical of her recollection. "I knew I'd done the right thing," she later recalled. "I never, ever doubted I'd done what I should have. Yet no one ever came to me and said, 'You were right.' The dean and the doctors are a fellowship. They always close ranks. I'm used to this."

THE trial of Michael Swango on seven counts of aggravated battery began on April 22, 1985, in the Adams County courthouse in Quincy, a modern redbrick-and-glass replacement for an ornate old courthouse that had been damaged beyond repair by a tornado. Perhaps fearing that local passions had already been aroused by the case, Swango's lawyer, Dan Cook, had moved unsuccessfully for a change of venue. Swango had waived his right to a trial by jury, so the judge assigned to the case, Dennis Cashman, would both preside over the trial and render a verdict.

Cashman, forty, had been a prominent local attorney before being elected to the bench as a Republican. He was well known in Quincy, both as the son of a prominent family—his father was president of a local savings and loan—and as the former city golf champion. Tall and sandy-haired, he hadn't changed all that much since his days as a star golfer at the University of Illinois. His demeanor was calm and measured, but he ran his courtroom with a firm grip. Sheriff's deputies, assistant state's attorneys, and defense lawyers alike had from time to time experienced his impatience and, occasionally, his wrath. Although Adams County voters tend to be conservative on matters of law and order, Judge Cashman was, if anything, known as being tough on law enforcement officers, keeping a close eye in particular on the sheriff's office.

The second-floor courtroom, the largest in the building, was packed that morning with local press and curious members of the public. Muriel had returned from Florida to stay with Ruth Miller, and was seated in the front row, just behind Swango and Cook at the defense table. Next to Muriel was Rita Dumas, who'd gotten off work at the Ohio State Hospitals in order to attend the trial. Swango's brothers didn't attend. Ed Morgan, the prosecutor from Columbus, sat inconspicuously near the rear.

Some of Swango's former colleagues among the paramedics, especially Krzystofczyk, worried that Swango was too smart to be convicted. The case was largely circumstantial: no one had seen Swango put anything in the doughnuts, the sodas, or the tea. The tea that had been tested for arsenic had languished in a locker over a weekend and had then been handled by several people before it found its way to the lab. It could easily have been tampered with. Chet Vahle, the assistant state's attorney in charge of trying the case, had already conceded in court that the paramedics were "a bunch of amateurs who were trying to do their own undercover investigation." And health department investigators had initially diagnosed the paramedics' illness as a viral infection, not poisoning.

Vahle opened the trial. "Mr. Cook, your honor, the People of the State of Illinois will show by the testimony of witnesses and introduction of evidence that between September 14, 1984, and October 19, 1984, the defendant, Michael Swango, administered a deadly poison, arsenic, to certain members of the Adams County Health Department ambulance crews.... After consuming the offered food or drink, the victims became violently ill within 30 to 45 minutes. The illnesses, which included the immediate symptoms of nausea, vomiting, stomach cramps, dry heaves, a feeling of weakness, hot flashes, and thereafter symptoms of resounding headaches and general malaise were common to all of the victims." Vahle continued that the sample of tea had tested positive for arsenic, and that a hair sample taken from paramedic Brent Unmisig, who had been poisoned twice, "contained a level of arsenic which is indicative of an unnatural accumulation."

Vahle also addressed the issue of motive, noting that the police investigation "established that the defendant was captivated and entranced by injury and death, by mass trauma of unsuspecting victims." He mentioned Swango's reaction to the McDonald's massacre, and pointed out that Swango had said it would be "nice to walk into the emergency room and start blowing people away." He cited Swango's admiration for suspected serial killer Henry Lee

Lucas. Finally, he quoted Swango's remark to Grover that "sometimes I feel I have an evil purpose in life."

"We believe that the evidence will show that the defendant's
statement was accurate, and that he's guilty of the offenses of aggravated battery as charged," Vahle concluded.

In Swango's defense, Cook emphasized that it was the obligation of the state to prove Swango guilty beyond a reasonable doubt.
He stressed that no one could directly link Swango to the tainted
tea, no one had seen him tamper with it, and no one had even seen
Swango inside the hospital the day the paramedics became suspicious the tea had been poisoned. "The issue cannot be based upon
guesses, hunches and baseless opinions," Cook concluded.

The prosecution's star witnesses were the paramedics, who testified in detail about the events of the previous September, and how
suspicion of someone they had initially considered a colleague and
friend slowly took root. Unmisig, the first witness, described
Swango's actions and his illness, and told of witnessing Swango's reaction to the McDonald's killings and his description of the "ultimate call." "He had a serious look to him, and [was] in a hyper
state," Unmisig recalled.

Greg Myers testified that when Swango returned from Ohio
State, he was "more unsettled, more apprehensive." Lonnie Long
said he was "more on edge, more stressful," adding "he was truly intrigued by violent trauma and death." Krzystofczyk described the
scrapbooks, quoting Swango to the effect that "it just snowballed to
the point where it was an obsession, and he didn't feel like he could
stop." Another paramedic, Michael Alcorn, testified that he had detected resentment on Swango's part toward the poisoned paramedics and that Swango had told him, "Those guys need to be taken
down a notch."

Just outside the courtroom, in the corridor leading to the
judge's chambers, was an ice machine, which Swango passed each
day as he came into the courtroom. As the testimony continued,
and the evidence of poisoning and Swango's morbid interests
mounted, Judge Cashman ordered that the machine be padlocked.

Then the trial shifted to the investigative trail. Quincy police
detective Billy Meyer described the search of Swango's apartment,
and the discovery of the array of poisons and the numerous bottles

of Terro ant poison, many with their warning labels removed. One bottle of ant poison had been diluted, and the degree of dilution exactly matched the concentration found in the paramedics' hair samples. A clerk at Keller's garden and feed store pointed to Swango as the man who had purchased the ant poison, wearing a paramedic's uniform.

Gasser described his positive test for heavy metals. Dr. Jeorg Pirl, from the Illinois toxicology laboratory at the University of Illinois medical school in Chicago, testified that the tea sample contained arsenic, and that Unmisig's hair sample had a high concentration of arsenic. Although tests for arsenic in the other paramedics' hair samples were inconclusive, Pirl testified that heavy vomiting had likely reduced the residue of arsenic in their systems. The victims' symptoms were all consistent with arsenic poisoning.

But the most important witness was Swango himself. He had been scribbling notes furiously throughout the trial, avoiding eye contact with his former colleagues. Now he took the stand in his own defense, waiving his Fifth Amendment right against self-incrimination. He was neatly dressed in jacket and tie, as he was throughout the trial. His delivery was measured and earnest. He described his background, his outstanding record in high school and at Quincy College, and his promising medical career. Swango flatly denied poisoning or attempting to poison anyone. The linchpin of his defense was that he had experienced a serious ant and roach problem in his apartment, and had purchased the ant poison both in Columbus and Quincy for the purpose of eradicating the pests. He testified that they were an unusual "reddish-type ant."

The other items in his apartment, he said, simply reflected his interest in chemistry. He'd purchased an advanced chemistry set while in Columbus, and most of the materials came from that. He read the books on terrorism and paramilitary actions, he said, to better understand his father's work in Vietnam. Swango said that his father had been involved in "guerrilla warfare" there. He had collected the castor beans and articles on ricin for his college paper on the murder of the Bulgarian exile.

He stressed that while others might find his reading habits or sense of humor distasteful, it was a free country and he shouldn't be on trial for his thoughts or reading material. His remarks about the

McDonald's massacre were "a joke." The "ultimate call" was a "gross exaggeration" of what he'd said, which in any event reflected a "gallows-type black humor." His fantasy about killing children in a pediatrics ward, too, was "the gallows, black humor type that I have already described regarding going up to the—I believe the pediatrics ward—I'm not sure if it was specifically that hospital—and I believe killing babies with a .357 magnum, sir." His interest in violent death simply reflected the fact that "I myself would want to participate in the bad calls I've noted because I feel that I would be as capable as anyone handling that call." He said he had no memory of telling Monty Grover that he had an "evil purpose" in life.

When Swango completed his testimony, Cook called one other crucial witness for the defense: Kevin O'Donnell, president of O'Donnell's Termite and Pest Control, a local Quincy exterminator. The inspector said that at the request of Swango's lawyer, he had inspected Swango's apartment on Eighteenth Street and had indeed detected numerous of the "reddish-type" ants Swango had described.

There was only one problem with what at first seemed to be independent corroboration for the most important element of Swango's defense. On cross-examination, the inspector said that the species of ant in Swango's apartment wasn't native to central Illinois—or, indeed, to any northern part of the country. It was found only in the Southern states, particularly Florida. In any event, the species was never found indoors, unless someone deliberately put it there.

At Christmas, Swango had visited his mother and half brother in Florida.

Each day after the trial, Muriel Swango had returned to Ruth's house and given her a detailed account of that day's proceedings. She had been shocked by much of what she heard, but she insisted that she believed Michael when he said that these stories were gross exaggerations and he was innocent. Anyone could have tampered with the tea or poisoned the paramedics' drinks and food, she maintained. But gradually her defense of her son had become less impassioned, less certain. After hearing Michael's defense and listening to the testimony of the exterminator, she returned to Ruth's house and said simply, "I know now he's guilty." Muriel didn't cry or otherwise express any emotion, but Ruth could tell that her world had collapsed.

The prosecution and defense rested on May 2 at four P.M. Judge Cashman deliberated overnight, and then summoned the participants the next morning for the verdict. "This is a difficult case," Judge Cashman began. "No question about it. It's difficult from the standpoint of the People. It's difficult from the standpoint of the Defendant, and Lord knows it's difficult from my standpoint." After reviewing the elements of the case that had to be proved beyond a reasonable doubt, the judge continued, "I do not want to make this seem dramatic because it's not my intention to do so, and rather than leave the outcome in doubt, I'm going to state my findings as to each charge."

Swango folded his hands tightly together and closed his eyes.

"[The] first thing I'll say is that I have considered all the physical evidence and the testimony of the witnesses, and I have assessed their credibility as to each charge. . . . I have looked at all the evidence from every angle, I assure you of that. I have looked at it from every perspective. I have determined that certainly in this case all the evidence is not circumstantial. There is direct evidence." With that, Judge Cashman announced that on count 1, aggravated battery of Mark Krzystofczyk, "I find the defendant, Michael Swango, not guilty." A murmur went through the courtroom. Krzystofczyk groaned to himself—this was just what he had feared.

"As to count 2, aggravated battery of Allen Dingerson [another paramedic who became ill], I find the defendant, Michael Swango, guilty."

Swango covered his face with his left hand, and kept it there while the judge continued with the remaining five counts of aggravated battery. As to Brent Unmisig: guilty on two counts. Greg Myers: guilty. Fred Bennett: guilty. When he finished, the judge said, "To recapsulize, I found the defendant not guilty on one count. As to all the other charges, I find the defendant guilty."

Judge Cashman made clear that the only reason he found Swango innocent of the charge related to Krzystofczyk was because his illness was less severe, and thus less certainly the result of arsenic poisoning. "The bottom line in this case," the judge concluded, "is there are many tracks, and every track leads to the defendant's door, and I'm convinced beyond a reasonable doubt on those charges that I found him guilty of that he is in fact guilty, and on the one I found him not guilty of, I'm not necessarily convinced that he's not guilty, but I certainly have an obligation, and I have carried out that obligation, and the defendant is found not guilty on that one because the People failed to prove it beyond a reasonable doubt.

"I stayed up late last night, I assure you of that, Dr. Swango. I looked at every piece of evidence. I went over it again and again. I spent perhaps ten hours of deliberation. I didn't keep track. I didn't watch the clock, but I didn't get much sleep, and when I woke up this morning my decision was just as firm as when I went to bed."

Because of the nature of the charges and the possibility that Swango might still poison others, Vahle moved that his bail be revoked and he be confined in the county jail until sentencing.

"It's indeed a sad day," Judge Cashman responded, turning to look directly at Swango. "You have the mind and the intellect to do great deeds, but yet you haven't. On the one hand you have performed great deeds, but on the other you have clearly performed evil deeds. As much as it hurts me to do so, it's clearly obvious to me that every man, woman, and child in this community or anywhere else that you might go is in jeopardy as long as you are a free person, Doctor.

"What makes it worse," the judge continued, "is that there is no explanation. . . . It would sure help if I knew why, but there isn't any why. There is no explanation why you would do these things to your friends and co-workers, and if you would do these things under those circumstances, I have every reason to conclude . . . that you might do them to anyone else. I think that you could and are very capable of it. . . . Those people deserve and need my protection, and I'm going to give it to them. I hereby revoke your bond.

"It is indeed a sad day for me, Doctor," the judge concluded. "I don't like what I had to do, but certainly it had to be done for the people of this community. I hereby recess."

The judge stood and prepared to leave, but as he did, Swango handed a foam cup to Rita Dumas across the rail separating him from the spectators. A jail attendant, fearing the cup might contain poison, leaped up and knocked it out of Swango's hand. But the cup was empty. Inside it, Swango had written, "I love you Dumas. Hang in there." Dumas broke down in sobs as Swango was handcuffed and led from the courtroom by sheriff's deputies.

JUST outside, Swango met briefly with Dan Cook and then spoke to Muriel about the possibility of an appeal. He insisted on his innocence and said he needed her to pay for it. But Muriel had been badly shaken by the evidence and the verdict. This time, she refused to give Michael what he wanted. "I don't have the money," she said. "Anyway, I was there" for the trial, Muriel went on, looking her son squarely in the eye. "I know you're guilty. The evidence showed you were guilty."

Michael, furious, abruptly turned away, leaving his mother standing alone in the corridor.

CHAPTER SIX

THE WEEK AFTER the verdict, Muriel Swango called Judge Cashman's office and scheduled an appointment with him. Cashman wasn't looking forward to the visit. Though he considered it part of his job to explain his decisions, and had met parents and other relatives of people he'd convicted before, they almost invariably gave him a hard time.

Thus, it came as something of a surprise to him when Muriel came into his chambers, took a seat, and began the conversation by saying, "I understand why you reached the decision you did, and I have no quarrel with the verdict." But she obviously felt the need to talk, to try to explain her son, and she stayed for an hour. She told Cashman that she wanted him to know that Michael was "a very troubled young man." She said that he had bitterly resented his father's long and frequent absences. Still, "Mike never caused me any type of unusual problems"; he "got along well with others and was well-adjusted." It was only toward the end of his college career, after he had returned from the Marines, that Muriel began to worry. "He became easily agitated. He was always working. He never slept," she said. She had found his behavior "bizarre." Even so, she had initially believed in his innocence, and the notion that he might poison someone was "completely out of character." Something inside him "must have snapped," she concluded.

Judge Cashman found Muriel to be composed and dignified, and thought she was taking her son's conviction as well as could be expected. Still, she indicated that since Michael's arrest she hadn't been feeling well, and she had felt even worse after the guilty verdict. Perhaps it was the stress, the judge thought.

DURING the summer, the Adams County probation department prepared a presentencing report to guide Judge Cashman in imposing a sentence. Since Swango himself continued to maintain his innocence, the report was unable to offer insight into any possible motivation. "If this arrest had not occurred," the report stated, Swango "believes he would currently be working as an emergency room physician at a hospital." Swango "believe[d] his upbringing was normal and stable" and said he was "close to his mother" and had "regular contact" with his brothers. He said his father's return from Vietnam "caused personal problems for him" and "alcohol became a problem." He listed his "hobbies" as "running, exercising, reading, participating in and watching sporting events" and said he "does not smoke or drink." He had refused to be examined by a court-appointed psychiatrist.

Muriel, too, had told the probation officer that Michael had "a normal childhood." But she said that he had a difficult relationship with his father. Her husband's return from Vietnam had been "extremely traumatic for him. [Virgil] was never the same person after he returned home," and he had turned to "serious alcohol abuse." The couple had separated; Michael "tried to get his father to curb his drinking and reconcile" with his mother. "There was an estrangement" between Michael and his father, Muriel explained, "because his father resented Mike trying to get him to straighten up."

The presentencing report also reviewed Swango's sterling academic record, noting that he had been class valedictorian in Quincy, had near-perfect grades at Millikin and Quincy College, and had received his medical degree from SIU. But the report suggests how difficult it was even for court officials to get information from Ohio State. Even after Swango had been convicted of poisoning his co-workers, the only description of the problems at Ohio State in the report is a brief, sketchy account of the Rena Cooper incident: "an incident occurred whereby a patient on a floor he was working [on] had a 'respiratory arrest.' The patient was placed in intensive care for one day. His supervisor told him to take two days off, away from the floor." The result was that as Judge Cashman approached the task of sentencing, he knew little about the most serious incidents involving Swango.

Cashman convened a sentencing hearing on August 23. Swango called several character witnesses, including his half brother and his girlfriend. Both testified that they had no qualms about leaving their young children alone with Swango and had done so on many occasions. Dick also told the court, "I personally don't feel that he is guilty." But pressed on cross-examination, he said "I was not here during the trial, and therefore, I really don't know whether Mike is guilty or not guilty." Muriel didn't attend the sentencing hearing.

A few days before her testimony, Rita had broken her public silence about the case and spoken to an Associated Press reporter. She had refused to cooperate with the OSU police investigation and had agreed to answer questions only with a lawyer present. Dumas had been on duty the day Ricky DeLong died, but she had gone off duty hours before his death. "I love Michael, I do," she told the AP. "I never, ever doubted that he was innocent, because I know his nature. He wouldn't do something like that." It was she, Dumas said, who complained about the ants in Swango's apartment and told him to do something about them.

As a character witness, however, Rita did not repeat her claim about the ants. She testified that she began dating Swango in July 1983 after they met at the Ohio State Hospitals, and said, "I do not feel I would have survived had he not been there for me." During the fall of 1983, she explained, "I went through some very, very difficult times in my life. . . . And even though Michael and I had not been dating for a long period of time and we were not seriously considering a long-term relationship at that time, he was very supportive. He would not let more than four or five hours go by, usually it was about three, that he would call and make sure that I was all right, make sure that I was still hanging in there, so to speak. And I do not think that I would have survived that period in my life had he not been there and been so supportive."

But the witness who made the greatest impression on Judge Cashman, though probably not in the way he or Swango intended, was Robert Haller II, the vice president of National Emergency Service in Toledo, who had hired Swango as an emergency room doctor while he was awaiting trial. Even though Swango had persuaded Haller to hire him without ever disclosing the fact that he was facing charges of poisoning his fellow paramedics, Haller traveled from Toledo to support Swango's bid for leniency.

On the witness stand, Swango's lawyer asked Haller whether he would "have any problem" hiring Swango again, even after his conviction. "I wouldn't personally," Haller replied. "But because of the press received in Ohio, and I can speak for most of the hospital administrators, they would have a hard time getting him credentialed."

"But you personally, based on your knowledge, would have no problem?"

"I would have no problem at all, as well as the hospitals that he worked in. They wouldn't have a problem themselves. But it's the public that comes to the hospital that would find it, you know, which would create a problem."

Cashman was startled almost to the point of disbelief by this testimony—the willingness to rehire a convicted poisoner, the disdain for a "public" that would "create a problem."

Chet Vahle, the prosecutor, rose to cross-examine Haller.

"Mr. Haller, did Dr. Swango tell you about these charges when he applied for work with your firm?" Vahle asked.

"No, he did not."

"And just exactly when did you advise the hospitals about these charges?"

"To be quite honest, it hit the paper before we were aware of it. It first broke in the Cleveland *Plain Dealer*. And we found out the day that it was going in the newspaper."

"Did you consider that to be a breach of trust in the application process?"

"No," Haller explained, "because on the application there is a question, if they have ever committed a felony, and at that time he had not been tried. So I, you know, don't feel that it had any bearing on his ability nor had he violated anything in terms of the application that he filled out."

After some further colloquy, Vahle asked, "What I'm getting at is that you as an employer of doctors wouldn't be bothered by the fact that the doctor had been charged with six counts of poisoning?"

"We were concerned about it, sure."

142

BLIND EYE

"And even though he has been convicted, you would rehire him?"

"Yes," Haller replied. "Based on what he did for [the] company, the patients that he treated, if it were up to me, I would."

Cashman shook his head in disbelief. Haller's willingness to rehire Swango seemed so bizarre that the judge discounted the testimony. It seemed inconceivable to him that any doctor or medical administrator would ever hire Swango again.

Swango had spent weeks preparing his own statement to the court, which he had carefully written out in longhand. Now he rose and addressed the judge, reading from his prepared text.

He began by again asserting his innocence. "I am fully aware that I have been found guilty in a court of law. And with all due respect to the Court, I wish to state once again that I am innocent of these charges." Without being specific, he attributed his interest in death and violence to his relationship with his father, "one of the most unique and talented men to ever come out of Quincy, Illinois." Noting their respective military careers, and especially his father's "involvement in the endless guerrilla war in Vietnam" and "close ties to the military and intelligence communities in Vietnam," he said that "I naturally was very interested and concerned with what he was doing." He continued, saying that "I deeply regret, your Honor, that my possession of items reflecting that natural father-son relationship led this court . . . to its verdict."

After reviewing his sterling record of accomplishments, Swango made an eloquent, almost tearful, plea that he be allowed to pay his debt to society. Citing his "faith in God" and "[the] support of my family and friends," he said he was left with one overriding question: "What can I do, Judge Cashman . . . to convince you and show you that I still have a great wealth of good and caring to return to this society and that I should be allowed . . . to resume that service to society?

"After graduation from medical school I took the Hippocratic Oath and I have never nor would I ever violate the sacred trust of the doctor-patient relationship. . . . In no way, shape, or form, under no conceivable circumstance am I now, or have I ever been, or will I ever be, a danger to any human being on the face of this earth." With that, Swango folded his notes and sat down.

Judge Cashman thanked Swango and remarked that his position was "quite eloquently stated." Nonetheless, he continued, "as I sit here today, I have never been more confident in my own mind that you were proven guilty beyond a reasonable doubt of these offenses than any other case I have had occasion to preside over." Though Swango had begged for the court's trust, Cashman pointed out that Swango had already violated it by finding employment as a doctor in Ohio, and then using his Christmas visit to his family to transport red ants back to his apartment. "You fabricated evidence in this case in an effort to show that somehow you had an ant infestation in your apartment," the judge noted. "I found that evidence to be totally implausible and perhaps you are so smart that you didn't quite accept the fact that someone might be smart enough to see through that. I don't know. . . In fact, your intelligence is so well documented that it is hard for me to understand how a person that smart could leave such a trail of guilt."

Cashman said he had no explanation for Swango's crimes. "The only explanation I can come to is that inside of Michael Swango there must be another person. There has to be two Michael Swangos. . . . Here there is no reason for what you have done that I can see. You are doing these things to co-workers for no apparent reason. There was a little evidence about maybe some petty jealousies or maybe a desire to work more and therefore if you made people sick you would get to work more. Well, I don't think that is much of an argument . . . there is no real answer to what has happened here and I don't understand it and probably never will."

Cashman noted that if Swango's behavior had not been so inexplicable—if, for example, the battery had occurred during a "barroom brawl where the individual was intoxicated"—he could order appropriate treatment and consider probation, as Swango had requested. But "probation is not appropriate. The protection of the community is more important because there is no way I can know of when and why you might do something like this again. Just on a whim."

The judge sentenced Swango to five years in prison, the maximum sentence, saying that "you deserve the maximum under the law because there is no excuse for what you have done."

• •

AFTER sitting though Swango's trial, Ed Morgan, the Franklin County prosecutor, told *The Plain Dealer:* "The verdicts indicated to me that we are now investigating a man who is obviously a very sick individual and has to be considered a very dangerous individual. It indicates to me and my office that we are on the right track in pressing the investigation and we will continue the investigation." Morgan realized, nonetheless, that Swango was a formidable adversary. The doctor had been a poised and seemingly earnest witness— in Morgan's opinion, smooth and good-looking; he could see why women fell for him. Had Swango opted for a trial by jury, the prosecutor wasn't sure he would have been convicted. But the courtroom testimony, especially the evidence of Swango's fixation on death and disaster, convinced Morgan that he very well might be dealing with a psychopath. He returned to Ohio convinced that Swango had committed crimes at Ohio State, probably murder.

In June, Morgan hired an experienced homicide detective Patrick McSweeney, to investigate Swango full-time on behalf of the prosecuting attorney's office. Morgan and McSweeney set up an office at the Ohio State police headquarters, where they joined efforts with Eley, the medical board investigator, and Herdt, who remained in charge of the overall investigation. They frequently consulted the Franklin County coroner, William Adrion, and an Ohio State University toxicologist, Daniel Couri. To minimize the earlier frictions between the police and hospital personnel, all interviews with doctors, nurses, and other hospital employees were coordinated through Michael Covert, who had replaced Donald Boyanowski as the hospital's executive director.

Finally, interviews with eyewitnesses got under way in earnest, though not without continuing problems at the hospital. Arranging interviews through Covert was time-consuming. Robert Holder, as Chief Herdt had predicted, had taken a new job as a special assistant to Tzagournis. Out of concern for patient confidentiality, Holder insisted on a subpoena before providing any documents, which was also a cumbersome and time-consuming process.

Some relatives of possible Swango victims, such as the parents of the young gymnast Cynthia Ann McGee, had quietly accepted monetary settlements from Ohio State. The investigators were angered to learn that as a condition of the settlements, Ohio State had required the families to remain silent, even to the police, unless they obtained a subpoena. As McSweeney later described the process, "Everyone on the OSU staff was hesitant. Appointments were broken. We made it as convenient as possible. We'd go at two A.M. if that's what they wanted. Not one of them showed up on time. Once we waited three hours for a doctor to show up. They sent some doctors away [out of town] when we wanted them. I got the impression that they thought we were just dumb cops and they were the saviors of mankind. I've dealt with hospitals for years on homicides, and I've never seen anything to compare to the treatment we got at OSU."

Still, McSweeney, Harp, and the others were able to interview and in many cases videotape the statements of such critical witnesses as Rena Cooper; her roommate, Iwonia Utz; the head resident on duty that night, Rees Freeman; and numerous other doctors and nurses. After scouring the record of every patient who had died in the hospital during Swango's rotations, they were able to identify five suspicious deaths, plus the possible poisonings of the doctors at Children's Hospital, and interview the doctors and nurses involved. The results were startlingly at odds with the conclusions of the hospital's own investigation.

McGee, the gymnast, had not died of a "pulmonary embolism," as Goodman reported, apparently relying on a hearsay account of the autopsy results. On January 14, the head resident had asked Swango to draw a blood sample from McGee. At about 11:15 P.M., Swango told a nurse he was going to draw the sample. He was seen heading toward her room carrying a syringe and culture bottles. At about midnight, a nurse found that McGee had "a pale, dusty, bluish look" and called a code, to which Swango didn't respond. The code was unsuccessful, and McGee was pronounced dead.

Another doctor reported that six days later Swango had been among a group of doctors making evening rounds on the neurosurgery floor, but had been alone with patient Ricky DeLong while the others examined DeLong's roommate. Swango had called out to them, "I think your patient is dead," which had come as a shock since DeLong had seemed to be in stable condition. Swango had later written on the patient's progress notes that he was "pro-

nounced dead at 1803 hours. Family notified. . . . Franklin County
Coroner's Office notified of death. They will assume jurisdiction
and perform autopsy." Swango called DeLong's wife and told her
DeLong had died of a heart attack. When she became distraught, he
repeated the information to her mother. Family members came to
the hospital, met with Swango, and requested an autopsy. They
completed an autopsy form given them by Swango. But the form
was never filed and no autopsy was performed.

Similarly, in the highly suspicious death of Rein Walter, who
started gasping and lost consciousness ten minutes after a visit from
Swango, Swango signed the death certificate, citing the cause as cardiopulmonary arrest. There was no autopsy.

And in the case of Ruth Barrick, whose death had so upset
Nurse Anne Ritchie, Swango filled out a form on which he stated
that "This is not a Coroner's case" and "The Coroner will not assume jurisdiction," Again, he had ensured that no autopsy would be
performed.

Far from being routine, as Goodman and Whitcomb had indicated in their respective reports, the other deaths had seemed mysterious to the hospital's medical staff at the time they occurred.
When the investigators interviewed Dr. Marc Cooperman about the
death of Charlotte Warner, he told them,

"The first problem that I had with her case, that I didn't understand was the results of the autopsy . . . and that demonstrated what
they called multicentric thrombosis. Basically what happened is she
had developed clots in all of her major arteries. She had clots in the
arteries in her heart, in the vessels to the intestine, in the vessels to
her kidneys, to her liver, and to her lungs. And I could never understand why this type of thing would have happened to somebody
who had undergone a straightforward surgical procedure five days
earlier and was walking around having no problems. And so it always bothered me."

In early 1985, when Cooperman learned that castor beans had
been found in Swango's apartment in Quincy, he consulted some
toxicology texts at the medical school library. When he discovered
that ricin poisoning causes, in his words, "blood clots, thrombosis, and thromboembolism throughout the vascular system," and
thus might explain Warner's baffling autopsy findings, Cooperman

called his attorney, and they decided to notify the coroner. Cooperman thus became the first—and only—doctor at Ohio State to initiate contact with an investigative authority outside the hospital.

When asked about Evelyn Pereny, the gallbladder patient who also experienced bizarre bleeding, even from her eyes, Dr. Gary Birken told the investigators that such bleeding typically occurs in poisonings. He said that Swango had examined Pereny before she experienced the bleeding and "total body failure."

In the now notorious case of Rena Cooper, there was none of the ambiguity or conflicting testimony that had caused Dr. Whitcomb to dismiss the whole affair as a grand mal seizure. Karolyn Beery, the student nurse whose testimony had been belittled as unreliable, was even now, a year after the incident, quite certain that she had seen Dr. Swango, from a distance of only three feet, standing by Cooper's bed. "It looked like he was putting something in her IV," she now told the OSU police. "I knew he was putting something in. You can just tell." John Sigg, the first nurse to respond to Beery's calls for help that night, testified that Beery told him when he arrived that she had seen Dr. Swango with a syringe doing something to Cooper's IV. He recalled that Cooper, too, told him, "The doctor put something in my IV."

But the most telling interviews were of Cooper and her roommate, whose earlier accounts had been dismissed as unreliable, if not delusional. Utz, the roommate, said she was alert and perfectly capable of remembering what she had seen. She remembered quite clearly that a doctor came into the room and "he gave her a shot or something . . . and I just started screaming for the nurse . . . I started screaming like mad." Utz described the doctor as young, with blond hair and glasses, wearing a white coat. Moreover, she said she recognized Swango as the doctor when she saw pictures of him on television after his arrest in Illinois.

Cooper said she was wide awake that evening and not suffering any aftereffects from her anesthetic. She remembered that a blond-haired person had come into her room and, using a syringe, had injected something into her IV. She was lying on her side, so she couldn't see the person's face, but she thought it was a man. She said nothing about the "yellow pharmacy jacket" that had figured so prominently in the doctors' earlier exoneration of Swango, and seemed puzzled by questions about it. She testified that as a "blackness" spread through her body and she realized she could not speak, she deliberately rattled the bed rail in order to attract attention. That is, she was *deliberately* shaking the bed rail; she wasn't suffering a "seizure." She recalled writing the notes because she couldn't speak with the tube in her mouth and throat.

Morgan went to some lengths to determine the basis for the hospital's conclusion that Cooper had been paranoid and thus potentially delusional. It appeared that another doctor had reported that Cooper had accused the OSU neurologist Dr. George Paulson of trying to burglarize her home, and this was the basis for the conclusion that she was suffering "paranoid ideation." But in her interview with OSU police, Cooper vehemently denied ever accusing any doctor of such a thing. While her house *had* been burglarized, she hadn't suspected Dr. Paulson, who in any event wouldn't have known where she lived. (Dr. Paulson, too, said that to his knowledge Cooper had never made any such allegation, and said he wasn't the source for the report.) Thus, the diagnosis of Cooper's mental state appeared to rest on the flimsiest of hearsay and, as far as Morgan was concerned, was completely unjustified.

The investigators also interviewed the three doctors who had spoken to Swango about the incident: Freeman, the head resident; Carey, the chief of surgery; and Whitcomb, who headed the hospital inquiry. Freeman, the first to speak to Swango, testified that "I confronted him [Swango] and did question him and he said he was not in the room. Nor did he see her [Cooper] just prior to the incident."

Dr. Carey reported that "I asked him whether, in fact, he had done anything to Mrs. Cooper, or injected anything in her I.V. and he said 'no.' I explained to him that there had been an incident report suggesting that he had and he said, 'no.' He was in the room at the request of one of the two patients, and I don't remember which one, to get her slippers for her, and he had gotten the patient's slippers, whether it was Mrs. Cooper, or the other person in the room, I don't remember. But that's all he had done. And he hadn't done anything with the intravenous line."

Dr. Whitcomb made this statement to the OSU police when he was interviewed on February 15, 1985: "He [Swango] told me that he was in the room, as I remember now, that he was in there to draw blood. That was the reason for him to have been in the room and that he either had a brief conversation with Mrs. Cooper, or some contact with her and left the room and the next thing he remembers was to recognize that there was a resuscitation effort going on in that room." (This statement differs from the account Whitcomb earlier gave Meeks.)

Thus, the testimony indicated that Swango had given three inconsistent accounts: that he wasn't in the room; that he went in to get slippers; that he went in to draw blood.

As for the diagnosis of Cooper's respiratory arrest as a grand mal seizure, Dr. Brakel, who witnessed it with Dr. Freeman and helped resuscitate Cooper, said the symptoms didn't indicate such a seizure, but were instead "consistent with a paralyzing drug"—specifically, the anesthetic Anectine, to which Swango would have had ready access while he was in the hospital.

Armed with the witnesses' accounts, Morgan, Herdt, and the other investigators turned to the physical evidence. To their dismay, none of the syringes used by Swango had been saved, nor had any of the patients' IV tubes. And, of course, Nurse Moore had thrown away the syringe discovered by Risley after no one showed any interest in it and she was told Swango had been cleared.

Through the coroner's office, the investigators did have tissue and fluid samples from all the patients on whom autopsies had been performed. The bodies of the three patients who were not autopsied—DeLong, Walter, and Barrick—were exhumed. But just as Morgan and prosecuting attorney Miller had feared, detecting the presence of poisons or paralyzing drugs proved a daunting and frustrating task. Given the supplies found in Swango's apartment in Quincy, they tested for arsenic and nicotine and also tried to come up with a test for ricin. Because it was readily available in the hospital and could have caused Cooper's symptoms, they also tested for Anectine.

None of the samples tested positive for arsenic, which was not surprising since the only victims who showed any symptoms of arsenic poisoning—the doctors at Children's Hospital—had vomited heavily, and also had apparently been poisoned on only one occasion. Two patients, Warner and Pereny, showed symptoms consistent with ricin poisoning, but there was no test for ricin, although the OSU toxicologist worked for months to find one. None of the samples tested revealed any residue of Anectine, which was suspected in the Cooper incident and in the deaths that didn't involve massive bleeding. But Anectine passes quickly out of the body, often leaving no trace.

However, Coroner Adrion did make a startling discovery when he performed an autopsy on the corpse of Ricky DeLong: gauze had been stuffed into his trachea, causing suffocation. Adrion changed DeLong's official cause of death to "cardiopulmonary arrest due to gauze in trachea causing partial occlusion." On July 8, he ruled the death a homicide.

But Ohio State brought in a pathologist from Phoenix, Arizona, and had him examine DeLong's body. This pathologist said that an undertaker might have placed the gauze in DeLong's throat, and Ohio State used this possibility to lambaste Adrion's conclusion that the death was a homicide.

The investigators, and now the coroner, too, were dumbfounded. For the evidence did not support Ohio State's contention: the gauze bore markings indicating a hospital use, and more significantly, the investigating staff interviewed the mortician who had embalmed DeLong's body, and he said that not only hadn't he left any gauze in DeLong's body but that he didn't even use that kind of gauze. After Ohio State made its claims, Adrion convened a meeting of the investigative staff and asked for a secret vote on whether the verdict of homicide should be changed. The verdict stood.

It seemed that wherever Morgan turned, someone at Ohio State was trying to thwart him. Evidence hadn't been collected or had been discarded. The Goodman and Whitcomb investigations had been disastrous. Swango himself had never even been subjected to a formal interview, nor was any attempt made to reconcile the three inconsistent versions he'd offered of his involvement in the Cooper respiratory failure. Every doubt was resolved in favor of Swango and against the credibility of everyone else. Morgan was so upset that he discussed with Miller whether there was sufficient evidence to consider seeking an indictment of Ohio State officials for obstruction of justice. But they discarded the possibility as unwar-

ranted, politically dangerous—and unsatisfying, given that Swango
was the real target.

On *that* score, Morgan's pessimism grew as the months passed
and the search for physical evidence proved fruitless. All he had was
a strong circumstantial case based on eyewitness testimony. But
given that Ohio State had already dismissed most of that testimony
as unreliable, a good defense lawyer would easily establish a reasonable doubt of guilt. Although he firmly believed Swango was guilty
and a continuing menace to society, Morgan concluded that pursuing criminal charges would end in failure. Herdt and the other investigators reluctantly agreed.

Morgan's frustrations with Ohio State were evident in an extensive report he prepared during January and February 1986, two
years after the incidents involving Swango in the OSU Hospitals.
Morgan concluded that, while "numerous University Hospitals employees can place Dr. Michael Swango at or next to the bedsides of
patients who suffered unexplainable respiratory arrests," investigators found "a total absence of evidence tending to prove a specific
intent to cause serious physical harm or death attributable to Dr.
Swango." The hospitals made "no effort" to preserve the various syringes and other physical evidence involved in the incidents. Nor
were autopsies conducted in three suspicious cases, and

it should be noted that neither the departments of neurosurgery or general surgery conducted a "morbidity and
mortality conference" to review *any* of the five suspicious
deaths discussed in this report. . . . Obviously, if such a
conference occurred it could have led to the discovery of
physical evidence and/or additional witnesses or statements by Dr. Swango regarding his treatment procedures.

One of the most critical factors present in any criminal investigation, [Morgan's report continued] is the
amount of *time* that develops between the occurrence of
the criminal act and the subsequent investigation. It is obvious that the unusually long delay between incidents and
investigation as detailed in this report adversely affected
any hope to uncover admissible evidence. It cannot be
overemphasized that eight months had passed before the

Ohio State University Police had even heard the *name* of
Dr. Michael Swango. . . . Thus, it is not surprising that
toxicological testing done one- to one-and-a-half years
after the suspected poisoning would not result in positive
findings. . . .

In summary, there is no question that there exists
circumstantial evidence demonstrating a pattern of possible assaults and/or criminal homicides and this circumstantial scenario also includes a motive. It can be proven
that at the time the series of questionable respiratory arrests began, Dr. Swango was in danger of being terminated as a neurosurgery resident and he had been notified
of this fact.

Yet, in the absence of evidence of intent, "it was within Michael
Swango's *job description* to be with these patients and to treat them
using drugs and syringes."

Since under Ohio law, conviction on the basis of circumstantial
evidence requires that evidence to be "wholly inconsistent" with
"any reasonable theory of the defendant's innocence," "it is the recommendation of this writer that there be no criminal prosecution
of Dr. Michael J. Swango at this time."

Morgan gave the sixty-page draft to Miller to review, and Miller
suggested they show it to Jennings, Ohio State's president. Morgan
personally delivered it, and Jennings thanked him and shook his
hand. By the end of the day, lawyers were on the phone to Miller
with one demand: delete all the names, including those of all the
doctors involved. The report was released on April 1, 1986, with
doctors identified only by number.

As far as Morgan could tell, his report landed with a thud. The
press showed scant interest in his conclusions. He believed that
most reporters didn't bother to read it. As for Swango himself,
Morgan thought, "I'll never hear of him again."

Charles Eley had been involved in the investigation on behalf
of the Ohio State Medical Board. Though all the board's activities
are confidential, it is known to have investigated whether Dr. Carey
or anyone else at the medical school should have notified it of
Swango's suspicious activities, or at least of his arrest in Illinois.
Eley prepared a report about thirty pages long on the matter, but he

was ordered to turn over his only copy to the board. No action against anyone at Ohio State was taken.

Michael Swango's licenses to practice medicine were suspended, by Ohio on February 12, 1986, and by Illinois on March 19.

As Morgan was winding up his investigation and putting the finishing touches on his report, Swango began a campaign to rehabilitate his reputation by agreeing to be interviewed by correspondent John Stossel for the ABC news program *20/20*. The program aired on February 13, 1986, the day after his license was suspended in Ohio. It was the first national exposure Swango received.

Swango was interviewed at Centralia Correctional Center in southern Illinois, where he had begun serving his five-year term on August 27, 1985, and he was calm and collected, occasionally asking the producers for a glass of water. He was neatly dressed in a coat and red tie.

20/20 cohost Hugh Downs introduced the segment thus: "Dr. Michael Swango's case is an unusual one. The plot could have been lifted from a TV murder mystery. There is a mix of ingredients— poison tops the list. There's circumstantial evidence, and an ending that leaves room for a sequel."

Swango was even more adamant than before Judge Cashman that he had been wrongly accused and convicted. "First of all, I'm innocent," he began. "I could never do any of the things that were— that have been alleged that I have done. I think my whole life speaks for that, everything I've done in the past, my work both as a paramedic and a doctor, and I simply could not have done those things."

"Why do all these people think you did?" Stossel asked.

"I don't know. I think that some people think I did because they have been misled by evidence that was—that has no integrity. . . ."

Stossel brought up Swango's defense that there were ants in his apartment, and Kevin O'Donnell, the pest-control expert, said on camera, "This ant is never found indoors, particularly in our area. There were about a thousand of them, milling around aimlessly in the kitchen and the living room, and it appeared in my opinion that they had been dumped there."

Swango replied, "You know, I don't know anything about ants.

All I know is I had an ant problem, and I took care of it as best I could." As he had in the past, he explained the scrapbooks of death and disasters which "unfortunately are part and parcel of, you know, a paramedic's end of medicine in general." As for the recipe cards for poisons, "I'm a scientist. I'm a physician. And part of the curriculum is poisoning, toxicology, the symptoms and how to treat these various illnesses."

Asked specifically about whether he put something in anyone's IV tube at Ohio State, Swango replied, "I deny any criminal behavior or any violation of the Hippocratic Oath in working in Ohio or working anywhere."

"The judge said that maybe there are two of you," Stossel continued, quoting Judge Cashman.

"I think the judge is wrong," Swango replied. "The judge—the judge is very wrong."

"He also wanted you to get psychiatric help. Did you ever think of seeing anyone?"

"Absolutely not. He said that, thinking that I was guilty. I'm not guilty. I didn't do these things."

Stossel pointed out that because of the time he'd already served in the Adams County jail during his trial and before sentencing, and with time off for good behavior, Swango might be released in another year and a half. "Do you know some people are scared of you, now that you're getting out?" he asked.

"I'm sorry about that," Swango replied. "There's certainly no reason for anybody to be scared, none whatsoever."

Judge Cashman, for one, wasn't so sure. That Christmas he received a handwritten card wishing him and his family "a safe Christmas."

It was signed "Michael Swango."

CHAPTER SEVEN

MICHAEL SWANGO was released by the Illinois Department of Corrections on August 21, 1987, after serving two years of his five-year sentence. He remained under corrections department supervision for an additional year. Rita Dumas's support had been unwavering throughout his imprisonment. She now gave friends a new explanation for Michael's conviction: that he had been "framed" by Wayne Johnson because the coroner had feared that Swango, who was far more skilled, would supplant him.

Swango and Dumas moved to Hampton, Virginia, a town on the Chesapeake Peninsula near Newport News and Colonial Williamsburg. Both Rita and Michael wanted to begin a new life, away from Quincy, Columbus, and their past. Rita later told friends she had always wanted to live near the ocean, as well.

But Swango proved unable to escape his past. He applied for a medical license from the state of Virginia, and met with the state's licensing committee on August 12. Citing his felony conviction and the suspension of his Illinois and Ohio licenses, the committee voted to reject his application.

Instead of practicing medicine, Swango went to work as a counselor for the Career Development Center, which helped students get into medical and other professional schools. While he was working there, three of his colleagues came down with symptoms suspiciously similar to those experienced by the paramedics in Quincy: sudden nausea, vomiting, and severe headaches. One of them was hospitalized. And despite Swango's relationship with Rita Dumas, a second woman accused him of stalking her after she spurned what she deemed to be sexual advances. She soon became one of the three to experience similar symptoms.

Colleagues were already wary of Swango. His obsession with violent death and accidents had survived his confinement in prison. He carried clippings of disasters in a large paper bag and was often seen working on his scrapbooks. Then coworkers discovered that Swango had converted a basement room at the center into living quarters, and was frequently spending the night there. He left in May 1989.

Acting on a complaint from another employee at the counseling center, the Newport News police launched an investigation of the mysterious illnesses. They soon traced Swango to Columbus, Ohio, and spoke to prosecutor Morgan's office. Morgan sent them a copy of his report on Swango's activities at Ohio State. The Columbus inquiry also led to a tip to *The Columbus Dispatch,* which reported that Swango was now under investigation in Virginia. After a friend sent the *Dispatch* article to Swango and Dumas, Swango called the Newport News police and, in an effort to clear himself, asked to be interviewed. No charges were filed, but the investigation into Swango's past seems to have prompted him to begin legal proceedings to change his name. On January 18, 1990, by order of the Circuit Court of York County, Virginia, Swango legally changed his name to David Jackson Adams.

Still using his original name, Swango next found work as a lab technician at Aticoal Services, a company that tested samples of coal to be exported to France from the United States. He also worked part-time as a paramedic at a nearby hospital and began taking courses to be certified as an emergency medical technician. No one questioned his references or called anyone in Quincy for further information.

Aticoal's president, William C. Banks, found Swango to be pleasant and hardworking, an exemplary employee. Swango introduced Banks to Rita Dumas, and Banks thought they made a charming couple. Not long after, Swango asked him for some time off to get married. On July 8, 1989, he and Rita were finally married, nearly six years after meeting at Ohio State.

Despite his past, Swango had a semblance of a normal, stable life, with a well-paid job and a wife. Yet almost immediately after the wedding, problems surfaced. His relationship with Rita, which had survived so many external strains, rapidly deteriorated. She later confided that she realized almost immediately after marrying Swango that she had made a terrible mistake. Despite his years of purported devotion, he now showed scant interest—either romantic or sexual—in her. He wouldn't sleep in the same bed, and lived almost entirely in one room of the apartment, its den. He was constantly working on his computer and ignored Rita. She also complained that he stole money from her account and refused to contribute any of his earnings toward household expenses. But the breaking point may have come when a clerk at a nearby video rental shop became pregnant. Rita was certain that Michael was the father. In any event, she thought he had been cheating on her with other women. In January 1991, only a year and a half after marrying, Rita and Swango separated, later stating in court that they intended to "discontinue permanently the marital cohabitation." Rita resumed use of her maiden name, Brodegard.

As Swango's marriage unraveled, some Aticoal employees became violently ill. Banks himself had to be hospitalized after suddenly feeling dizzy, nauseated, weak, and sweaty. Another executive lapsed into a near coma after experiencing similar symptoms, and also had to be hospitalized.

Meanwhile, Swango resumed his quest for employment as a doctor. By early May 1991, Swango, or Adams, as he now legally was named, was in contact with doctors at Ohio Valley Medical Center in Wheeling, West Virginia, about a job opening there. He had to reveal his real name so it would accord with his medical school record and references; the hospital's chief of medicine, Dr. Jeffrey S. Schultz, later told the Illinois police that Swango claimed that his Illinois medical license had been suspended on account of a "single felony/battery conviction resulting from an altercation occurring in a restaurant."

At the time there was no national clearinghouse for information about doctors convicted of crimes or found liable for malpractice. The American Medical Association kept a "master file" intended to track errant doctors, and the American Federation of State Medical Associations maintained a list of doctors whose licenses had been suspended by state boards. But neither had any de-

tails of Swango's arrest and conviction. In any event, there's no indication Dr. Schultz made any attempt to contact them. Instead he
wrote the state's attorney's office in Quincy, saying that "we are
considering offering him a position" and "we want to be fair to this
young man." The letter continued, "Frankly, the severity of his punishment seems out of proportion to the offense committed, based
on his description."

Dr. Schultz also checked with the Illinois Department of Professional Regulation, the body that had suspended Swango's license,
and learned that he had not, in fact, been convicted of battery because of any "altercation" in a restaurant, but had been convicted of
six counts of poisoning. Dr. Schultz confirmed this in a phone conversation with the state's attorney in Quincy.

It is apparently a measure of Swango's persuasiveness, not to
mention one doctor's evident willingness to take the word of another, that the revelations from Illinois did not bring negotiations
between Ohio Valley and Swango to a halt. Schultz wrote Swango a
letter offering him the opportunity to document his version of
events. Swango responded in a letter dated May 20:

> Dear Dr. Schultz,
> I received your letter of 5-10-91 on Thursday, May
> 16, and I've been working constantly since then to try to
> locate and obtain, as soon as possible, the copies you re-
> quested. . . . I'm so happy to tell you that via numerous
> phone calls and FedEx, I've been able to get copies of
> what you need, I've enclosed three sets of copies, so peo-
> ple can have them right away. . . . As we discussed during
> my interview, I'm prepared to accept a position right
> away—and am truly looking forward to coming to Wheel-
> ing and joining your Residency program.
> Thanks again.
> Sincerely,
> David J. Adams, M.D.

Among the documents Swango provided was a prison discharge "fact sheet," which explained the battery as a brawl. "Re-
leasee struck a blow with his fist," the document said. Similarly, a
"docketing statement" contained this description of the case:

Appellant was convicted in a bench trial of (felony)
battery, violation of Chapter 38, Illinois Revised Statutes,
Section 12-4—intentional application of physical force to
an individual with resultant bodily injury caused by said
force. In this case, the force was a blow struck by appellant's fist.

Appellant was sentenced to a term of six months, to
be followed by eighteen months probation. . . .

Swango also submitted a 1989 letter from the governor of Virginia, Gerald L. Baliles. Written on the letterhead of the Common-
wealth of Virginia, Office of the Governor, it said,

Dear Mr. Swango:
I have before me your application for Restoration of
Civil Rights which will restore certain rights forfeited as a
result of your felony record.

Reputable citizens who are familiar with your conduct since your conviction(s) advise me that you are leading an upright, law-abiding life and they recommend that
your civil rights be restored. Relying on these recommendations, I am removing your political disabilities. . . .

I am pleased to convey my actions to you and wish
you much success in the future.

These and other documents prompted Dr. Schultz to write
again to Quincy authorities, this time saying that Swango had "submitted copies of court documents which would appear to support
his story." Schultz asked for "a brief letter" indicating "the nature of
his difficulties which led to his revocation of his medical license."
He attached copies of the documents Swango had submitted.

Quincy authorities were both alarmed and amazed. The docketing statement was an outright forgery—a crime in itself. (The
state of Virginia verifies that Swango's civil rights were indeed restored, on December 31, 1989.)

Scott Walden, the Adams County state's attorney, immediately
sent Schultz copies of Swango's sentencing order and of the appellate court opinion rejecting his appeal. He also sent copies of the
materials to Judge Cashman, urging that he, too, contact Schultz. In
his note to Cashman, Walden wrote, "As you can see, Swango has

gone to great lengths to cover up what he has done—even to the point of falsifying documents."

The flurry of documents and calls from Quincy finally persuaded Schultz to reject Swango's application. But there's nothing to suggest that doctors at Ohio Valley took any further steps to alert other doctors and medical residency programs to the possibility that Swango might apply. In any event, the rejection did nothing to discourage Swango, who was soon applying for other resident positions.

IN 1986, while Swango was still serving his prison term in Centralia, Dr. Michael Prince Brody was suspended from practice at John F. Kennedy Memorial Hospital in Indio, California, after an anonymous caller alleged that Dr. Brody had submitted false references and concealed his past. When the hospital investigated, it learned that five years earlier, Dr. Brody had been suspended by Bayshore Hospital in Pasadena, Texas, where he was a staff obstetrician, after a series of bizarre incidents that culminated in his being admitted to the emergency room with a stab wound. Brody claimed to have operated on his own abdomen with a pocket knife.

Dr. Brody had been suffering a drug problem for years. Nurses reported that he took Dexedrine by day and Valium at night, and had actually fallen asleep while performing surgery on a patient. They often had trouble locating him, and he frequently refused to see patients. Long before the stabbing incident, Bayshore Hospital administrators had concluded that he "personally abused analgesic, sedative and stimulant drugs, including amphetamine compounds, benzodiazepine compounds and opiate compounds," according to a later report. Before being hospitalized for drug treatment, Brody "had been regularly seeing patients, treating patients, and making decisions with regard to the welfare of patients while suffering from an adjustment disorder with mixed disturbance of emotion and conduct, mixed substance abuse, and psychological factors affecting physical conditions," the report continued.

In 1980 Brody did not respond to an urgent summons to show up for the delivery of a baby girl. Nor had he arranged for another doctor to cover him in his absence. The infant, Andrea Ferris, suffered brain damage from loss of oxygen and was subsequently

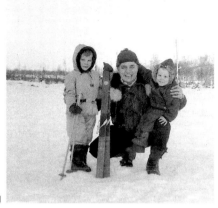

Michael (right) had little contact with his father, John Virgil Swango, a career military officer who seemed happiest during the nine years he spent in Vietnam. The family moved sixteen times before he retired. Here they are pictured at snowy Fort Richardson, Alaska, in 1957, when Michael was three. Michael's older brother Bob is at left.

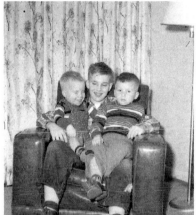

Michael (left) with his half brother, Richard Kerkering (center), and Bob. Richard later left the Swango home to live with his father, but Michael stayed closer to him than to his other brothers.

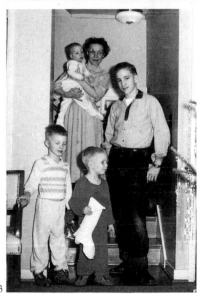

Michael said his mother, Muriel, "held the family together." She favored Michael, who she said was "gifted," with a private school education and music lessons, but rarely bestowed any affection on any of the four boys, Richard, Bob, Michael, and John, the youngest.

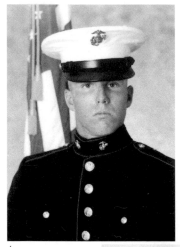

After Michael returned from the Marines in 1976, he was obsessed with fitness, dressed in military fatigues, and, when criticized, dropped to the floor to perform push-ups.

Classmates at Southern Illinois University's medical school found it fitting that Swango was alone in all his yearbook photos. He made few friends, and some classmates tried to have him expelled. His nickname was Double-O Swango, which meant "License to Kill."

4

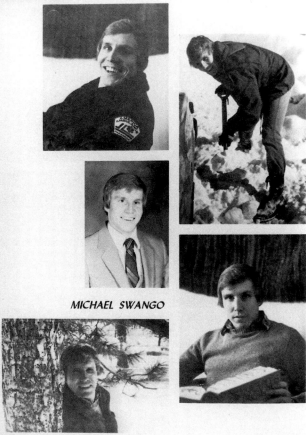

MICHAEL SWANGO

5

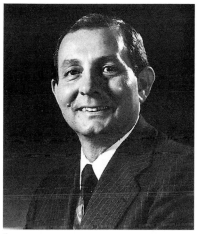

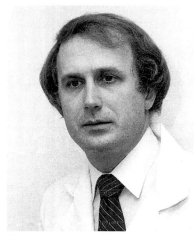

6   7

Above left: Confronted with eyewitness reports that Swango had tampered with a patient's IV tube and nearly killed her, Ohio State College of Medicine Dean Manuel Tzagournis asked for a report, then ultimately ordered that Swango be allowed to complete his internship.

Above right: Dr. Joseph Goodman, the Ohio State neurosurgeon in charge of investigating Swango, attributed the reports to the "nurses' grapevine" and concluded the rumors were unfounded and "out of hand."

When police searched Swango's apartment in Quincy, Illinois, in October 1984, they found a virtual poison lab, with a book bearing a skull and crossbones amid vials, needles, bottles, and handwritten recipes for poisons. These are two photographs of the evidence. The recipe cards, shown at right, include formulae for ricin, botulism, supersaturated cyanide, and fluoroacetic acid.

8

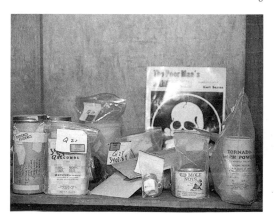

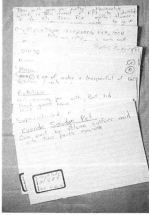

9 Kristin Kinney met Swango at a life support class in Newport News, Virginia. "He'll give me all his attention and take good care of me," the popular, vivacious nurse told her parents.

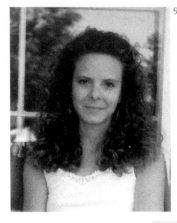

Like many who met him, Kristin was attracted to Swango's all-American looks and demeanor. Kristin and Michael became engaged in 1992, just after he was accepted to a residency in internal medicine at the University of South Dakota.

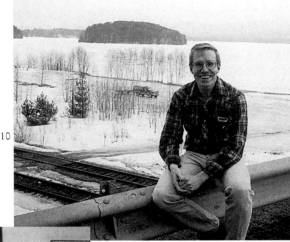

10

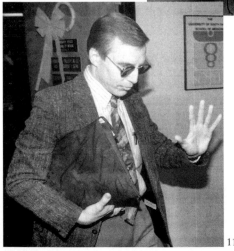

When news broke in South Dakota that Swango was a convicted poisoner, he dismissed the reports as a "media hoax." But horrified hospital officials rushed to suspend him, and South Dakota governor George Mickelson said he was "incredulous" that Swango could ever have been hired as a medical resident. Here Swango ducks the press after a hearing to protest his suspension.

11

12

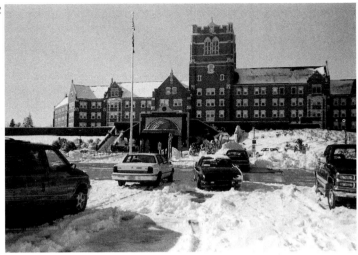

The VA hospital in Sioux Falls, South Dakota

When she returned from South Dakota, Kristin had stopped wearing her engagement ring. But Swango told Kristin's mother, "I want to get everything back on track with Kristin."

13

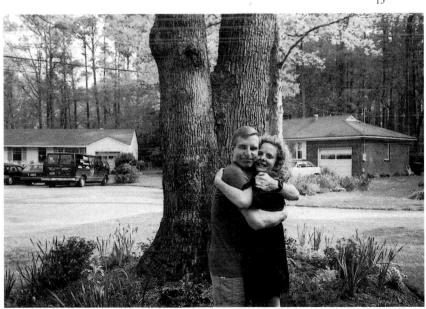

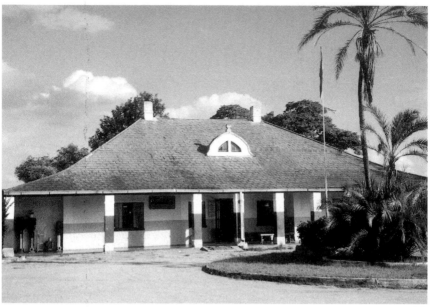

14

The remote Mnene Mission Hospital in the African nation of Zimbabwe seems little changed since its founding in 1927 by Lutheran missionaries. Church officials could hardly believe their good fortune when they recruited Swango, who they thought was dedicated to the poor and afflicted and had an outstanding résumé.

OPPOSITE:

Top: Doctors at Mpilo Hospital in Bulawayo, Zimbabwe, at first embraced Swango's assertion that he'd been a victim of reverse discrimination against whites at Mnene. Only later did the fact that he was living in the hospital, with access to patients at all hours, seem sinister.

Bottom: At this Zimbabwean farmstead, five brothers and sisters, now orphans, are trying to support themselves by farming. Both their father and their cousin died unexpectedly while being treated by Swango at Mnene.

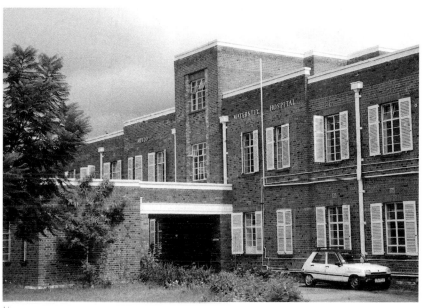

15

16

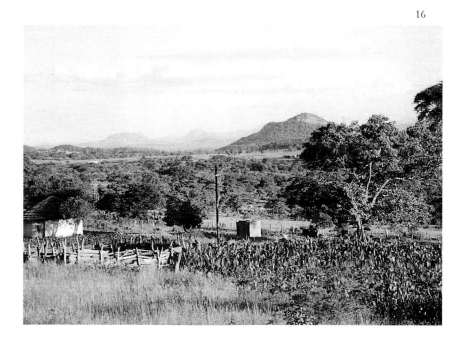

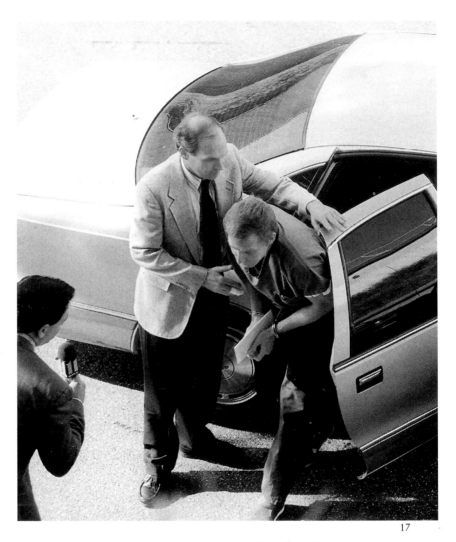

17

Swango arrives for arraignment at the federal courthouse in Union-dale, New York, on Long Island. He agreed to plead guilty to fraud charges and was sentenced to forty-two months in prison in June 1998 for gaining admission to a medical residency at the State University of New York under false pretenses.

awarded $119 million in an out-of-court malpractice settlement, at the time the largest ever awarded in Texas. Brady's hospital privileges at Bayshore were suspended. But after he agreed to undergo psychotherapy and substance abuse treatment, they were reinstated.

A month later came the episode in which Brody said he had operated on himself with a pocket knife. His hospital privileges at Bayshore were now revoked, this time for good.

But this was hardly the end of Dr. Brody's medical career. No one at Bayshore reported him to state medical authorities, to the American Medical Association, to the Federation of State Medical Boards, or to any other investigative authority. Brody moved on to Hospital in the Pines, in Lone Star, Texas, where he again failed to respond to calls to deliver a baby. This time both mother and child died. The hospital reached an undisclosed settlement with surviving family members, and Dr. Brody resigned. Again, no other disciplinary action was taken.

When Dr. Brody applied to renew his Texas medical license in 1982, he responded no when asked whether he had ever been disciplined by a hospital, even though Bayshore had revoked his privileges. His license was renewed. Brody left Texas, was licensed in California, and was hired at JFK Memorial in Indio. His license to practice in Texas was still in effect when JFK suspended him.

Brody's is hardly an isolated case. This and other examples of doctors moving from state to state to escape disciplinary action and license suspension were the focus of a June 23, 1986, episode of ABC's *Nightline*. Asked on the show why he hadn't reported Dr. Brody, a spokesman for Bayshore Hospital said simply, "It's, I don't think, up to me to report these kinds of things to the state board of medicine."

The medical literature, not to mention the popular press, has been full of accounts of incompetent physicians. In 1986, *The New York Times* quoted medical officials to the effect that "five out of every 100 doctors are so incompetent, drunk, senile or otherwise impaired that they should not be practicing medicine without some form of restriction." A medical director of the Kaiser Foundation Health Plan testified in Congress in 1986 that 3 to 5 percent of the nation's 425,000 practicing physicians have an "impairment of some degree from a wide variety of causes."

Even when hospitals or state licensing boards take action
against incompetent doctors, they usually do so quietly, often in
confidence, as they did with Swango. The result, concluded Robert
Adler, counsel to the U.S. House of Representatives Subcommittee
on Health and the Environment, charged with regulating the medical profession, is "a group of 'rogue' physicians who are free to
leave the immediate hospital or jurisdiction and continue their practice elsewhere."

While *Nightline* brought the Brody case to the attention of a
national audience, and eventually to that of lawmakers in Washington, the problem of "rogue" doctors would no doubt have gone un-
addressed had the medical community itself not reacted as strongly
as it did to an Oregon case. In 1981, several of Dr. Timothy
Patrick's colleagues at Columbia Memorial Hospital in Astoria,
Oregon, alleged that he was incompetent and recommended that
his hospital privileges be suspended. These same doctors had earlier
invited the surgeon to join them in their practice at a local clinic. Instead Patrick started a competing practice of his own. After they
tried to revoke his hospital privileges, Patrick sued the doctors,
claiming they were trying to maintain a monopoly by shutting
down his practice. A federal district court jury agreed with Dr.
Patrick, and awarded him $650,000, which under federal antitrust
laws, was trebled to nearly $2 million in damages.

The result outraged the medical profession, and not because
Dr. Patrick had been mistreated by his fellow physicians. Many doctors felt the verdict threatened the peer review process. As they saw
it, doctors who tried to discipline a colleague for incompetence had
instead been punished themselves.

Peer review, the evaluation of practicing physicians by other
physicians, is the foundation of the disciplinary process within the
medical profession, and has been at least since 1760, when doctors
were first licensed in the United States. The notion is that only doctors can evaluate the quality of patient care, a principle that the
American Medical Association has championed with near-religious
zeal. This deeply ingrained tradition was no doubt part of the reason that Ohio State doctors resisted calling the police to investigate
Swango, and they openly acknowledged their fears of being sued.

In the wake of the Patrick verdict, doctors argued vociferously
that his case and several similar ones were making it all but finan-

cially ruinous for doctors to try to dismiss an incompetent physician. When the Patrick case went to the U.S. Supreme Court, the AMA argued that "doctors who seek to discipline other doctors they consider incompetent should not be put at risk of huge damage awards for which insurance is not available, whenever a jury can be convinced their motives were not pure," according to *The New York Times.* And the AMA lobbied for federal legislation exempting doctors from the nation's antitrust laws, to eliminate the possibility that doctors could be sued for terminating another doctor's privileges or suspending a license.

But the AMA's sudden interest in strengthening the peer review process by insulating doctors from liability struck many as disingenuous, for the profession's efforts to police itself had always been lax. While the logic of peer review has never been seriously questioned, its effectiveness has. In a 1988 study, Timothy Jost, a law professor at, of all places, Ohio State, concluded that "there is substantial evidence that, despite its potential, the medical staff [peer review] system has traditionally operated quite laxly." It is "never a comfortable task to sit in judgment of one's peers with whom one works on a day-to-day basis. A physician in this position must always deal with the temptation to give the benefit of the doubt and gloss over a colleague's errors."

State medical licensing boards are largely an extension of the peer review process. Though the boards may include at least token nondoctors, they are dominated by physicians. They suffer from all the problems of peer review boards in hospitals, not to mention restricted budgets, lack of time for contested hearings, and inadequate investigative staffs.

These problems all surfaced in Ohio. In April 1985, in the wake of the Swango case and the Ohio State Medical Board's failure to take any disciplinary action against anyone at Ohio State, *Plain Dealer* reporter Gary Webb published an exhaustive seven-part series on the effectiveness of the Ohio board, which showed that the lapses in the Swango case were hardly exceptional. Among the series' conclusions, all of them backed up with numerous examples:

- The Ohio board allowed doctors convicted of felonies such as drug trafficking, insurance fraud, forgery, theft, sexual assault, and drug abuse to remain in practice.

- The board allowed physicians with serious alcohol or drug problems to remain in practice—even perform surgery—while they were undergoing treatment, withdrawal, and psychotherapy.
- The board allowed doctors diagnosed as suffering severe mental problems to remain in practice for years while their cases wended their way through the board's hearing process.
- The board routinely allowed doctors convicted of felonies to continue practicing for years while their cases dragged on in appellate courts.
- Even when a physician repeatedly violated the law, the board seemed loath to pull his or her license; board members worried that the physician would be unable to earn a living.
- While ignoring some physician crimes, the board kept its small staff of six investigators busy digging up evidence against nurse-midwives, physician's assistants, health-food stores, chiropractors, acupuncturists, masseuses, manicurists, and others suspected of practicing medicine without a license.

The Plain Dealer also chastised the board for the "use of secret hearings and deals negotiated privately with the offending doctor," noting that virtually everything about the board's procedures is confidential.*

The *Plain Dealer* series made clear, as have numerous academic and legislative studies, that "the effectiveness of state licensing boards at weeding out incompetent physicians has always been inadequate," as legislative counsel Adler put it in a 1991 survey of the boards. Yet any congressional move to replace or modify peer review has been summarily dismissed because of opposition from the medical profession.

Doctors' outrage over the Patrick verdict was rooted in the notion that a jury had slapped the Astoria physicians with a $2 million

* The board repeatedly rebuffed my requests for information about their investigation of Swango and Ohio State's handling of the matter, on grounds of confidentiality.

verdict simply because they had blown the whistle on an incompetent surgeon. This was the view pressed on Congressman Ron Wyden, Democrat of Oregon, by doctors in Oregon and by the AMA. He echoed these concerns in a speech on the House floor: "Regardless of the guilt or innocence of the Astoria doctor, cases like this demonstrate that if this country wants physicians to come forward and prevent truly bad doctors from hurting people, there must be legal protection for them from the possibility of multimillion-dollar litigation, years in court and financial ruin."

But while momentum to protect whistle-blowing doctors gained force, the actual facts of the Patrick case were ignored, as Wyden's comment—"regardless of the guilt or innocence of the Astoria doctor"—makes obvious. A jury, the Ninth Circuit U.S. Court of Appeals, and the U.S. Supreme Court all eventually found that Dr. Patrick was competent, had not behaved negligently or recklessly, and was actually being hounded out of business by rival doctors' vindictive use of the peer review process. The doctors had begun their campaign against Dr. Patrick only after he rejected their offer of a partnership in the Astoria clinic and set up a rival practice. The principal basis for the charge of incompetence, and the attempted revocation of his hospital privileges, was that Dr. Patrick had left a patient in the care of one of his colleagues. Even then, Patrick himself was only ninety minutes away, but no one had called him. The Court of Appeals noted that "there was a great deal of testimony that Patrick was quite a good surgeon."

If anything, the Patrick case seems a glaring example of how doctors can manipulate and abuse the peer review process to further their own economic interests and prevent competition. It should have been grounds for questioning peer review. As the Court of Appeals noted, "There was substantial evidence that the defendants acted in bad faith in the hospital's peer review process."

Yet the case instead became a national symbol for the persecution of doctors trying to use peer review to root out incompetence. The case was cited by Congressman Wyden when he introduced legislation on March 12, 1986, to immunize physicians engaged in peer review.

The AMA has for years been trying to exclude the medical profession from antitrust liability, a move which, among other things, would free doctors from the laws banning price fixing and restraint of trade and would all but certainly drive up the cost of medical care. The Wyden bill, cloaked in a concern for protecting the peer review process, was a significant step in that direction—and was quickly recognized as a Trojan horse by others in government. The proposed legislation attracted fierce opposition from the Federal Trade Commission, the Justice Department, the House and Senate Judiciary Committees, and the House subcommittee overseeing the FTC—all bodies involved with overseeing the nation's antitrust laws—which saw it as a gambit to escape antitrust restrictions.

Wyden's bill would have died quickly without the support of California representative Henry Waxman, a powerful Democrat who was chairman of the House Subcommittee on Health and the Environment. It so happened that Dr. Brody, who had been highlighted on *Nightline,* had surfaced in California, Waxman's state. Wyden had added to his proposed law a provision that required doctors, in exchange for immunity, to report to a national clearinghouse actions taken against incompetent doctors. Hospitals would be required to check with the clearinghouse before they hired or extended hospital privileges to a physician.

The "Brody" reporting provision establishing a national data bank cost Wyden the support of the AMA. Testifying in a hearing on the bill, a member of the AMA's board of trustees, Dr. Raymond Scalettar, complained that "the national clearinghouse would be duplicative and unnecessary. There is no need to create a new body and source of data. . . . Such data will include an extremely large amount of complex and possibly misleading information." But Wyden defended his approach of addressing the problem of rogue physicians in the same legislation that granted physicians immunity from the kind of liability faced by every other profession.

"Well, I tell you, I think . . . it is in the public interest to tie the two together," he said. "If we don't tie the two together, it seems to me that we are setting up a situation where rights are being given in particular to physicians and to medical providers. I am very much in favor of doing this. It is something I have put in many, many hours behind. I am in favor of those rights. But I am not in favor of giving those rights without some responsibilities which are in the public interest."

With vigorous lobbying from the medical profession, however, crucial elements of the national data bank on incompetent physicians were watered down. The penalty for failing to comply was minimal, nothing more than a "presumption," in any medical malpractice action against a hospital, that the hospital had knowledge of any information available through the data bank. But the AMA still opposed the bill, largely because of the national data bank.

In essence, the final bill provided that persons engaged in peer review activities "[could not] be held liable for damages under any federal or state law" as long as they complied with the act. In return, the proposed bill required state medical boards to report to a national data bank each time a physician's license was suspended for incompetence or misconduct. All "health care entities" were required to report actions "adversely affecting the clinical privileges of a physician," as well as any instance in which they "accept[ed] a surrender of clinical privileges while the physician was under investigation."

Thus, had the law been in effect in 1986, or made retroactive, the Ohio and Illinois state medical boards would have been required to report the suspension of Swango's medical license to the national data bank.

The combined opposition of the AMA and virtually every governmental organization involved in antitrust enforcement seemed certain to doom the measure. But at the last minute, just four days before the Ninety-ninth Congress was due to adjourn, Waxman displayed the legislative dexterity for which he is renowned. By tacking the bill onto an omnibus piece of health care legislation that already contained eight other bills, he ensured that it would undergo minimal scrutiny.

The bill, titled the Health Care Quality Improvement Act of 1986, was passed by the House of Representatives on October 17. It was sponsored in the Senate, which held no hearings at all on the immunity or reporting measures, by then senator Al Gore, and was passed unanimously on October 18. When President Reagan voiced misgivings and indicated he might not sign the legislation, Representative Wyden took his case to the public in an opinion piece in *The Washington Post*. Although the establishment of a national data bank to keep tabs on incompetent doctors made up only a small part of the legislation, and although it had been watered down because of opposition from the AMA, it was this provision that Wyden stressed.

After reviewing the Brody case, he wrote:

> There are many other cases like this one. The House Energy and Commerce health and environment subcommittee heard testimony indicating that three to five per cent of the doctors in this country account for most of the malpractice. There are 450,000 physicians nationwide; in other words, a moderate estimate indicates there may be 18,000 doctors regularly malpracticing.
>
> The need for legislation is clear. There is no effective national system for keeping tabs on doctors who are truly incompetent. Physicians have told the health subcommittee, on which I sit, that they are now afraid to speak out when a colleague malpractices. Hospitals can't take action against physicians they know are incompetent because they fear the legal consequences. The result: the incompetent doctor continues to practice, inflicting poor care and soaring costs on the unsuspecting.

President Reagan signed the bill into law on November 14, 1986. The National Practitioner Data Bank was inaugurated in September 1990. Although the AMA had rather audaciously proposed that it be in charge of the data bank, it remains under the supervision of the Department of Health and Human Services, administered by a private company in Virginia.

DURING the summer of 1991, while he was still living in the Newport News area, Michael Swango enrolled in an advanced life-support course at Riverside Hospital. One day when he drove into the parking lot in his 1987 red pickup truck, he noticed an attractive young woman getting out of another red truck. He pointed out the similarity of their vehicles and introduced himself, using his real name. She said her name was Kristin Kinney. She was twenty-five years old, with beautiful long reddish-blond hair.

Kinney worked as a nurse in the intensive care unit at Riverside. She had recently returned from a stint as a "traveling" nurse in

Naples, Florida, where she had made some close friends and enjoyed the work. But she returned to Virginia because she was dating Dr. Jerome Provenzano, a medical resident there. Swango told
her he was a chemist. The two spoke occasionally during the
course, but otherwise had little contact. Kristin was soon engaged
to Dr. Provenzano, and she wasn't interested in dating Swango.
Still, when the course ended and students filled out evaluations that
asked for "the best thing about this course," Swango responded
"Kristin Kinney."

Kristin had been living with her mother and stepfather, Sharon
and Al Cooper, but moved into her own apartment that summer.
Sharon was an emergency room nurse, and Kristin had followed in
her footsteps. Using fake names to preserve confidentiality, the two
often traded stories about their patients. Once, Kristin told her
mother about a patient who had tried to commit suicide by shooting himself in the head. He hadn't died, but would remain dysfunc-
tional for life. The emergency room doctor had complained
vociferously, Kristin had reported. "If you want to commit suicide,
shoot yourself in the chest," the doctor had proclaimed with exas-
peration. "Don't shoot yourself in the head."

Kristin had a lively, and at times wicked, sense of humor. Because of it and her reddish hair, her mother and friends sometimes
compared her to comedienne Lucille Ball. She was especially irreverent toward doctors. Once she was giving mouth-to-mouth resuscitation to an emergency room patient while a group of medical
residents stood by. After struggling to stabilize the patient, she
turned to them and asked, "Does anyone here want to play doctor?"

Though Kristin initially resented her mother's new husband,
Al, a retired Navy pilot—she called him Alpo, after the dog food—
she and her stepfather had developed a close rapport. She confided
in him about her relationship with Provenzano, saying that she was
having doubts about the engagement. Provenzano would come
home from his long stints at the hospital too tired to pay much attention to Kristin. She complained that he'd turn on the stereo and
ignore her. She wasn't sure she wanted to marry a doctor. They
seemed too consumed with their work to have much time left for a
family.

Then one evening Kristin called her parents to report that

she'd met someone else, someone who promised "he'll give me all his attention and take good care of me," as she told the Coopers. The young man she'd met in life-support class, Michael Swango, now formally divorced from Rita, had been calling her, asking her to at least meet him for a cup of coffee. She'd finally agreed, even though one of her best friends, a nurse at Riverside, warned her to stay away from him. He'd applied to work at the hospital, but had been rejected because of "something in his past." But the friend wasn't any more specific, and Kristin, who could be stubborn at times, preferred to trust her own judgment. She met Swango for coffee. She learned he was a *Star Trek* fan and loved Tom Clancy novels. He was soon calling her every night, showering her with attention and begging her to call off her engagement to Provenzano. Now, Kristin told her parents, "I have a big decision to make."

"Why don't you get away for a while?" Al Cooper suggested. So Kristin checked into a Holiday Inn on the ocean in Virginia Beach to think things over. The next day, Al called her there. "Have you made up your mind?" he asked her.

"Yeah," she said. She paused, then added, "Michael showed up." Swango had tracked her down there and persuaded her to break the engagement. She told her stepfather she cared deeply for him and that he was a wonderful person. She assured him that Michael had a good job as a chemist.

The Coopers were initially wary. Kristin, for all her vivacity and natural beauty, had not had good luck with men. She'd married a classmate from nursing school during her senior year, and he turned out to be a handsome rogue, cheating on her with other women. They were divorced two years later. Then she began dating someone who became so possessive that, after she broke off the relationship, she had to obtain a court order preventing him from seeing her. She was so afraid of him that she bought a nine-millimeter pistol and took target practice at a shooting range. She became a good shot, and kept the gun in her truck, even after she moved back to Virginia from her stint in Naples.

Not long after Kristin broke off her engagement, the Coopers let themselves into her apartment, as they often did, and were waiting for her to return when the phone rang. Sharon answered, and told the caller she was Kristin's mother. "I love your daughter!"

Swango exclaimed. "I'll be good to her." Sharon couldn't get him off the phone, even though Al was growing annoyed. Swango went on and on about how wonderful Kristin was and how much he loved her. Sharon tried to ask him a few questions, but didn't make much headway. She couldn't deflect him from singing Kristin's praises. When Sharon finally got off the phone, she told her husband, "This is either the most wonderful thing in the world for Kristin or he's some kind of nut." But Swango seemed so sincere, she couldn't really believe he might be the latter.

A few weeks later, Kristin called her parents with a revelation about Swango. "Guess what?" she said. "The one thing I didn't want to have happen. Michael is actually a doctor."

Al was startled. Hadn't Michael told her he was a chemist? "So he lied to you?" Al asked.

"He didn't want to scare me away," Kristin explained.

"What are you going to do now?"

"I guess it's too late, isn't it?" she asked.

DR. Anthony Salem, director of the internal medicine residency program at the University of South Dakota in Sioux Falls, was sifting through completed applications in September 1991 when one letter captured his attention.

"My situation is somewhat unusual," the letter read. "My medical career was interrupted by a personal tragedy in 1985. . . . Under circumstances unrelated to medicine or medical practice, I was convicted of battery in the State of Illinois. I appealed the conviction vigorously, but without initial success in the courts. Upon completion of my probation, I began to rebuild my personal life and my medical career. In August 1989 I received a Restoration of Rights/Removal of Political Disabilities from the [then] Governor of Virginia, Gerald Baliles. This is essentially a pardon for the conviction in Illinois, and restores any and all rights."

The letter was signed "Michael Swango," not Adams.

Intrigued, Dr. Salem looked through Swango's completed application. His credentials looked excellent; Salem was especially impressed by his internship at Ohio State, accompanied by the 1984 certificate signed by Tzagournis and Carey. Unlike Ohio State or Iowa, the University of South Dakota medical school did not enjoy a prestigious national reputation, though it was highly regarded in the northern Plains states. Given the remote location and harsh weather, it wasn't easy to attract and retain competent doctors in the Dakotas, and USD tried to accept and train residents who showed some promise of remaining in the state. Increasingly, that had meant recruiting foreigners. So Swango's application was highly attractive, except for the curious matter of the battery conviction. Salem wondered what had happened. He was almost certain that a felony conviction would bar Swango from being admitted to the program, but he thought he'd follow up, mostly to satisfy his own curiosity. He suspected that Swango might have been convicted of some kind of domestic violence.

Dr. Salem was known as thorough and meticulous, detail-oriented almost to a fault. On September 18, he called the Illinois Department of Registration and Education, the Ohio State Medical Board, and the American Medical Association.

Illinois reported that Swango's medical license had been revoked for "disciplinary reasons." Ohio reported the same information. Neither licensing agency provided any details, saying only that Swango had been convicted of a felony. The AMA was even vaguer, responding over a month later that Swango had been subject to unspecified "action by two licensing boards." All of this was consistent with what Swango had already revealed in his letter, and did nothing to signal any more serious problems. It also failed to satisfy Salem's curiosity.

The next day, Salem had an associate contact Swango in Virginia, asking for more information about the battery conviction, and Swango provided a one-page supplement to his earlier letter and application. This time he abandoned the fictions he had created when he applied to the Wheeling, West Virginia, residency program, fictions that had ultimately backfired. Not only was he using his real name, but he acknowledged that the battery was a case of poisoning, not a restaurant brawl. He explained that during the summer of 1985, he and his fellow paramedics had become suddenly ill at work. (Swango himself, of course, had not been ill.) To his "utter surprise," several weeks later he was arrested and charged with putting something in their food and drink. He claimed the accusations were made by his coworkers, who were jealous of the fact that he was a physician, and he added that the physical evidence of poison had come from a state laboratory "later closed by the Governor of Illinois and the State Police due to gross incompetence and numerous deficiencies." He offered to provide further information if requested.

Now Salem was even more intrigued, and instead of rejecting the application outright, he called Swango on the phone. Swango was at his most charming and persuasive. He eagerly elaborated on the letter, weaving a sophisticated fabric of truth, half-truth, and outright fabrication to support his claim that he was a victim of a gross miscarriage of justice. Swango shrewdly premised his story on the notion of jealousy and hostility toward doctors—a scenario likely to appeal to other physicians, who increasingly saw themselves confronted by hostile forces.

Salem came away from this and several subsequent phone conversations persuaded that Swango was not only a remarkably candid young man, but also a courageous one. Increasingly, Salem found himself liking him.

Still, he thought it unlikely that Swango could be a serious candidate, because USD policy was not to hire residents who couldn't later be licensed to practice medicine in South Dakota. Salem assumed that a felony conviction would preclude licensing. Hearing this, Swango himself offered to research the question, and reported back to Salem that nothing in South Dakota law precluded him from being licensed if he showed he had successfully completed a three-year residency. Without consulting anyone else in South Dakota—such as, for example, the university's lawyers—Salem accepted Swango's assertion and invited him to Sioux Falls for a round of personal interviews. (While Swango's assertion may have been technically accurate—no law specifically bars a felon from practicing medicine—as a matter of policy South Dakota treats felony convictions as a bar to licensure on the grounds that the underlying crime constitutes unprofessional conduct.)

Five internists, including Salem, interviewed Swango on October 3. They asked about his experience and knowledge of internal medicine and his willingness to practice in South Dakota; Dr. Salem asked him again whether he could be licensed to practice in the state. Swango emphasized that South Dakota was one of a "handful" of states where, if someone "turns their life around," they can be licensed to practice. Incredibly, no one asked any other questions about his conviction on battery charges. Swango was seemingly earnest, sincere, persuasive. Salem's positive impressions were substantially reinforced by the meeting. It never occurred to Salem, or anyone else who interviewed Swango, to contact police or judicial authorities in Quincy.

But the next day, when Swango was interviewed by participants in the family practice program, to which he had also applied, things didn't go so smoothly. Dr. Bruce Vogt, the residency program coordinator at an area hospital, asked about the battery charges, and seemed more skeptical of Swango's explanation. When he asked for Swango's permission to interview his parole officer, Swango seemed uncomfortable, and finally refused. The group told Swango on the spot that they wouldn't consider his application any further. After the meeting, Swango lobbied Dr. Vogt, asking if there was any way he could apply for a "transitional" residency program directed by Vogt. Vogt told Swango it was possible, but he would probably be wasting his time.

But no one who participated in the family practice interviews conveyed the group's decision or misgivings to Salem or anyone else in internal medicine. This wasn't so surprising, because the two residency programs often competed for the same applicants and tended to keep decisions to themselves.

Then Salem learned from the Federation of State Medical Boards that Swango had had his licenses revoked by Illinois and Ohio, which Salem already knew; that his application for a license had been rejected by Virginia; and that he had legally changed his name to David Jackson Adams. The name change troubled Salem, but Swango explained on the phone and in writing that he had changed his name to "get a fresh start" and had since reverted to using his real name. "Perhaps most importantly," he wrote, "I realized that I did not want there to be even the appearance of any attempt to conceal my past difficulties."

To gain a residency appointment in South Dakota, Swango had to go through the same national match process that had gotten him accepted by Iowa and then Ohio State.

The University of South Dakota's internal medicine residency ranking committee met on February 24, 1992, to rank the seventeen applicants still under consideration for the eight positions in the program. Four doctors attended, including Dr. Salem and Dr. Vogt, who had participated in the family practice discussions. For the first time, Dr. Vogt told the group that the family practice group had declined to rank Swango. But Dr. Salem argued persuasively on Swango's behalf; since Salem had had by far the most contact with him, and the other doctors trusted Salem's judgment, they decided to rank Swango. However, there was little expectation that he would rank high enough to gain a match and hence an appointment. Dr. Vogt ranked Swango last or close to last. So did one of the other doctors. Another ranked him only several names from the bottom. But Dr. Salem must have given him a fairly high ranking, because when the results were totaled, Swango ranked eleventh of the seventeen candidates. Of the six applicants ranked behind him, five were foreign doctors. The other showed evidence of mental instability.

The results of the national match program were announced on March 18, 1992. Swango was accepted to a residency in internal medicine at the University of South Dakota.

NOW that Swango's future seemed secure, he and Kristin became engaged, in May 1992. He took her shopping for a ring, and she chose a small diamond in an antique shop. Kristin loved old jewelry and antiques. The Coopers finally met Swango that same month, at a dinner at Gus' Mariner Restaurant, located on the beach. Swango was neatly dressed, poised and charming. Sharon thought he treated her daughter like a queen. He held her hand throughout the meal and told the Coopers how much he loved her. Kristin beamed with appreciation, and her parents thought she'd never looked better. She showed them her new ring, and said she'd be moving to South Dakota with "Mike-O," as she called him. But they weren't planning to be married right away.

During dinner, Al asked Swango to tell them about his background and education. He mentioned his many awards and achievements, his medical degree, his internship at Ohio State. But Al noticed there was a gap of about three years, from 1984 to 1987, and he asked Swango what he was doing then. "I'll tell you about that

later," Swango said mysteriously, though he gave no hint it was anything awkward or embarrassing. "It's not important." He said nothing about any previous marriage.

The Coopers also asked about Swango's parents. He told them
about his father's military career, and that he had died. He said
nothing about his mother, so Al asked about her. Swango paused,
then said, "She's in a nursing home."

"Where?" the Coopers asked.

"In Missouri," Swango replied. He seemed uncomfortable, and
volunteered nothing further.

"When was the last time you saw her?" Al continued.

Swango paused. "I haven't."

Kristin jumped in to defuse what was rapidly becoming a tense
conversation. "It's a really sad story," she said. "He'll tell you about
it sometime."

In fact, after Muriel complained to Judge Cashman just after
Michael's conviction that she wasn't feeling well, her physical and
mental health had deteriorated rapidly. She had confided in Ruth
Miller that having two sons reject her when she refused to fund the
appeal was even worse than Mike's arrest and conviction. Still, she
never broke down or showed any self-pity, preferring to keep her
feelings to herself.

After the trial, Muriel had moved back to Florida to be near her
youngest son, John, but a thank-you note to Louise Scharf in
Springfield not long after Michael's sentencing had been oddly written and barely coherent. Muriel soon entered a nursing home in
Palmyra, Missouri, not far from Quincy; she was diagnosed as suffering from Alzheimer's disease. But family members were convinced she was suffering from "a broken heart," as Scharf put it.
"She never got over the fact that Mike was found guilty."

The Coopers, of course, knew none of this. After their dinner,
Kristin walked with them to their car and asked them what they
thought of Mike. It was obvious she wanted their approval, and
they gave it. Al said, "If you can deal with the gap [in his résumé],
then I think you've got a winner."

But both Coopers were more troubled than they let on, and
more by the fact that Swango had never visited his ailing mother
than by the mysteries in his background.

As they reached their car, Al said to Sharon, "I hope he is what he says he is."

IN late June, just before Swango was due to arrive in Sioux Falls, Dr. Salem decided he should review Swango's file one more time. This was, after all, the first time he knew of that the university had admitted a convicted felon to its residency program. As Salem went through the materials, everything seemed to be in order—verification of Swango's degree from SIU, the dean's letter indicating the problem with his OB/GYN rotation, the certificate of completion of his internship at OSU. . . . Suddenly, Salem recognized that he'd gotten a copy of the OSU certificate from Swango himself, and had never gotten direct verification from Ohio State. So he had his secretary send what he considered a routine inquiry, asking Ohio State to verify the internship and for any other information the school maintained on Swango.

More than a month later, on August 7, Salem received a letter from Ohio State. Incredibly, even though the University now knew that Swango had been accepted to another residency program and would be working in a hospital, it said nothing about the medical school's investigation of him or about the reopening of the case by Morgan's office in 1985. It did not send either the Meeks or Morgan reports, both documents of public record. Instead, an associate to Tzagournis at Ohio State replied that both Swango and the University of South Dakota would have to "execute waivers and hold-harmless agreements" before Ohio State would release any information.

Salem thought the legalistic demand was absurd. Since Ohio State raised no red flags about Swango, Salem considered the university to have verified the certificate. He put the Swango file away.

At no point in this process does it seem to have occurred to anyone at the University of South Dakota to check whether the recently inaugurated National Practitioner Data Bank had anything on Swango. But since the act establishing it wasn't retroactive, the suspension of Swango's licenses in Illinois and Ohio wouldn't have shown up. And as the act was being interpreted, hospitals *could* query the data bank before hiring residents; no query was *required*. In any event, the university concluded in an internal report prepared in December 1992: "Apparently, there is no medical clearing house for information concerning criminal charges such as these. Neither the AMA nor the FSMB [Federation of State Medical Boards] had anything other than information of record."

SWANGO seemed elated by his acceptance at South Dakota. He lavished attention on Kristin, taking her to plays and concerts, the kind of cultural events she'd never experienced. The two spent so much time alone together that the Coopers only saw them once more before they left for South Dakota. Swango mentioned that his favorite movie, which had recently won the Oscar for best picture, was *The Silence of the Lambs,* starring Anthony Hopkins as a diabolical killer. He'd insisted that Kristin see it with him, and he himself had seen it three times. "That's the sickest movie I've ever seen," Al said, and Kristin chimed in that she found it "disgusting."

"No, no, you're wrong," Swango exclaimed. "It's a great movie."

Michael and Kristin left for South Dakota at the end of May, taking both their trucks. The night before, Sharon had an anxiety attack. She called Kristin. "I don't want you to go," she said, near tears at the prospect of her daughter moving so far away, with a man she barely knew.

Kristin dismissed Sharon's concerns, saying she wanted to go: "This is a chance for Mike to get ahead with his career."

But Sharon wasn't reassured. She didn't know why, but she felt frightened. The day Kristin left, she couldn't stop crying.

CHAPTER EIGHT

SIOUX FALLS, located on a bend in the Big Sioux River close to the Minnesota border, is a city of about 100,000 people, the largest in South Dakota, with modest houses, small, well-tended lawns and shady trees, a small historic district near the downtown, and a low crime rate. People there tend to be polite, unassuming, inconspicuous about their wealth, and accustomed to the long, harsh winters. Kristin Kinney quickly became one of the most popular nurses in the intensive care unit at the Royal C. Johnson Veterans Memorial Hospital, where she began working as soon as she and Michael moved to town. She was vivacious, cheerful, full of greetings and encouragement for the patients and irreverent comments for the doctors. "Did someone piss in your Wheaties?' she asked one doctor. "My God, you are so grumpy," she told one of the most dour surgeons. Word of these remarks brought visits from nurses on other floors, curious about the newcomer willing to stand up to the medical staff. Just about everyone called her by her initials, K.K.

Though she was by nature talkative, Kristin initially said nothing about her engagement to Swango or the reasons she had moved from Virginia to South Dakota. Not even Lisa Flinn, a nurse who conducted Kristin's orientation and often worked the same twelve-hour shifts as she did, knew that Kristin had any connection to Dr. Swango, the new resident who was doing a rotation in internal medicine at the VA hospital. But one day Swango responded to a code on the floor, and after the patient was stable, Flinn noticed that Swango stayed around and chatted with Kristin. "Who is that guy, anyway?" Flinn asked. "I don't think I've met him."

"Oh, that's Dr. Swango," Kristin replied. Only several days later did she tell Flinn that she was engaged to him. Flinn thought Kinney was just being modest, trying not to impress anyone with the fact that she was soon going to be married to a physician, something likely to set her apart, both socially and financially, from the other nurses in the unit.

Flinn and Kinney became close friends, and gradually Kristin confided more about her life to Lisa, who was older and more experienced. Beneath the vivacious surface, it was obvious that Kristin suffered the lingering effects of a difficult childhood. Her mother had taken refuge, with Kristin in a shelter for battered women before her parents divorced. But Kristin had gone to live with her father in order to finish high school with her friends. A heavy drinker, prone to violent outbursts, her father was someone she both loved and feared, and after graduating, she had moved back with her mother. Kristin had suffered a disastrous first marriage, then a bout of Crohn's disease, a digestive malady characterized by cramps, diarrhea, and weight loss and thought to be brought on by stress. Kristin spoke mostly in generalities about her past, but Lisa knew enough to recognize the symptoms of child abuse. Thank goodness, she thought, that Kristin had finally met someone like the nice new resident, Dr. Swango.

Swango was almost as popular on the ICU floor as Kinney. He was much more skilled in emergency medicine than most of the other new residents; he was even teaching a course in advanced cardiac life support. The nurses didn't want to think of themselves as provincial or prejudiced, but they also liked the fact that English was his native tongue. It was difficult, especially at first, dealing with the many foreign-born doctors who were showing up in the university's residency program. And, at age thirty-seven when he moved to Sioux Falls, Swango was older than most of the other residents, and seemed mature.

Swango displayed none of the idiosyncrasies that had attracted such attention from the paramedics in Quincy. Eager to put his past behind him, he seemed to have turned over a new leaf in Sioux Falls. Most of the nursing staff found him handsome, calm, and reassuring. Several of them nicknamed him the Virginian, after the 1960s TV series hero played by James Drury, because Drury's character was so cool and, of course, he had come from Virginia. Swango seemed pleased by the comparison and liked the nickname.

Swango quickly developed a reputation for being good in emergencies, and always seemed to show up when codes were called. Flinn noticed him at several code emergencies; they seemed to excite him. Kinney sometimes mentioned that Michael had phoned her at work, and if she was having a bad day in the ICU—an unusual number of emergencies, accidents, or deaths—he'd say she was "lucky" and that he envied her. But no one in Sioux Falls knew about Swango's scrapbooks, and he didn't make any of the comments about sex and disaster that had haunted him at his trial in Quincy. Flinn and the other nurses didn't give Swango's comments to Kristin much thought. He was interested in emergency medicine, so it seemed to follow that he'd be interested in their work in intensive care.

When Swango finished his month's rotation at the VA hospital, he brought in a cake and a card, thanking the nurses for "all your help." The gesture caused grumbling among the other new residents, who complained that Swango was just currying favor with the nursing staff and trying to make them look bad by comparison.

Once Swango moved on to Sioux Falls' other university-affiliated hospitals—Sioux Valley and McKennan—the nurses at the VA didn't see much of him. Occasionally he joined Kristin and some of the other nurses after work at Chi-Chi's, a popular Mexican restaurant, but usually Kristin went alone. Now and then he and Kristin showed up at a potluck dinner or other social event hosted by someone on the staff. Kristin wrote her parents, assuring them that the relationship with Michael was good, that they were happy and had made new friends. But no one was invited to visit them at the small one-story house they rented on East Fifth Street. Swango was too busy with his residency, and Kinney was also taking courses to finish her bachelor's degree, besides working extra shifts to earn more money.

In October, things were going so well for Swango in South Dakota that he applied to join the American Medical Association, using his real name, giving his address in South Dakota, and revealing that he was again practicing medicine. For someone trying to conceal his past, it was a highly risky step. Unlike the University of

South Dakota, the AMA official in charge of his file, Nancy Watson, wrote the courthouse in Quincy to obtain a copy of his conviction. To her surprise, her letter prompted a call from Judge Cashman, who was dismayed to learn that Swango was applying to join the AMA and, evidently, was again practicing medicine. "Do you know who this guy is?" he asked Watson, somewhat incredulously.

"Not really," she replied. Judge Cashman told her about the bizarre events in Quincy, and also told her about the suspicious deaths and ensuing investigation at Ohio State.

Shocked, Watson wrote Swango to say that because his licenses had been revoked in two states, his application would have to be referred to the AMA's council on ethical and judicial affairs for further investigation. As soon as he received the letter, Swango phoned, leaving a message for Watson that he was withdrawing his application. Evidently he was hoping to forestall any further questions. But Watson mentioned what had happened to several other people on the AMA staff, one of whom happened to know Dr. Robert Talley, the dean of the University of South Dakota medical school.

To the extent he'd had doubts about Swango, Dr. Salem's concerns were eased by just about everything he'd heard since the new resident arrived in Sioux Falls. Swango seemed to be popular with the staff; he was extremely hardworking; he was courteous, even ingratiating, around Dr. Salem, who had been so instrumental in his admission. Whereas he had performed poorly at Ohio State, all of Swango's evaluations during his first five months were favorable. The few problems that did surface were strictly of a personal nature, according to Salem, and that was only to be expected in a new resident.

So Swango's past had all but faded from Salem's mind by four P.M. Wednesday, November 25, 1992, the day before Thanksgiving, when he received a call from Dr. Talley, wanting to know about Swango. Talley reported that he'd just received a call from the AMA, alerting him to the fact that Swango had had "problems" in his past.

"I know," Dr. Salem replied. "I've heard all about them in Illinois."

"No," Dr. Talley said, "this was an issue of suspicious deaths at Ohio State."

Salem was startled. He'd been prepared to tell Talley the story of how Swango had been unjustly convicted of poisoning co-workers in Illinois, but deaths in Ohio? "I have absolutely no knowledge of anything like that," he said.

Salem suddenly felt all his misgivings about Swango return. He was shocked and worried. He looked quickly at the residents' schedule and assured Talley that he would personally supervise Swango for the next three days. They agreed that since it was the eve of a holiday, they would say nothing immediately, but that Talley would contact the dean at Ohio State, Tzagournis, on Friday to find out what the AMA official had been talking about.

Salem spent an uneasy Thanksgiving worrying about his earlier failure to follow through on the letter from officials at Ohio State. After the holiday, Talley spoke with Tzagournis. Talley later wrote a confidential memo summarizing the conversation, which he sent to Dr. Salem:

> I have contacted an acquaintance of mine who was dean at the time Michael Swango was an intern at Ohio State. Manny Tzagournis states that Michael Swango was aware of the following areas:
>
> 1. That a nurse felt he injected something into a patient which was deleterious.
> 2. He was told of this instance and he would be investigated.
> 3. He was reassigned to non-clinical duties during the investigation.
> 4. He was told he could go back to work as the investigation was resolved to everybody's satisfaction "at the time" and no disciplinary action was taken.

Talley and Salem had yet to formulate a plan for dealing with Swango. Then matters were taken out of their hands. That night at ten P.M., on the Discovery Channel, *The Justice Files* aired a segment on Swango that used the footage from the earlier *20/20* broadcast on which John Stossel interviewed Swango in prison. At 10:20 P.M. Dr. Salem got a call from a panicked staff member at the VA hospital. Five minutes later, he heard from a doctor, who, recognizing

Swango, was shocked by the disclosures. Salem rushed to his office
to review all the files on Swango, trying to determine if he had falsified anything or distorted his record. By e-mail, he revoked
Swango's pharmacy privileges and suspended his residency. Just
after midnight, he returned home and watched a tape of the *Justice
Files* episode. For the first time, he realized that the conviction in
Quincy of his fellow physician had been no miscarriage of justice.

On Tuesday morning, the Sioux Falls *Argus Leader* was emblazoned with the headline "Medical Resident Suspended": "A first-
year resident practicing medicine at three Sioux Falls hospitals was
convicted of poisoning six co-workers in Illinois and spent $2\frac{1}{2}$
years in jail," the newspaper reported. "Swango is also suspected in
the death of at least one patient at an Ohio hospital."

Swango's coworkers were suddenly reluctant to talk to the
paper. "There's a concern knowing that he has poisoned six of his
co-workers in the past," one unidentified resident told the *Argus
Leader.* "You don't know what he's capable of doing. He seems like
a very nice person, but the thing that's always worried us is he
couldn't look us straight in the eye. A lot of times that made us concerned that maybe he was dealing with some problems of his own."

At nine A.M., Salem called Swango to tell him not to show up
for work at the hospital, and to set up a meeting with him at two
P.M. Swango asked to bring his fiancée. Meanwhile, Salem notified
the medical school's board members, and the hospitals launched a review of the files of all patients whom Swango had treated.

When Swango arrived for the meeting, accompanied by
Kristin, he was neatly dressed in a jacket and tie. He seemed puzzled by all the controversy and eager to clear things up. Rather than
summarize the *Justice Files* story, Salem put the tape in his VCR and
had Swango and Kinney watch it in its entirety. Then he asked for
an explanation. Kinney had turned ashen and said nothing. It was
obvious to Salem that she had not seen the program, and knew little
of the history it presented. Under the circumstances, Swango remained remarkably calm and poised. He still seemed puzzled. He
had no idea he had been investigated at Ohio State, he insisted. And
he continued to maintain that the poisoning conviction was a miscarriage of justice fueled by disgruntled coworkers, some of whom
appeared on the program. Salem thought it was at least possible that

Swango didn't know about the investigation at Ohio State. But everything else he said seemed to be flatly contradicted by the show. Salem said Swango's suspension would remain in effect.

Salem didn't report Swango's suspension to the national data bank created by the Wyden legislation. Presumably, because Swango was a medical resident, not licensed anywhere to practice medicine, he wasn't a "physician" within the law's definition, and the reporting requirement did not apply—a glaring loophole in the law.

The next day, the university sent Swango a certified letter giving him until four P.M. Friday, December 4, to submit his resignation. If he failed to do so, the letter said he would be dismissed.

ONE of Kristin's friends in the ICU, Linda Wipf, was in a patient's room with the TV on when she heard the announcer say, "Coming up, a local doctor accused of poisoning." Wipf wondered who that could be. South Dakota had experienced the odd case of a physician charged with using drugs, but nothing like this. When the news resumed she looked up and saw Swango's face. "That can't be," she thought. "It's got to be a mistake."

She hurried back to the nurses' station. Everyone was talking about the news. Kristin hadn't come in that day, but that afternoon, after the meeting with Salem, she called in tears, saying that Michael had been suspended. Through her sobs, it was hard to get a coherent story, but she indicated that although she knew he had been in prison in Illinois—either for a bar brawl or after being framed in the poison case—she'd known nothing about the allegations at Ohio State. Lisa Flinn dispatched another nurse to be with Kristin, so she wouldn't be alone and would have someone to talk to.

Later Kristin spoke to Flinn; she said she trusted her own judgment about Swango, no matter what the media said. Swango was a "good person"; he "really cares about people"; he really liked to practice medicine; and "he would never do anything to hurt another human being, not the Mike I know," she insisted. Flinn asked whether she wasn't afraid to be around Swango, given the nature of the charges. No, she said, she was angry and upset, but not at Swango. She felt the media were defaming his character and ruining his career. "There is no one who is more caring than Mike," she said.

•   •

IN Virginia that evening, Sharon Cooper was taking a bath when she heard the phone ring. Al answered it. She was still toweling off when he came into the bathroom and said, "You'd better sit down."

"What?" she asked, alarmed by his tone.

Al Cooper explained that he'd just spoken with Swango in South Dakota. "Michael just told me about this incident from his past," he said. "It's all over the news there in South Dakota that he poisoned people."

Sharon felt sick, faint, as if she might pass out.

"It's okay," Al said, trying to reassure her. "Michael says it's all a media hoax."

"Where's Kristin?" Sharon demanded. She had an impulse to jump in the car and go get her daughter.

"She's fine, she's okay." Al went on: Michael had explained that he'd been in prison, but hadn't poisoned anyone. He'd pleaded guilty to battery because he'd been "led astray" by his lawyer, who said that if he did plead, he wouldn't be given any prison time. But then a harsh judge had sent him to prison anyway.

Al hadn't asked Michael what he had pleaded guilty to. He was skeptical of the story, but he didn't want to arouse Kristin's doubts, for fear that to do so might put her in jeopardy. Nor did he want Sharon to panic. At least they finally knew what accounted for the missing years in Michael's résumé, the ones he'd said weren't important. They couldn't believe that Kristin had known the truth, or she wouldn't have considered dating him.

But now it was too late. Sharon immediately got on the phone to Kristin. "Mom, everything's okay," Kristin insisted. "Michael assures me this is just a media hoax"—the same words Michael had used with Al. When Sharon asked Kristin to come home to Virginia, she refused. She told them she loved Michael and that she needed to support him while he fought his suspension.

Though he was worried about Swango, Al admired her fortitude. "I commend you for standing by your man," he told her. Sharon, too, once she realized Kristin was determined to stay with Michael, tried to be supportive. "I know this is rough," she said to her daughter. "But remember, God doesn't send you more than you can handle."

Then Michael spoke. It wasn't clear whether he'd been listen-

ing all along on an extension. "This will all blow over," he assured
the Coopers. "This is just a temporary setback."

THE discovery of a convicted poisoner in their midst naturally
caused an uproar at the University of South Dakota and in the hospitals where he had worked. South Dakota governor George Mickelson said he was "incredulous" that such a thing could have
happened: "I think the public is going to have an extremely difficult
time understanding this, and I don't blame them."

Hospital officials rushed to reassure the public. On December 3,
only two days after the news broke, the three Sioux Falls hospitals where Swango had worked issued statements that a review of
patient files had uncovered no mysterious deaths or other irregular-
ities that could be linked to Swango. Sioux Valley Hospital had reviewed fifty patient files; the VA had reviewed 129; McKennan
simply issued a statement saying it had found "no problems." But
no statistics appear to have been compiled to determine whether
during Swango's tenure the number of deaths or codes at any of the
hospitals exceeded the norm.

The South Dakota board of regents convened on December 10
and 11 to consider a report by the medical school on how Swango
had been hired and what steps needed to be taken to prevent such a
thing from happening again. Dr. Talley said bluntly that the admission process was "shallow and failed." He said doctors at the medical school had "trusted their personal evaluations" and let them
override the felony conviction, yet he hoped doctors there "would
continue to judge people on an individual basis."

The medical school's own report to the regents found it difficult to assign any individual blame for Swango's admission. It noted
that "all sources are unanimous in their assessment of Swango as an
open, enthusiastic, good-natured person. He appeared to be trust-
worthy."

Nor did it fault Dr. Salem, whom it praised for being "open and
empathetic"—but though these qualities tend to be valued in South
Dakota, where people often say they are more trusting than residents of many more-urban states, they are the very qualities that
had enabled Swango to slip past the admissions process. Although
Dean Talley offered to assume full responsibility for the affair, the

report noted that he was never consulted or involved in the hiring of residents, nor would he be in routine residency matters.

Still, the report noted that the admission of an admitted felon was not routine, and implied that the dean and legal counsel should have been consulted, which might have led to questioning the Illinois authorities and to doubts about Swango's eligibility to be admitted to practice medicine in South Dakota. And although Dr. Vogt had summarized the family practice group's rejection of Swango, the report also faulted those doctors for not "sharing" their information with the internal medicine committee. It further faulted national organizations for not maintaining any "medical clearing house" concerning criminal charges against physicians. The report's writers appear to be unfamiliar with the Wyden legislation or the national data bank.

Although one of the regents denounced the university's decision on Swango as "shocking" and another characterized it as a "drastic mistake," the regents recommended only that admissions procedures be reviewed and detailed guidelines prepared. Neither Talley nor Salem was blamed. On the contrary, the regents said that Talley shouldn't let "this one blemish" lessen his "eagerness to serve the people of the State of South Dakota."

By the comparatively tame standards of Sioux Falls, the Swango story triggered a media frenzy. Television crews camped on Swango and Kinney's small lawn, aiming bright lights at the house during the night. Kristin was afraid to turn on a light in the house, for the instant she did, indicating someone was home, reporters would start banging on the front door. She and Swango checked into a local hotel for a few days to escape the attention. But wherever Swango went, camera crews dogged him.

The Swango story dominated local call-in radio shows, and even inspired Swango-themed doggerel. In mid-December, KXRB disc jockey Dan Christopherson sang his own lyrics to the tune of "Rudolph the Red-Nosed Reindeer":

> *Swango the troubled doctor*
> *USD says out he goes*
> *And if you saw his rap sheet*
> *All of us would say "Oh, No!"*

> *All of the administrators*
> *Prefer their patients not be maimed*
> *They won't let Michael Swango*
> *Play any more doctor games.*

Finally Swango broke his silence. He compiled a handwritten list of all the local reporters on the story and began calling them to issue a prepared statement. The *Argus Leader* headlined its December 7 edition with "Swango: 'I'm a Good Doctor.' " Swango stressed that he had been open and honest with university officials at the time he applied. "I was fully open concerning my conviction eight years ago," he said in the prepared statement. "If the university wishes to change their requirements so that that cannot occur again, so be it. But I was accepted into this program after full disclosure, with every intention of completing a successful residency." He pleaded with the public to let him bury his past. No one should "crawl into a hole and waste away . . . my conviction was eight years ago. Let it rest.

"I truly regret all of the problems and all of the difficulties that this has caused everybody, certainly most of all myself, but obviously everyone in a medical community is affected by something like this. And I will say that no one in this town has any reason to hang their head at all, because of the decision or because of my performance."

In an appearance on radio station KSOO, he added, "I know of course that I'm innocent, but whether I could convince everybody of that is certainly— I don't know that. But I truly believe that the people who have known me in Sioux Falls, who know what I think of this community and especially the medical community, and have worked with me, and have helped me treat patients and care for patients, I think they know that I'm a good doctor and I'm a good person."

Swango also hired a local lawyer, Dennis McFarland, to challenge his dismissal from the residency program. McFarland represented him at formal suspension hearings in December, to no avail. A review committee upheld the dismissal on the grounds that Swango had withheld information and distorted the facts of his conviction when he applied for a residency. At McFarland's recommendation, Swango called Vern Cook, an administrator at the VA hospital who coordinated doctors' orders and prescriptions in the cancer ward, one floor below the ICU where Kinney worked. Among his other duties, Cook was president of the hospital's union, the American Federation of Government Employees, and McFarland had suggested that Swango challenge his suspension on the theory that he was a federal employee by virtue of his work at the VA hospital, and thus entitled to federal employment protections. "Do you know who I am?" Swango asked Cook on the phone, and asked if he could come for a visit.

Of course Cook knew Swango, given all the recent publicity. He had already noticed him among that year's group of residents. He admired the fact that Swango worked incredibly long hours, often staying at the hospital late into the night, long after his shift had ended. Cook, too, worked long hours. And Cook had noticed that Swango always took three or four of the pumpkin bars with cream cheese frosting that Cook's wife made and he brought to the hospital two or three times a week, almost as if he were hoarding them. Cook also knew Kinney from the hospital; he was crazy about her. He often thought that if he had another sister, he'd want her to be just like K.K.

Swango met with Cook three times before Cook agreed to represent him. He seemed relieved that Cook didn't press him for details about his past. Cook never asked whether he was guilty of the poisoning charges or had harmed anyone at Ohio State. Cook didn't want to know. Swango certainly didn't seem like the kind of person who would poison someone, but Cook's primary concern was simply that the VA had treated him unfairly, whatever had happened in his past. He agreed to take Swango's case, and they were soon poring over the case law and having long strategy meetings at Cook's house, often attended by Kinney.

Cook and Swango became close friends. Cook was a Vietnam War veteran, a former Green Beret who had participated in the CIA-led Phoenix Program while Swango's father was in Vietnam. He also had a reputation, mostly from his union work, for being resentful of authority. Cook was impressed by the breadth and depth of Swango's intellect, his seeming ability to speak knowledgeably about nearly any topic. The only person he'd met who was remotely like Swango was a captain in Vietnam, who had gotten Cook to read and discuss the philosopher Bertrand Russell.

Swango was fascinated with Cook's experiences in Vietnam, often comparing them with what he knew from his father. Swango told Cook his father had worked in the CIA, but Cook couldn't remember meeting him. Swango wanted to know all about the secret operations, intelligence work, special operations. He was especially interested in what Cook felt when he killed someone, asking him about it repeatedly. Cook thought it was impossible to convey the experience in words, but he tried. He hadn't loved killing people, but he had loved the war. He felt he was skilled at what he did. His whole life had been the Army and the Green Berets, and even his family was sometimes forgotten.

Swango seemed to identify with Cook's experiences, often saying how he had missed his father growing up, and how Virgil had shown little interest in the family he'd left behind in America. He said he couldn't understand why his father had never explained his absences in terms Michael could understand. Cook thought Michael felt equal parts admiration and bitterness toward his father. He said almost nothing about Muriel. He never mentioned having any brothers.

Gradually, Swango opened up to Cook in a way he hadn't with others in South Dakota. He talked of his fascination with disasters, occasionally sending Cook some of his newspaper clippings. Sometimes Swango couldn't resist following sirens to the scene of a fire or accident in Sioux Falls. He seemed fascinated with serial killers Ted Bundy, a former law student who allegedly killed nineteen women, culminating in the murders of two Chi Omega sorority women at the University of Florida in 1978, and John Wayne Gacy, arrested in 1978, a building contractor who volunteered as a clown and killed an estimated thirty-three young boys. Swango was riveted by a television special on serial killers. Cook didn't make much of these interests, since Swango had so many. Nor did he know that Swango had ever been linked to any suspicious deaths.

Swango's and Cook's conversations often lasted until four or five in the morning, occasionally all night. Cook's wife would be getting up for work and he and Swango would still be talking at the dining table, legal papers and notebooks spread out before them.

Cook was struck by how restless Swango often was. His mind
would leap from topic to topic. One thing they did not discuss was
Swango's medical career. Cook didn't want to hear about it, and
Swango seemed all too willing to ignore it.

At the ICU, everyone tried to rally in support of Kristin. The
charges against her fiancé had sown considerable confusion among
the nursing staff, especially since the hospital itself never made any
attempt to explain what had happened. (It did make a staff psychiatrist available for anyone who wanted to talk about their reactions.)
But the nurses took their cue from Kinney, who was adamant that
Swango had been framed and now was being persecuted. No one
could believe the way the media were hounding her and Swango;
every time he appeared in public, it seemed, he'd be shown on television trying to flee the cameras. Though Kinney's spirits weren't as
high as they had been before the news broke, she seemed to be re-
acting well, carrying out her duties as before and still displaying her
quick wit and sense of humor. She even joked about the media and
their tactics. She changed to the night shift, which offered a 25 percent pay raise, and worked weekends in order to help support
Swango now that he wasn't working and was incurring legal costs.

But privately, even some of Kinney's closest friends were becoming concerned about Swango. Stories of odd behavior were beginning to circulate. One of his fellow residents was in the hospital
as a patient, and she awoke in the middle of the night to find
Swango sitting at her bedside, watching her. She was overweight,
and she hadn't liked the way other residents had teased her. But
now something about his gaze frightened her. She would no doubt
have been even more alarmed if she knew about one of Swango's
bizarre comments in Quincy: he'd said that he hated fat people, and
had fantasized about slicing them with razor blades attached to the
tips of his shoes.

Even more worrisome for Kinney's friends were reports that
Swango began dating another nurse at Sioux Valley soon after moving to Sioux Falls. Swango had apparently given her the phone number of a 7-Eleven convenience store where she could leave messages
for him. Residents at Sioux Valley reported to nurses at the VA that
they overheard Swango calling Kinney to say that he was tied up
with an emergency and couldn't be home until late, or had to cancel

plans. They knew those claims weren't true, that there was no emergency. Then there came reports that a nurse at Sioux Valley thought she was being stalked by Swango, and might even file charges. Talk of the stalking was so rife that Linda Wipf decided Kristin had to be told. Kristin rejected the notion out of hand. She burst into tears and said, "Oh, what else are they going to dig up on him?"

No one else said anything about these things to Kinney. They wanted to protect her, even as they worried that Swango might not be the person she so fervently seemed to believe he was.

But as the weeks went by and nothing further developed, a sense of normalcy returned. The press attention tapered off. When the ICU nurses planned their annual potluck Christmas dinner, the possibility that Kinney and Swango wouldn't be invited—or that Kinney would be invited but Swango wouldn't—never even occurred to anyone. On the contrary, the other nurses encouraged Kinney and Swango to come, saying they needed to get out of the house.

Still, the party had a slightly surreal quality. The nurse at whose home it was held was married to a police detective, who insisted on following Swango from room to room to make sure he didn't try to poison the food. At the same time, people were fascinated by Swango. Some guests who were on their way out when they saw Swango arrive returned and stayed for hours. He was the center of attention, seemingly eager to discuss the charges and his efforts to vindicate himself. He insisted he wanted to get back into the South Dakota residency program and, with help from his lawyer, thought he would succeed. If not, he'd practice medicine somewhere else. He was too good a doctor not to be practicing somewhere, he said.

Kristin and Michael had come to the party after attending a performance of Handel's *Messiah.* Everyone else had dressed casually, but Swango wore a black jacket and tie, and Kinney wore a long black evening gown. They made an elegant couple. People thought Kristin had never looked more beautiful. She had told a fellow nurse that her difficult childhood had made her a stronger person. Perhaps, the nurse thought, she was right.

IN early January, after the holidays, Al Cooper got a phone call from Kristin. He knew immediately that something was wrong.

Her voice was wavering, and she seemed near tears. "I found something in the back of a picture," she said.

"What?" Cooper asked.

She explained that she'd been cleaning around a framed copy of Michael's medical diploma when something fell out from behind the backing in the frame. "It's a recipe card," Kristin said, taking a deep breath. "It looks like there are poisons on it."

Al Cooper felt a stab of fear. "My God, are you all right?" he asked.

But Kristin seemed to have collected herself. "I'm okay," she said. "I'll ask Mike about it when he comes home."

The Coopers heard nothing the next day, so Al called his stepdaughter. "Kristin, I'm coming to get you," he said.

"No, no," she insisted. Michael had explained that the card had belonged to his father. She didn't say anything more, but Al's mind was racing with questions, even though he and Sharon still didn't know that Michael had been convicted of poisoning people. What was the card doing in the frame? Why would Michael save such a thing? What would his father have been doing with a recipe for poisons? But Kristin seemed withdrawn, unwilling to talk. He wondered if Swango was listening to the conversation. The Coopers and many of Kristin's friends had noticed recently that when they called, Swango always answered the phone, never Kristin.

Despite her assurances to her parents, Kristin's friends at work became concerned. Kristin had stopped laughing and joking. She had become withdrawn and seemed depressed. When Lisa Flinn asked her what the matter was, she said nothing, but then finally said, "I found something." She wouldn't tell Lisa what it was, but she said she now thought it possible that Swango was guilty. At about the same time, she confided her doubts about Swango's innocence to another nurse, Eric Barnes. And one evening she just showed up at Vern Cook's, without Swango. She sat down on the couch and curled up next to him, as his sister had done when she was a child. She cried and cried, and told him that she wasn't sure she could trust Michael. She said she couldn't believe how little she really knew him, even though he was her fiancé and they had been living together for over six months.

Whenever she confided any of her own concerns to Michael—such as when she asked for an explanation for the poison recipes—

he reacted angrily, even threatening to leave her. Every day, it seemed, she learned new facts that needed different and convoluted explanations. Compounding her emotional woes, her health deteriorated. She confided in Lisa Flinn and others at work that she had begun to experience severe headaches and nausea. They attributed her symptoms to the stress she was living under.

Then, on January 13, Kristin became violently ill in the lobby of a local clinic. She experienced intense nausea, headache, and disorientation, and she passed out when she got home. These are the classic symptoms of arsenic poisoning.

Though Kristin never expressed any suspicion that she was being poisoned, she was feeling increasingly desperate, and as if she had nowhere to turn. She began confiding her thoughts to a written journal. The first entry is dated January 14, 1993:

> I don't know where to begin. I don't know how to help myself. I don't know who to talk to. I can say only so much to Michael before the pain is too much for him. Anyone else in my life is too far away, and it gets too tiresome to try to explain and make someone else understand when I struggle to figure it out myself. I know I'm tired. Michael at times must be exhausted trying to make lawyers, the schools, the press, and the public understand. To look at the volume of papers on my kitchen table and listen to the twists and turns it seems impossible to make any sense out of this. Every day there are new "wartime strategies" to listen to and critique. Michael explains new things to bring up in the appeal and I don't get it. He becomes angry. Maybe my headache has fried my brain. Every day there are new developments and I sit and listen to him rehearse how he will present it. Will it work? I don't know.
>
> I hope writing this will help. Maybe I won't get any more migraines. I still feel numb and drugged from this one. It has been the worst ever and I can't stand many more.
>
> I was in the lobby of Central Plains clinic. I felt the color leave my face and sweat begin. I got tears in my eyes. I began wandering to find a restroom. I was dry heaving and my vision was getting blurry. I was hanging on to the staircase railing and latched on to some woman and pleaded with her to help me. I was vomiting in the bathroom. I kept thinking, I feel like a horse who broke their

legs in great pain and no way for it to heal and someone will come soon and shoot me and it will be all better.

Michael was angry the whole day, I think because I am weak and can't control these headaches. He got me home. I passed out and he was gone. . . .

When things were overwhelming at home when I lived with my father, I would get in trouble so I could spend time in school suspension. It was quiet there. No yelling. No nothing. No one talked to you and you couldn't say a word. I loved it. Time out. You didn't have to deal with anyone or anything—for a few hours, anyway. I can't find anything like that now.

I don't want to find another job. I just want to be left alone. But one must not be weak and I have to get us through this financially.

Michael's anger toward Kristin often seemed to trigger memories of abuse at the hands of her father. In certain passages, references to Michael's displeasure are intertwined with explicit accounts of physical abuse she experienced as a teenager. After one such passage, Kristin wrote of her conflicting feelings toward her father: "So full of love—but a desolate, empty feeling."

In entries dated January 15 and 19, 1993, she continued to complain of depression. "I feel I don't belong anywhere," she wrote. "It's a constant empty feeling that mysteriously and wonderfully disappears when I'm taking care of someone ill. I hear over and over from my patients, 'You're always so happy.' 'I love when you take care of me.' Why can't I feel okay at other times?" Another entry describes a memory of going into her father's closet, reaching for his gun, and pointing it at her head, but being unable to pull the trigger. "During the episode this morning I still wished I had done it. Why do I feel so strong sometimes—most of the time—and it seems instantly I'm beyond the point of [no] return?"

On January 22, Kristin wrote of her admiration for actress Audrey Hepburn, who had become an ambassador for UNICEF. "I would also love to be helping—maybe I will soon," she wrote. But then she returned to her plight:

Michael hates the weekends and I worry about him while I'm at work. He says he feels like things aren't happening . . . it's two days where he knows he wouldn't possibly hear any news about getting out of here. This place was once an area of opportunity. Now—well, you can imagine how it feels now. Not so nearly the same as jail, but a reminder, I'm sure. He wants out, but can't right now. I don't know how I feel about being here. I want out—to go to another country—but at the same time I feel paralyzed.

Vern Cook sensed during this period that something had come between Michael and Kristin, though neither was specific about what it was. Kristin began seeing a marriage counselor in Sioux Falls, Carol Carlson, who insisted that Michael also attend the sessions. Kristin mentioned trouble in the couple's relationship in a journal entry dated January 28:

> It's been two long months since all of this began. I can feel Michael growing more anxious to move on. We haven't heard when the date for the appeal is. He continues to write to organizations and send resumes and such but hasn't heard anything yet. I admire his perseverance. I am very nervous about our future. Sometimes I feel like I'm pulling away from him. He keeps repeating how he could be leaving me. I feel like I'm waiting for another bomb to go off. In a way I wish it would hurry up and happen but I don't know how I'll deal with it.

February was a difficult month, part of what Kristin described as "the longest and coldest winter in my life. –14 degrees tonight. Colder in more ways than one." Her migraines and nausea continued. One afternoon she called her friend Lynette Mueller, who was a nurse on duty at the ICU, asking if she could leave work and meet her somewhere. Mueller was worried about Kristin, so she asked the head nurse for permission to leave, and went to Champs, a local sports bar. Kristin was sitting in a corner wearing dark glasses, and said she was afraid of being recognized. She seemed terribly unhappy. "I need out," she told Mueller, asking if she might stay with her and her husband at some point. Kristin said Michael was talking about finding a job as a doctor in a foreign country to escape all the controversy. Kristin said she'd like to do some missionary work, to help people. She was thinking of going with him, but felt she needed some time away from him to think. Mueller thought Kristin was torn by indecision, uncertain whether she was really in love.

Kristin spent the weekend of February 27 alone. Michael had driven to West Virginia, for unspecified reasons. She wrote in her journal, half-seriously, that she was grateful for that day's World Trade Center bombing because it diverted Michael and "gives [him] something to do."

That Friday evening she watched the tabloid television program *A Current Affair*, which did an episode on Swango's poisoning people in Quincy. She seemed to take the program in stride. "It was mostly on his past and very little of the present situation," she wrote. "Michael didn't see it." But then, later the same evening, she wrote that "I found some things (papers) that disturbed me and I panicked. My mind was racing so fast."

Kristin began taking pills to calm down—possibly the antidepressant Prozac, which she was taking—and called Carlson, the marriage counselor. Talking helped, but the next day she was trembling with weakness and anxiety, and called in sick. Saturday evening she drank a few gin and tonics to calm herself. She remembered nothing more.

The Coopers had been calling Kristin all day, but there was no answer. Alarmed, Sharon Cooper had called Lisa Flinn at the hospital, asking if she knew where Kristin was. She didn't. Kristin hadn't shown up to work the weekend shift. The Coopers were distraught.

Late Saturday night, the Sioux Falls police picked up a young woman walking naked on East Fifth Street. At the time the temperature was three degrees. It was Kristin Kinney. She was admitted for observation to Charter Hospital, a psychiatric facility, where she awoke Sunday morning. She was released on Tuesday.

Kinney wrote in her journal the next day, Wednesday, that "everyone should do a stint in a psychiatric hospital just to walk on the other side. I met some interesting people. I couldn't talk about the situation for fear it would end in the papers. I was numb. I couldn't think. I just sat at my window most of the time and watched six inches of snow fall, looking for an answer. I didn't find one."

Whatever Kristin had found in Swango's documents that so upset her, and that she felt she couldn't talk about in the psychiatric facility, she was determined not to allow her doubts to undermine her devotion. Perhaps, as with her father, she couldn't reconcile her love for Michael with her growing doubts and the evidence of his cruelty. "I got out Tuesday morning," she wrote. "Michael came to get me. He's so good to me. God, this past three months have been hell. But I love him so much. I don't know what will happen or where we'll end up, but I know that I love him."

When Kristin returned to work, she told Lisa Flinn that she needed to talk to her in private, so they went to the small room the nurses used for their breaks. "I need to know," she began, somewhat haltingly, "I need to ask, if I ever need a place to come to or go to, whatever time, day or night, can I call you?"

"Of course," Flinn replied. "You know that you can." Then she asked, "Are you feeling like it's not safe anymore where you are?"

"No," Kristin replied. But she said she'd been experiencing some "strange things," and told Lisa that she'd been found by police that weekend walking around in the cold without a coat. She suggested to Lisa that the incident might have been triggered by smoking too much, though she had no memory of smoking that day. The notion might have been suggested by a diagnosis at Charter of possible nicotine poisoning. Besides being the primary addictive ingredient in cigarettes, nicotine is also a potent poison; in high doses, it can cause paralysis, coma, and death. Symptoms of nicotine poisoning include confusion, muscular twitching, weakness, and depression, all of which Kristin had experienced. But Lisa found this explanation puzzling, since Kristin hardly ever smoked, and couldn't have had much more than a pack of cigarettes even if she had chain-smoked that Saturday. And despite Kristin's denial, Lisa was convinced that she was feeling so threatened and unsafe around Michael that she was having bizarre, even delusional experiences.

Neither Kristin, nor Lisa, nor anyone at Charter knew that nicotine had been among the poisons discovered in the search of Swango's apartment in Quincy.

ON March 21, Al Cooper was taking a routine treadmill stress test during a physical exam when he collapsed from a heart attack. He was rushed to the hospital for multiple bypass surgery. The emergency seemed to energize Kristin, giving her something to focus on other than Michael's troubles in South Dakota. She called her mother to say she'd fly back immediately to be with Al, and something in her voice told Sharon that she was desperate to get away from South Dakota. A nurse herself, Sharon knew she'd need Kristin's help more once Al was back from the hospital, but Kristin insisted on coming immediately for the surgery. She also asked to pay for her ticket with a credit card Sharon had given her for emergencies. Her mother said of course. She knew Kristin had to be short of cash, for she had never used the credit card before.

When Kristin arrived in Virginia, her mother was shocked by the change in her appearance. She had lost weight. She seemed exhausted. She complained of headaches and nausea. She was using a nasal inhaler to take Stadol, a prescription painkiller. She looked at her mother with tears in her eyes and said, "Why have I gone through so much in the short time I've lived?"

All Sharon could say was "I don't know." But, she added, "Remember, I'm here if you need me."

Sharon also reminded her daughter that if things got too bad, she could seek professional counseling. "Promise me you will," she insisted, and Kristin agreed.

Al's surgery was successful, though he remained in the hospital for several weeks of recovery. Kristin spent hours with him, cheering him up and telling him how much she loved him. The Coopers couldn't tell whether the cause was being away from Michael, or helping her mother care for her stepfather and feeling needed, but Kristin seemed to regain her bearings and good humor. Her aunt offered to rent her an apartment she owned in Portsmouth if she moved back, and Kristin said she'd consider it. The Coopers didn't want to put any pressure on her, but they were desperate to get her out of South Dakota and away from Michael Swango.

One day Kristin turned to her mother and said, "I have something to tell you. Promise you won't tell anyone." When Sharon agreed, Kristin said that when she went to Michael's apartment the first time, she was shocked to discover that he was living in the bathroom. He had a mattress on the bathroom floor, a TV, a few clothes, a frying pan, and a fork. That was it. His underwear was so worn and dirty that Kristin immediately took him shopping for some new clothing.

Sharon was shocked. "Didn't that scare you a little?"

"Yeah," Kristin replied, "but if you knew everything. . . ."

"Like what?"

"I'll tell you sometime," Kristin said.

WHEN Kristin returned to South Dakota in late March, she had made up her mind to leave. "I'm feeling more ready to get out of here and strong enough to do it," she wrote in her journal. She gave notice at the hospital and told her friends she was returning to Virginia. Some of them worried that she wouldn't have a support group to turn to in a new location. "I need to know that you're going to be safe," Lisa Flinn told her. But Kristin assured her she'd be close to her parents.

Her friends at work noticed that she had stopped wearing her engagement ring. When Lisa asked her about that, Kristin said only, "I just can't right now," and didn't elaborate. But she made it clear that Michael would not be following her to Virginia, and that she would spend some time away from him. Even though that year's March Day had come and gone, and Michael hadn't landed a new residency, Kristin hinted that he had new job prospects and would be moving somewhere else. When Michael left for several days of job interviews, Kristin was secretive about the trip, telling Lisa "I'm not going to tell you where." Lisa thought Kristin was afraid to say anything.

Kristin wrote in her diary, "I won't miss Sioux Falls"—a place she described as a "black cold hole of depression"—but "I will miss a lot of the people I work with." A couple of days before she left, her friends held a going-away party for her at Chi-Chi's, the Mexican restaurant. Michael came, along with six or so people from the hospital. Everybody drank margaritas, and both Kristin and Michael seemed in good spirits. But when Linda Wipf got out her camera and started taking snapshots, Michael leaped in front of her. "Who's gonna see this?" he demanded. "I just want it for my photo album," she assured him.

On April 9, Kristin packed her belongings in her pickup and left for Virginia.

SWANGO had planned to stay in Sioux Falls to pursue the appeal of his dismissal. The Waco massacre on April 19, 1993, when federal

agents stormed and set fire to the Branch Davidian complex, diverted his attention; he was glued to CNN with Vern Cook. Then
job possibilities elsewhere seemed to be opening up. Swango told
Cook that he was looking into two possible medical residencies,
one in psychiatry and the other in pediatrics. Cook wasn't so sure it
was a good idea for Michael to pursue a position as a physician. He
thought it too likely that what had happened in South Dakota
would recur once the local media learned of his past. But if Swango
was determined to remain a doctor, Cook stressed two things: "Use
your own name" and "Don't take a job in pediatrics."

"Can you imagine if something happened to a child? They'd
crucify you," Cook warned him. Michael was upset at the suggestion, saying he "loved" children.

Less than two weeks after Kristin's departure, Swango came to
tell Cook good-bye. He said he'd packed his things and was ready
to leave. Cook didn't know where Michael was going and didn't
want to. If law enforcement authorities questioned him, Cook
didn't want to have to betray Swango's whereabouts.

Michael told Vern that he'd always admired Vern's writing tal-
ent. The two had worked so well together that Michael vowed to see
him again. "We are going to get together and we are going to write a
book," he told him emphatically. "Perhaps a novel."

Swango hugged Cook and went out to his truck. But then he
came back and hugged him again. He left and came back a second
time. Swango had tears in his eyes. "I wish you were my father," he
told Cook, and then he left for good.

CHAPTER NINE

THE COOPERS were delighted by Kristin's return to Virginia. She looked better the minute she arrived, bounding out of her truck, wearing shorts and a fanny pack. "Isn't this silly?" she said. "Anyone could see I was carrying a gun." Her nine-millimeter pistol was plainly outlined in the small pack. The Coopers thought she had to have been frightened, to be carrying the gun.

Sharon noticed immediately that Kristin wasn't wearing the engagement ring, and asked her about it. "That's on hold for a while, I guess," Kristin replied, but didn't elaborate. Sharon was relieved.

Kristin moved into her aunt's apartment in Portsmouth. She immediately resumed work as an ICU nurse at Riverside Hospital, where she was rehired by an old friend. She volunteered at a homeless shelter in inner-city Norfolk, where she befriended a young woman with a new baby, showing her how to care for the child and taking her shopping. She also spent more time with her stepfather, now well on his way to recovering from his heart surgery, and with Sharon, who enjoyed hikes with her daughter in Mariners' Museum Park. She stopped complaining about the headaches. It was almost as though the horrifying experience in South Dakota had never happened.

Suddenly, all that changed. On April 22, Swango showed up in Virginia and moved in with Kristin. They came over to see the Coopers the next day. Al was out, and Sharon greeted him at the front door. Swango looked as if he'd gained some weight, which surprised Sharon, since he'd always been so determinedly trim and fit. "You look like you've put on a few pounds," she said.

Swango nearly went berserk, ranting and pacing rapidly back and forth in the living room. "I don't know why you say these things about me!" he shouted, proceeding to denounce her treatment of him. Sharon sat in stunned silence until he calmed down. When he stepped briefly out of the room, she turned to Kristin. "What's wrong?" she asked. But Kristin looked petrified. "Just be quiet," she said.

When Swango returned, Sharon tried to make conversation. "What are you going to do?" she asked.

"I want to get everything back on track with Kristin," he said. It was the last thing Sharon wanted to hear.

After Swango's return, the Coopers rarely saw or heard from Kristin. It was almost as though she were back in South Dakota.

DR. Alan Miller, director of the psychiatric residency program at the State University of New York at Stony Brook, on Long Island, sifted through the many completed applications for the program the school had received during the spring of 1993. SUNY–Stony Brook was one of the medical schools that hadn't filled its quota on Match Day that year, a situation that triggered an onslaught of résumés from medical school graduates who had similarly failed to connect with their favored choices. A distinguished psychiatrist, the former state commissioner of mental hygiene under New York governor Nelson Rockefeller, Dr. Miller had stepped in for what he thought would be a temporary stint as part-time director, after his predecessor resigned. He was somewhat dismayed, though not surprised, by the quality of the applicants.

At most medical schools, psychiatric residencies were becoming increasingly hard to fill. With many insurance companies limiting coverage for psychiatric care, and with an increased effort to control medical costs, psychiatrists' job opportunities and incomes had shrunk. Fewer medical school graduates were choosing psychiatry as a specialty, and applications had dwindled, even at SUNY–Stony Brook, launched in 1972 as the crown jewel of New York State's system of publicly funded medical schools.

The medical school rises like a modernist slab from the fields of rural Long Island; with a lavish budget, it initially attracted many top specialists. But many of SUNY–Stony Brook's psychiatric residency applicants now were foreign, mostly graduates of Indian and other Asian institutions. He suspected many were simply using psychiatry as a way of getting into the United States to practice medicine.

Then an application caught Miller's eye: a graduate of an American medical school, with an excellent transcript, who had also been a Marine Corps sergeant. He pulled the application from the pile and made a note of the name: Michael Swango. Out of that year's 190 applicants, he easily ranked among the candidates invited to the campus for interviews.

Swango arrived in New York on April 27 for an interview with Miller; the chairman of the department of psychiatry, Fritz Henn; and another professor. Swango was good-looking, charming, and articulate. Dr. Miller was immediately impressed. The conversation had hardly begun, however, when Swango made a startling disclosure. Looking at the three doctors earnestly, he said, "I have to tell you, I've served time in jail. I want you to know that."

Miller was taken aback. So this was why such an attractive candidate had failed to gain a match. "What was all that about?" he asked, curious to know more.

Swango explained that he'd been convicted of battery in Illinois after a barroom brawl got out of hand. He said he hadn't meant to injure anyone, but that, having been a Marine, he sometimes forgot his own strength. He quickly produced the restoration of civil rights signed by the governor of Virginia, which he said was the equivalent of a pardon. (While Virginia had restored Swango's right to vote and hold office in Virginia, it did not pardon him—it could not have pardoned him—for a crime committed in Illinois.) Dr. Miller found his statement disarming; it seemed so candid.

Before he left, Swango gave Miller three references. After making one or two calls, Dr. Miller was satisfied; he assumed the admissions staff would pursue the usual inquiries.* SUNY–Stony Brook

---

* Dr. Miller concedes that he did not check all three references. He said the one or two people he reached spoke highly of Swango and confirmed that he had gotten a bad rap in Illinois. One of these people may have been Robert Haller II, the National Emergency Service VP who'd testified at Swango's sentencing hearing and

did confirm that Swango had graduated from SIU and had satisfactorily completed a year's internship at Ohio State. None of the
SUNY correspondence triggered any mention of Swango's now notorious history; even the SIU dean's letter that mentioned his failure to graduate on time had now fallen by the wayside. Unlike
administrators at South Dakota, SUNY officials didn't contact the
Federation of State Medical Boards, so they weren't aware that
Swango's licenses had been suspended in Ohio and Illinois. As in
South Dakota, there's no indication anyone even knew the National
Practitioner Data Bank was in operation. Nor did it occur to anyone
to check with judicial or prison authorities or with the police about
the battery conviction that Swango admitted, or even to find out
what Swango had been doing in the years since his release from
prison. He told them nothing of his aborted residency in South
Dakota.

Dr. Miller and the other doctors who interviewed Swango
briefly discussed the fact that they were seriously considering admitting to their residency program a convicted felon who had
spent time in prison. But they gave the matter even less thought,
and were generally less apprehensive, than Dr. Salem had been at
the University of South Dakota. They had heard not one word
about poison. It seemed to them there had been a miscarriage of
justice of some sort, and that Swango's crime wasn't related to the
practice of medicine. In any event, as a resident he'd be under their
supervision. When all was said and done, Swango was still one of
their most appealing candidates. As Dr. Miller later put it, he and
his colleagues—all eminent psychiatrists—were "entranced" by
Swango.

On June 1, 1993, Swango was formally accepted as one of
twelve psychiatric residents at SUNY–Stony Brook.

AFTER a gap of two months, Kristin resumed her journal in May, an
indication that her revived spirits were beginning to flag in
Michael's presence. "I'm ecstatic that he has the offer," she wrote of
the Stony Brook acceptance.

---

whom Swango was continuing to use as a reference. Haller recalls some such conversation, but says he had by now changed his mind and believed Swango to be
guilty.

But the people don't know the nature of the battery, and the fear is overwhelming. I've had difficulty the last two days. I know in my mind it is unrealistic to worry about what could happen, but everything is too fresh from South Dakota. It would be a miracle for him to complete a residency without it ever coming up. I wish he didn't have to go through this. The majority of my anxiety is watching him deal with this. He does a terrific job hiding his anxiety but I can feel it constantly. This is an exhausting life.

Though the Coopers had seen little of their daughter or Swango, Kristin was eager to celebrate Father's Day with Al. The two couples met for lunch at Nick's Seafood Pavilion on Chesapeake Bay on June 20. The Coopers growing dislike of Swango only hardened as he talked incessantly, boasting that he had been accepted at two medical residency programs, and had chosen one in New York. He talked as though he'd just gotten out of medical school, hadn't been in prison, hadn't been dismissed in South Dakota, and had nothing to look forward to but a bright future. Kristin listened meekly, betraying none of the anxiety she had confided in her journal. She said almost nothing, which the Coopers thought was worrisome and out of character. It was as though Swango had gained some mysterious hold over her.

When Sharon heard that Swango would be moving to New York State, she asked Kristin, "Will you be going with him?"

"No, not for a while at least," she said.

Despite Swango's enthusiasm, Al Cooper was skeptical. "Michael, after all these problems, what if they hear about them?" he asked.

"What they don't know, they don't know," Swango confidently replied.

Later, when Al and Sharon returned to their car, they spoke of their unease about Kristin's demeanor. "Something's wrong," Al said.

Michael left for Long Island a week later. Kristin's ambivalence is evident in a journal entry written that day:

Michael departed for his residency. A month ago, I wanted him to go. I felt ready for him to go. I just wanted to get the separation over with. He's been gone five hours now and I miss him so much. I went to see the movie "Cliffhanger," and when I came out I looked for Mike-O at my side. I thought I was in Sioux Falls. I was so confused. I didn't know where I was. I started crying. I don't know where to stuff all this anger.

I feel so lonely here. I feel beaten, so beaten. I have so much to do I just don't feel like doing anything. I have $200 left in my checkbook. I'm financially drained and mentally as well.

Still, she added, "I know it will get better."

MICHAEL SWANGO'S residency began on July 1. He rented a room in Centereach, Long Island, from Carol Tamburo, a landlady who often rented to people connected to the university. He had introduced himself over the phone, and she had agreed to let him spend one night there without having met him. She quickly offered him a lease once they met. She found him charming and personable and was impressed that he was a doctor, though she found it odd that he insisted she call him "Mike" rather than "Dr. Swango."

For his first rotation, Swango—or Kirk, as he introduced himself to some people, Kirk being the name of the starship captain in *Star Trek*—was assigned to internal medicine at the sprawling, modern Veterans Administration hospital in Northport, Long Island, one of the two hospitals affiliated with the Stony Brook medical school. A nineteenth-century whaling port, Northport is a quaint town on the north shore of Long Island Sound that seems far from New York City, just an hour's drive away. Swango moved into a dormitory provided by the VA for hospital residents, and he also rented a storage room from the VA. Though he now had hospital privileges—he had even boasted to his landlady that he had access to "every medicine chest in the hospital"—no one thought to check his background with the National Practitioner Data Bank. Thanks to his recent work experience in South Dakota, Swango was more poised and skilled than most of his colleagues, and he garnered favorable reviews from the medical school faculty. Some of them teased Dr. Miller, saving, "Why is a guy this good in psychiatry? He should be in internal medicine."

One of Swango's first patients at the VA hospital was Dominic Buffalino, an organizer for the Long Island Republican Party, World War II veteran, and former construction supervisor for Grumman Aircraft. He had entered the VA hospital after he developed some lung congestion. Although his family thought he was suffering from little more than a severe cold, they did fear the condition might develop into pneumonia.

On July 1, the day Swango began his residency, Buffalino was resting comfortably, his condition stable. But he was running a fever, and an IV line was supplying antibiotics in an effort to curb his infection. His wife, Teresa, was visiting with him, as she had every day. The couple had never spent a day apart in their entire marriage. Several doctors had been in and out of the room, but then a young resident arrived, introduced himself as Dr. Michael Swango, and indicated he would now be the primary doctor in charge of her husband. Teresa found him pleasant and reassuring.

The next morning, Teresa was leaving the Buffalinos' home in nearby Huntington Station to return to the hospital when the phone rang. She went back inside to answer it. "I'm sorry to inform you your husband is dead," Dr. Swango said. "We didn't expect him to expire."

Teresa was stunned by the news. She began to sob hysterically. "Stay on the phone," Swango said. "Don't hang up. Talk to me." Finally Teresa was able to ask if she could come to the hospital. "By all means," Swango replied. "Come up here."

When Teresa and her brother-in-law, Andrew Buffalino, arrived at the hospital, Swango was waiting there to see them. They went into the room where Dominic's body still lay, and Teresa again lost her composure.

The rest of the day was a blur, but she later remembered hearing something to the effect that her husband had been paralyzed. She couldn't understand why someone suffering from pneumonia would be paralyzed.

AL and Sharon Cooper spent the first two weeks of July vacationing in North Carolina. They had begged Kristin to join them, but she insisted she had to keep working to make more money. They didn't understand why she'd had to use the credit card they gave her, and borrow money from them, loans she carefully documented in a notebook and promised to repay. They had no idea her savings had been drained by Swango.

On the evening of July 14, Kristin received a collect call from Michael. Her neighbor became concerned, because during the lengthy conversation she heard Kristin screaming, then sobbing.

Then Kristin called her mother. Sharon was immediately alarmed. Kristin wasn't herself. She was remote, distant. Her voice seemed flat. "Come stay with us," Sharon pleaded. "No, Mom, I'm fine," Kristin insisted. "I love you."

When she hung up, Sharon broke into sobs. "There's something terribly wrong with Kristin. I'm leaving, I'm going down there," she told Al.

"Stop it," he said, urging her to get a grip on herself. "She's twenty-seven years old. Give her some space."

Sharon got on the phone to her sister. "Please go see if Kristin is all right," she begged. But her sister, too, said she was overreacting. Kristin was a grown-up, and if she needed or wanted her mother, she'd ask.

Then the phone rang, and it was Michael calling from New York, the last person Sharon wanted to speak to. Michael said he'd just spoken to Kristin, and suggested Sharon call her. "She sounds like she's upset," he said.

"Well, apparently she's calmed down," Sharon replied. She told Michael she'd just spoken to her daughter.

"Are you sure you shouldn't go down there?"

Sharon said no, that Kristin had been very even-toned and collected by the time they finished speaking.

The next morning, after a restless night, Sharon said she had to see Kristin, and suggested she and Al drive over to give her their house key, in case she ever wanted to come stay with them. They arrived at her apartment in Portsmouth at about ten A.M. There was no answer, which was surprising, since Kristin was working the three P.M.–to–eleven P.M. shift at the hospital. There was no sign of her red truck, so it appeared that she was out.

The Coopers drove past some of her favorite places, and then drove aimlessly, hoping to spot her truck. They returned home that afternoon, then called the hospital. Kristin had called in sick. It was too hot and humid to go anywhere else, not that they had any more ideas about where to look. The mercury was over ninety degrees.

Exhausted from worry, Sharon went to bed early. She heard the phone ring at about nine P.M. and Al answered. Then he came into the bedroom, threw some clothes toward her, and said, "Get up. Kristin's in trouble."

"Why?" she asked, panicked. But Al had no explanation. All the police had said was that they should come to the Newport News police station.

Sharon and Al were nearly silent in the car. Sharon's mind was racing. What could Kristin have done? They were going to police headquarters, a jail. Had she been drunk? That was very unlike Kristin. Had she been arrested for a traffic offense? But did the police put you in jail for a traffic offense? It must be something more serious. Bank robbery? She knew Kristin was short of money.

"Honey, I don't think this looks good," Al said gently, but Sharon barely heard him.

At the station, they were greeted by a police officer.

"Can you tell me why you're detaining my daughter?" Sharon asked indignantly.

"We'll talk to you upstairs," he said.

They were taken on the elevator and shown to a second-floor room. The police officer avoided their gaze. They waited for what seemed hours, but was probably only a few minutes. A second police officer entered and introduced himself. "Your daughter has been found shot through the chest," he said.

"Where is she?" Sharon asked, tears welling in her eyes, thinking she had to get to the hospital. There was silence. "Take me to her!" she demanded.

"We can't," the officer said. "She's at the medical examiner's office."

Sharon was motionless. Life seemed suspended. Then the officer said he had a photograph, and she heard Al say he'd identify Kristin.

"No!" Sharon exclaimed. "I will."

The officer placed a photograph on the table in front of her. It was Kristin's face. Her head was leaning against a tree.

Sharon had seen enough corpses in her work as an emergency room nurse to know that her daughter was dead.

• •

KRISTIN left several notes. One, found at the site of her death, was evidently written as the effect of tranquilizing drugs began to be felt, for the writing trails off at the end. It read:

"I am—I am finally happy. My greatest joy in my life has been my work—I loved my patients and many loved me back. I never felt better than when I was taking care of a critical patient. I excelled and I cherished it."

Another, found in her apartment, was addressed to "Mom and Alp":

> Please be sure Mike-O gets some money to hold him until the end of July.
> I love you both so much. I just didn't want to be here anymore. Just found day-to-day living a constant struggle with my thoughts. I'd say I'm sorry but I'm not. I feel that sense of peace, "peace of mind," I've been looking for. It's nice.
>
>   Take care and go travel more.
>   Love,
>   K.K.

At the bottom, she added "I'll be seeing you!"
Another brief note was addressed to "Mike-O":

> I love you more! You're the most precious man I've ever known.
>
>   Love,
>   K.K.

A fourth note said, "I want Mike-O to have all of my belongings. Kristin L. Kinney."

WHEN the Coopers finally got home, still stunned, it was nearly two A.M. Sharon called Swango in New York; evidently still awake, he answered immediately. When she told him the news, he paused briefly, as if collecting his thoughts, then said, "I'm sorry. When's the funeral?" He said he'd be down the next day, and asked if he could stay in Kristin's apartment. Sharon was too numb to object.

Sharon and Al couldn't bear to see Kristin's things. Sharon called her sister and asked her to go over to the apartment before Swango got there. Kristin's aunt stayed briefly, and found the notes on the kitchen table. She also took Kristin's journal, in which the last entry was the sadly optimistic "I know it will get better."

At Kristin's funeral, there was an outpouring of sympathy from Sharon's and Kristin's friends in the nursing community, and many others. Swango mostly kept to himself, saying little and avoiding Kristin's friends. He talked mostly to Bert Gee, a respiratory therapist who had become a friend of Kristin's when she was working in Florida. Gee had evidently become much closer to Swango than the Coopers had realized. He stayed with Swango in Kristin's apartment.

Despite all that had happened, Sharon felt sorry for Michael. She did find it odd that he showed so little emotion. She went over to him after the funeral ceremony and put her arm around him. He said, "You know, Kristin would not have wanted this. She would not have wanted all these people here."

Expecting to comfort and perhaps be comforted, Sharon was taken aback by the hostility in his tone, and suddenly wanted to get away from him. "Here," she said, giving him a necklace that Kristin had loved. And, though she had little spare money herself, she gave him $200 in cash, in an attempt to heed Kristin's wish that he have enough money to get through the month of July. Swango took the gifts, but then said, "I would have thought Kristin would have handled this better."

"How dare you," Sharon retorted, hurt and angry. "I'm her mother."

IN South Dakota, Vern Cook had learned of Kristin's death from a reporter at the *Argus Leader*, which also ran a brief obituary. He was so devastated he had to leave work. That night, Swango called him with the news, the first time he'd heard from him since he left Sioux Falls three months earlier. Swango called again after Kristin's funeral, and Cook thought he was upset over her death. But their conversation quickly shifted to Swango's new residency on Long Island. Swango told Cook he was using a false name and had lied about his conviction, defying Cook's advice. Cook was furious with him. "Mike, what the fuck are you doing?"

Swango insisted that he felt he had no alternative—he had to lie and conceal his past, or he'd never complete a residency.

TWO days after the funeral, Michael left for Long Island. When the Coopers finally mustered the strength to visit their daughter's apartment, it was bare. Swango had taken everything. Sharon was left with virtually nothing to remember her daughter by, except her photographs and a lock of Kristin's hair. And Swango had placed scores of long-distance telephone calls from Kristin's apartment (including the lengthy call to Vern Cook), leaving the Coopers with an enormous bill.

As they struggled to make sense of their daughter's death, the Coopers learned from Kristin's neighbor about her reaction to the phone call from Swango the night before her death. They speculated that something Swango had told her—that he was dating someone else, or that he needed even more money—had brought Kristin to the breaking point. They also learned from Kristin's friends in Sioux Falls that she had been seeing Carol Carlson, the counselor, and they spoke to her about what might have been troubling Kristin. Carlson was no doubt guarded out of professional responsibility; still, she insisted that Swango wasn't to blame. "You know, Kristin could be manipulative, too," she said. Michael was "a wonderful person," and what the media were saying about him was entirely untrue.

The Coopers also learned that Kristin had turned to a therapist the day she died. She had been to see her for the first time the day before, and had come in the next day distraught. "Nobody is coming for me," Kristin had repeated over and over. If she told the therapist anything about her last conversation with Michael, the therapist didn't share it with the Coopers. By the time Kristin left her office on July 15, the therapist felt she was considerably calmer. She had been devastated, she added, by her new patient's death.

Sharon despaired of ever understanding what had happened. All she knew is that she, too, now felt that life was hardly worth living.

• •

BARRON HARRIS checked into the Northport Veterans Administration Medical Center on September 29, 1993, for what he and his wife, Elsie, expected would be relatively brief treatment for pneumonia. The sixty-year-old Harris was otherwise in good health and, when not working as a cabinetmaker, enjoyed spending time with his five children and two grandchildren. The couple had recently celebrated their twenty-fifth wedding anniversary.

After a brief consultation with a respiratory specialist, Harris was assigned to a resident. When Elsie Harris arrived, she found the doctor sitting attentively near her husband's bed in the private room. He had blond hair, clear blue eyes, an athletic build, and a broad smile that Mrs. Harris found immediately reassuring. He introduced himself as Dr. Michael Kirk.

Harris was impressed by the time and attention Dr. Kirk bestowed on her husband, behavior that contrasted with the harried indifference she'd seen in many other doctors. Several days later, when she arrived to discover that her husband's hands were tied to the bed rails, Dr. Kirk was reassuring. Her husband, he explained, had suddenly become "agitated" and he had given him a sedative. Harris was now sleeping peacefully. The doctor had ordered several tests—something to do with Barron's liver—but it would be several days before they had any results.

On her next visit, Mrs. Harris arrived to find that the blinds in her husband's room had been lowered and closed, darkening the room. Dr. Kirk was alone with her husband, and was in the process of injecting the contents of a large syringe into her husband's neck. "What's that?" she asked. "Vitamins," Dr. Kirk replied. He removed the needle and left the room.

Later, when a nurse arrived, Mrs. Harris mentioned that the doctor had given her husband a vitamin injection. "You must be mistaken," the nurse said. "Doctors don't give injections at all. That's the nurses' job."

Barron Harris remained under what seemed heavy sedation. Still, when his wife introduced him to the nurse at the end of the week, he was able to smile and wave. Elsie Harris was wholly unprepared to find her husband unconscious and on a respirator the following Monday.

"I hope it's nothing I did," Dr. Kirk said.

"What are you talking about?" she asked.

"He's in a coma, and I know he's not coming out of it," Kirk replied.

Elsie Harris began to sob. Pressed by Dr. Kirk, who argued that her husband had already suffered irreparable brain damage, she agreed to a DNR order: "Do Not Resuscitate." Despite her anxiety and grief, Mrs. Harris was struck by the change she perceived in Dr. Kirk. His solicitous concern for her husband had evaporated. His manner seemed cold, detached.

SHARON COOPER knew only vaguely that Swango was working as a doctor somewhere in New York. But then she received a letter from him. "I think of you so much," Swango wrote. "I know Kristin wanted us to stay in touch. . . . I can feel Kristin sitting by me. . . . She taught me to have a better bedside manner." Sharon was not interested in corresponding or otherwise "staying in touch" with Swango. But she noticed he had written his address on Long Island at the bottom of the letter.

She wrote back, saying she didn't think it was a good thing for them to stay in close contact. "You'd better let go of Kristin," she advised.

But Sharon couldn't put Swango or his letter out of her mind. She knew he was working as a medical resident under false pretenses, that he hadn't told anyone he'd been convicted of a felony and had been in jail. No one would want to be treated by a doctor with such a record. She couldn't shake the feeling that he had been responsible, directly or indirectly, for her daughter's death. She'd dedicated herself to taking care of sick people. If she did nothing now, she feared, more people—perhaps another vulnerable young woman like Kristin—might die. Should she contact the authorities? If so, who? She didn't know where to turn. Nor did she want to expose Kristin's death to more publicity and inquiries. It was all too painful. And she herself was afraid of Swango. She thought he would retaliate if he knew she had revealed his secret. She was in such turmoil that she was having trouble sleeping.

Finally Sharon wrote a letter to one of Kristin's close friends in South Dakota, with whom she'd been corresponding since Kristin's death. "I was glad that Kristin was away from Michael and I knew he couldn't hurt her anymore," she wrote. "She is in a safe place. But I'm worried [about] who Michael is. He's gone to another residency in New York." Then she wrote Swango's full address. She thought of the letter as a silent plea. Every day she thought to herself, "Please, God, let this message get through." Sharon was still so apprehensive that she told Al about the letter only after she'd mailed it.

When she received the letter, Kristin's friend quickly realized its significance. She went to see the dean, Dr. Talley, and told him that Swango was practicing medicine again in New York. Dr. Talley happened to know the dean of the medical school at Stony Brook, Jordan Cohen; he called Cohen to alert him to the possibility that Swango had been accepted into the school's residency program. He told him of the experience in South Dakota, the *Justice Files* segment, and the ensuing uproar.

When Cohen found that Swango had indeed begun his residency at Stony Brook, he called Fritz Henn, the department chairman, who in turn called Alan Miller to tell him that the "battery" Swango had told them about with such seeming candor was in fact a case of poisoning. Miller was stunned. He reached Swango at the VA hospital, and said, "I need to see you right away."

Swango arrived in about fifteen minutes. "I've just heard the following," Miller told him, then outlined the cases of poisoning and what he'd learned about South Dakota. Swango visibly blanched. He said, "It's true. That's what they did convict me of. I didn't do it, but they convicted me." He seemed genuinely remorseful. "I'm sorry," he said. "I feel bad." But he said he had felt he had no alternative but to conceal the reason for his conviction. Miller had to agree that Swango was probably correct. It was one thing to hire someone convicted of battery after a barroom brawl. But Stony Brook would never have taken such a risk with someone convicted of poisoning people. Miller told Swango that his residency was suspended, effective immediately.

Miller was upset, castigating himself for not having checked out Swango more thoroughly. He called Swango's references again in the wake of the disclosure, trying to figure out whether he had missed something. To his amazement one reference reiterated his belief that the whole thing had been blown out of proportion and that Swango was innocent.

The next day, Swango asked to see Miller again. He repeated how sorry he was. "What can I ever do with my life?" he asked, seeming near despair. "It's doubtful you can ever practice medicine," Miller replied, but then, moved by Swango's seeming contrition, he qualified his remark. Almost in spite of himself, he found himself feeling sorry for Swango. He seemed so sincere and heartbroken. "The only way would be for you to go somewhere that really needed a doctor, somewhere that was desperate," Miller said, thinking that Swango might go abroad. "And they would have to know everything." Swango had tears in his eyes as he left the meeting. If he was acting, it seemed to fool Miller, despite his skills as a psychiatrist.

That day the VA also automatically suspended Swango's hospital privileges and ordered him out of his quarters. It dispatched its resident investigator, Thomas Valery, a former Securities and Exchange Commission enforcement investigator, to oversee the removal of his belongings. Valery watched as Swango backed up his red pickup to the storage room and loaded his things, mostly books, into the back of the truck. Then he was gone.

That same day, October 20, 1993, the electrifying news broke in *Newsday*, which devoted its entire tabloid front page to the story: "Poison in His Past: Hospital Fires M.D. After Learning He Fed Ant Killer to Paramedics."

"A young doctor sent to prison for feeding ant poison to six paramedics in Illinois and investigated by authorities for suspicious patient deaths in Ohio was hired at University Hospital at Stony Brook, where officials now say he lied about his criminal past," the story began.

"He didn't tell anyone he was put in jail for poisoning anyone," said hospital spokeswoman Michaele Gold. "We just found out a little while ago he falsified documents and lied to us through his teeth."

When Elsie Harris arrived at the hospital that day to see her comatose husband, she asked for Dr. Kirk. "Have you read the papers? I'd advise you to go home and read them," a nurse said cryptically. Harris got a copy of *Newsday*. She burst into tears when she saw Swango—Kirk's—picture. Her daughter joined her, read the article, too, and cried. They drove back to the hospital and demanded days after Swango was suspended, Dean Cohen called Miller. "Alan," he began, which Miller thought was presumptuous, since the two barely knew each other, "I think it would be best if you resign as chairman of the admissions committee."

"That's fine with me," Miller replied. He pointed out that given his part-time status, he was bound to have to leave sooner or later. The school needed a full-time admissions director.

"I'm going to have to make a statement to the press," Cohen continued, and Miller recognized with some bitterness that he was going to be made the fall guy.

Cohen announced Miller's resignation on October 26. In his prepared statement, he said: "During all the years of our medical program here at Stony Brook, we have never encountered a case like Michael Swango; we believe that evidence shows that we are dealing here, at a minimum, with a pathological liar." Nonetheless, he went on, "we have determined that a critical error in judgment was made during the interview and selection process, a process supervised personally by Dr. Alan Miller. . . . In recognition of the serious, albeit unprecedented, lapse on Dr. Miller's part, he has resigned his duties as Program Director." Cohen later explained, "I felt the deviation from standard procedures was so egregious that there had to be accountability for that. It was a very unfortunate circumstance, but he was responsible for the quality-control process, and I felt it was essential that there be public accountability."

Then, only two weeks later, Cohen himself resigned. Before he left, he faxed a letter about Swango to the dean of every medical school in the country. Cohen wrote: "In reviewing our records, I was chagrined to find that [Swango] had again conned very experienced faculty with outright lies about his past. He is an exceedingly charming young man who can weave a very convincing story that elicits sympathy and compassion. I bring this matter to your attention because I think we must assume that he will try yet again to secure a residency position of some kind somewhere."

During the week after the news broke, Swango was seen several times in the Stony Brook area driving his red pickup. A group of nurses, one of whom he had begun dating even before Kristin's death, held a going-away party for him. It was only then that FBI agents began to look for him. Though the police had been notified an explanation, but none was offered. Then it seemed all the doctors in the intensive care unit were rotated. The new doctors knew nothing about Swango or what had happened to Barron Harris. Finally Harris did get to speak to the doctor in charge of the ICU, but all he told her was that Swango had nothing to do with her husband's condition, and that it was unlikely he'd ever recover. Harris was shocked and grief-stricken.

Barron Harris never regained consciousness and died on November 8. The cause of death was listed as cardiopulmonary failure, secondary to encephalitis.

As at Ohio State and in South Dakota, university and hospital officials rushed to reassure the public that whatever Swango's past record, nothing untoward had happened at their hospital. Only a week after Swango was suspended, VA chief of staff Thomas Horvath announced at a press conference that investigators were still going through records of the 147 patients known to have been treated by Swango, but that the inquiry so far had revealed "no suspicious illnesses or deaths." He emphasized that "the rate of complications did not change during Swango's tenure," and insisted that "as a first-year resident, he had no independent patient responsibilities"—even though Swango had in fact been alone with Buffalino and Harris and had had ample opportunity to inject others.

Medical school dean Jordan Cohen issued a statement saying that "we are also mindful of the natural concern the public has expressed about whether Swango had caused any harm to patients or staff while he was in our employ." Cohen emphasized that Swango's "patient care activities were closely and contemporaneously supervised by the teaching attending staff"; that the VA's "quality assurance" system uncovered "no untoward events"; and that a subsequent review of every patient's chart had thus far "revealed nothing that would lead us to conclude that any patient was harmed." Cohen later said, "There were some deaths, which is not unusual. Those were of particular concern, nonetheless. We looked carefully, scrutinized. There was no indication that there had been any unnatural events. That came as something of a relief."

There was some accountability imposed on the medical school, however, as there had not been in Ohio or South Dakota. Several of Swango's presence on October 19, a squabble over whether the Justice Department or the Veterans Administration would be in charge of any investigation had wasted valuable time. Finally the Justice Department took charge, but by the time agents arrived, Swango had emptied his storage locker. It didn't occur to anyone to issue a warrant for his arrest on charges that he had defrauded SUNY and the VA by making false statements in his application, which is a federal offense. In any event, Swango himself was gone.

AFTER the news broke on Long Island, the *Daily Press* in Newport News ran a brief article on Swango's unmasking and his earlier conviction on poison charges. The Coopers had to read it several times before it fully sank in. Poison? They had never heard anything about a poisoning conviction. "Oh my God!" Sharon exclaimed repeatedly. "It's real." Her worst fears were being borne out.

Al called the *Daily Press* reporter, who knew little more about the case and suggested he check at a local library for access to articles that had run in Illinois and Ohio. The next day, the Coopers traveled to the College of William and Mary library in nearby Williamsburg, which was able to provide copies of many of the articles on Swango. When she read them, Sharon felt as though she might faint.

The Newport News article mentioned that Swango had disappeared, so Al called the Norfolk office of the FBI. "I might have information on the whereabouts of Michael Swango," he told an agent. Ed Schrader returned the call and came to see the Coopers. He said the FBI was trying to develop a profile of Swango, and the Coopers answered his questions as best they could. Al told him that they suspected Swango would try to stay with Bert Gee, who lived outside Atlanta and had been so friendly with Swango at Kristin's funeral.

Soon after, Schrader called to thank the Coopers and said the FBI had discovered a storage shed in Portsmouth rented by Swango and would like to examine the contents. Absent an arrest warrant or probable cause for a search warrant, the FBI needed the Coopers' help. The Coopers went to the police and explained how Swango had taken all of Kristin's belongings, which they suspected were in the shed. But the police said they couldn't do anything, given

Kristin's note bequeathing all her possessions to him. Then the FBI asked the Coopers to file a civil lawsuit alleging that Swango had wrongfully taken their daughter's things. But Sharon refused. Kristin's note had said she wanted Swango to have all her things, and she felt that a suit maintaining otherwise would require her to make a false statement under oath. However, Schrader assured the Coopers that the FBI had the shed under surveillance and that the storage facility's owner had pledged to notify them should Swango try to remove anything.

Months later, the agent called to report that Swango's red truck had been spotted in Bert Gee's driveway, and the FBI had him under surveillance.

In fact, Swango was living with Gee, and on February 24, 1994, had taken a job as a chemist at a company called Photocircuits in Peachtree City, just outside Atlanta. Photocircuits makes computer equipment, but significantly, Swango, using the alias Jack Kirk, was working in its wastewater treatment facility, which feeds directly into the metropolitan Atlanta water supply. Given Swango's fascination with mass tragedy, and the books he had checked out of Quincy's library, including the one about poisoning a city's food supply, his new employment alarmed the FBI. Acting on the Bureau's tip, Photocircuits fired Swango on July 22 on the grounds that he had lied on his job application.

The action apparently alerted Swango that he was under surveillance. He and his truck disappeared, and Schrader had to call the Coopers to report that the FBI had lost track of him.

In November, a friend of Kristin's from her time in Florida, Tracy Dunlap, got a call from Swango, saying he was in Georgia but wanted to come to Florida for a visit. Dunlap was still working as a nurse in Naples. She'd never met Kristin's fiancé, but Kristin had spoken about him occasionally, never mentioning anything about his past or the trouble in South Dakota. Swango had called Dunlap several times after Kristin's death, complaining that the Coopers weren't being very supportive and that he needed someone to talk to.

The next day, when Dunlap got home after work, her answering machine was full of messages from Swango, calling from a pay phone in Naples. When she called the phone, Swango answered,

saying he'd been waiting there all day. He wanted to come over immediately. Somewhat apprehensively, Dunlap agreed.

Thinking it odd that Swango would have come to Florida so
quickly and sat all day by a pay phone, Dunlap called Al Cooper to
ask what he thought of Swango.

"Why?" Al asked. Dunlap said that he'd shown up and wanted
to stay with her.

"Get rid of him," Al told her, though he wasn't more specific
because he didn't want to frighten her.

Despite the warning, Dunlap and Swango sat up talking that
night until three A.M. He seemed so earnest and pleasant, and, after
all, he had been close to Kristin. "I felt so sorry for him," she later
told the Coopers. The next day Dunlap was moving into a house
with two friends. Swango helped her move, volunteering his truck,
and then he just stayed, sleeping on the pull-out sofa bed and using
one closet for his belongings. What Dunlap and her roommates had
expected would be a two- or three-day visit stretched into weeks.
Swango was pleasant, but increasingly odd. He was out most days,
saying only that he was doing "research" at the library. He'd never
join them at the pool or hot tub. He refused to eat anything from the
refrigerator, or share a pizza, even when they offered, preferring to
keep his food in his closet. Her roommates noticed that he kept numerous containers on the passenger side of his truck. Finally Dunlap
asked Swango when he planned to leave. "Well, I thought I'd stay," he
replied. But Dunlap said that might be a problem for her roommates.

Around Christmas, Dunlap spoke to Al Cooper again and told
him Swango was living with her. This time, he all but ordered her
to get Swango out of the house. But before she could say anything,
she got a call from one of her roommates, who was working as a
nurse in Fort Myers; the roommate told her to drive over immediately. She had met two visiting nurses from Long Island, who told
her about Swango and even showed her a picture that looked like
their long-term guest. Dunlap and her roommate hurried to the
Fort Myers library, where they pulled up articles about Swango from
Newsday. When she read them, Dunlap felt she might have a heart
attack.

Dunlap immediately called the FBI in Miami. But the agent she
spoke with expressed no interest in anyone named Swango; he sug-

gested they call the local police. Dunlap concluded that would be a
waste of time, since Swango hadn't done anything in Florida.

In any event, they were worried about their other roommate,
who was at home alone with Swango. They hurried back to Naples
and told Swango he had to move out immediately. They showed
him copies of the *Newsday* articles. "It's not true," he insisted, but
he didn't argue further. He packed his belongings into the truck and
left that night.

The next day, an FBI agent appeared at the hospital where
Dunlap worked, asking about Swango, but it was too late. Dunlap
had no idea where he'd gone.

Swango had driven back to Georgia and stayed with Bert Gee.
Three days later, at two A.M., he and Gee showed up at the storage
locker in Portsmouth. The night manager, who knew nothing about
Swango, let them in. Swango and Gee loaded the truck and left. No
one called the FBI.

Only on October 27, 1994—a full year after his dismissal from
SUNY–Stony Brook—did federal authorities issue a warrant for
Swango's arrest on charges of defrauding a federal facility, the VA
hospital, by gaining admission to the Stony Brook residency program on false pretenses. Because the FBI agents thought they were
investigating a potential murder case, it hadn't occurred to them to
seek a warrant for this far lesser offense until they took what evidence they had to the U.S. Attorney's Office on Long Island.
Swango was now officially a fugitive, but the action produced no
new leads.

Ed Schrader visited the Coopers with the disappointing news.
"We've lost him," he said, attributing the delays and mishaps to
squabbling within the FBI over who should be in charge of investigating the case. Schrader had checked with the FBI's Miami office,
which confirmed that it had initially ignored the call from Tracy
Dunlap. Swango "wasn't a priority," Schrader said, sounding bitter
and disappointed.

"If I were you, I'd forget about this," Schrader told the Coopers. "He's the kind of person who will just show up dead someday."
For Swango had vanished.

CHAPTER TEN

B<small>Y</small> N<small>OVEMBER</small> 1994, spring had finally come to the tropical regions of southern Africa, bringing welcome rains that helped relieve the severe drought that had afflicted most of Zimbabwe for nearly three years. Dr. Christopher Zshiri, the director of the Mnene Mission Hospital, was in good spirits, bounding out to greet the new doctor from America when he arrived with Howard Mpofu, the church official who had picked him up at the Bulawayo airport. Mpofu introduced him to Dr. Swango, whose blond hair and fair complexion reminded him of some of the Swedish missionary doctors who had come before. Zshiri noticed that Swango had something of a nervous twitch in his eye. Perhaps he wasn't used to the bright sunshine.

Swango was charming and talkative, and they all chuckled over Mpofu's account of Swango kneeling to kiss the bishop's ring. Still, Zshiri was a bit skeptical of the mission hospital's good fortune.

"Why are you coming from a rich country like the United States to the bush?" he asked as soon as Swango had deposited his belongings in his bungalow.

"I love Africa," Swango replied. "I love blacks. I can breathe out here," he said, gesturing toward the sweeping, rain-freshened view beyond the hospital.

"Is that so?" Zshiri responded. "You'll be earning one-twentieth of what you could make in the U.S."

"I don't mind," Swango replied.

Zshiri wondered. It did seem odd to him that a young doctor from the United States would want to come to this remote African

outpost. But Swango seemed so idealistic and earnest. Zshiri
thought that maybe he was becoming too cynical.

Though Swango had been looking for a job through an agency
called Options, a subsidiary of Project Concern International,
which specializes in placing American doctors in foreign countries,
he had been hired by the church directly through a Lutheran placement organization in Harare, which obtained a copy of his application from Options. Swango had supplied a copy of his medical
school diploma; a glowing letter of recommendation from Robert
Haller II, who had hired Swango as an emergency room physician in
Ohio ten years before and testified at his sentencing hearing in
Quincy; and a letter from Diann Weaver, a nurse who was married
to a friend of Swango's from America Ambulance in Springfield.
Both letters were dated 1994. The dates must have been altered,
since Haller and Weaver hadn't written letters for Swango since his
sentencing in 1985. Swango also rewrote the text of Haller's recommendation, making it far more positive than the original.

The new doctor didn't quite prove to be the godsend Zshiri
had hoped for. He seemed curiously inexperienced considering that
he'd graduated from medical school in 1983 and, according to his
résumé, had been practicing medicine in the United States since
then. Despite his impressive academic credentials and his internship
at Ohio State—a name recognized even in southern Africa—Zshiri
discovered that Swango had trouble with routine surgery and
seemed never to have delivered a baby. But Swango ascribed his lack
of experience to his specialization in neurosurgery, a skill for which
there was little demand at Mnene, and Zshiri had indeed heard that
American doctors were highly specialized. In any event, Swango
readily agreed to undergo a five-month internship at Mpilo Hospital in Bulawayo to improve his skills, concentrating on obstetrics
and gynecology.

Mpilo Hospital is a teeming facility on the outskirts of Bulawayo. It is still referred to as the "African" hospital, as opposed to
the United Bulawayo Hospitals, which, before Zimbabwean independence, were for white patients only. Though differences between the hospitals have supposedly been leveled, Mpilo patients
remain overwhelmingly black and poor. The hospital has been inun-
dated with AIDS patients and, at the time of Swango's arrival, was

woefully understaffed. There were only three residents working at the hospital rather than the usual six, which meant one of them was on duty for a twenty-four-hour period every third night. Swango's arrival provided welcome relief.

Swango impressed the superintendent at Mpilo, Dr. Naboth Chaibva, as sociable and eager to learn. He was assigned to work under Dr. Christopher King in obstetrics. Soon after, at a lunch for the medical staff, Ian Lorimer introduced himself to Swango, who said his name was pronounced "Swan." Lorimer, tall, good-looking, and athletic, was a resident in surgery, and Swango said he was eager to improve his surgical skills. He asked if he could accompany Lorimer on his rounds. Affable and outgoing, Lorimer welcomed the company. He was amazed to find that Swango had the stamina to accompany him on his twenty-four-hour shifts, then continue immediately with his own rotation.

Swango was never anything but helpful, attentive, and eager to learn, and quickly won over almost everyone on the medical staff. The one exception was Dr. Abdi Mesbah, who was almost instantly suspicious of Swango. An Iranian national, Mesbah criticized Swango's skills as a doctor, puzzled over the vague references to his past, and concluded that Swango must be a CIA agent. But other doctors attributed Mesbah's suspicions to his open anti-Americanism, and dismissed his spy theories as far-fetched.

Lorimer was impressed by Swango's general medical knowledge and his ability to handle trauma cases—the result, Swango told him, of his having successfully completed an intensive advanced trauma life-support course. (He made no mention of his work in emergency rooms or as a paramedic.) On the other hand, Swango seemed woefully inexperienced in even rudimentary surgical procedures, such as draining an abscess. Lorimer didn't feel he could allow Swango to undertake common but more complex operations, such as hernias and appendectomies. Still, he felt his new colleague was learning quickly. Lorimer's only real concern, and a minor one in the scheme of things, was the frequency with which Swango swore or, as Lorimer put it, "blasphemed." Lorimer and his wife, Cheryl, a former ballet dancer, are devout Presbyterians, and led a weekly Bible discussion and prayer group at Bulawayo Central Presbyterian Church. When Lorimer asked Swango to watch his language, Swango seemed startled that he might have offended, and never again took the Lord's name in vain in Lorimer's presence.

Indeed, Swango seemed so chastened that Lorimer invited him to join them at church on Sundays, and he was soon a fixture in the congregation. Along with the Anglican Cathedral, Bulawayo Central Presbyterian Church is a pillar of the local establishment, numbering prominent businessmen, lawyers, and doctors, including Dr. King from Mpilo, among its members. Swango and Lorimer became close friends, and not just because Lorimer was becoming Swango's spiritual mentor. In the long stretches of time they spent together at the hospital they spoke often—in Swango's case, incessantly—about books, about current affairs, about personal relationships, especially Swango's eagerness to meet a girl and, eventually, to marry.

Lorimer was amazed by how well-read Swango was, not just in popular best-sellers and detective stories, which Swango loved, but in the classics: all of Dickens, Jane Austen, Tolstoy. He often referred to Dostoevsky's *Crime and Punishment.* The medical staff, some of whom felt derelict in their own attention to matters outside their field, came to rely on his trenchant analyses of current events. On one occasion, Swango expounded at length on the conflict in Bosnia, showing, in Lorimer's view, an amazing command of detail and ability to make sense out of a bafflingly complex matter. Indeed, if there was anything slightly irritating about Swango, it was that he never seemed to stop talking. He sometimes followed Lorimer into the men's room so as not to interrupt a train of thought.

As the two became close, Lorimer, twenty-seven, naturally talked about his upbringing: his father was Irish; he'd been born in Zambia but moved to Zimbabwe when he was two, had grown up in Harare, the capital, and had graduated from medical school there. For his part, Swango said he, too, was twenty-seven years old. (In reality, he was now forty.) His father had been in the military, was a strict disciplinarian, and was absent from the home for long stretches. It was his mother, Swango said, who held the family together. He mentioned a couple of brothers, but Lorimer had the impression that Swango hadn't been in contact with them or with his mother in some time. But Swango didn't seem to want to discuss his past. He was vague about just where he was from, where the family had lived, where he was educated or had worked in the United States. Lying about his age no doubt made it easier to gloss over his past.

Lorimer didn't press, though he did ask what had brought a young doctor like Swango to Africa. Swango said he'd always wanted geographic variety in his career. He said he'd considered Latin America, the Caribbean, Asia; that Zimbabwe hadn't been on his list; but that when the Mnene opening was mentioned, it immediately appealed to him.

In any event, no one in Bulawayo was inclined to think ill of someone like Swango. The beleaguered white community there would no doubt have embraced any charming, handsome young white American doctor who had come to live in their midst. Depressed by years of emigration, the failure of white rule, and constant fear that their remaining status, privileges, economic security, and even physical safety could be shattered by dictatorial decree, most whites who met Swango were flattered that someone with his stellar credentials—someone who could seemingly live anywhere—not only chose to come to their community, but was constantly extolling its virtues: the friendliness of the people he met; the ideal climate; the satisfaction of working in a hospital where he was truly needed and could make a contribution.

Swango not only attended the Presbyterian church on Sundays but also joined a weekly Bible study group led by Lorimer and enrolled in a sixteen-week Christian-marriage course also taught by the Lorimers. He played volleyball every Thursday evening, usually at the home of Ted Mirtle and his wife, Margaret, Cheryl Lorimer's parents, and played table tennis on Tuesday evenings in a league that met at the Catholic church. He seemed eager to meet women and to have a girlfriend. He told friends of the Lorimers, "I really like that girl with the ginger hair," referring to Rosie Malcolm, who also attended the Bible-study sessions. They jokingly told her to "watch out" for Swango unless she wanted a boyfriend, but he never directly asked her on a date. In May 1995, when the internship ended and it came time to return to Mnene, he told the Lorimers he wasn't all that excited about returning to such a remote location, but would honor his commitment. But he pledged to stay in touch, and

said he'd like to return permanently once he completed his stay at
the mission hospital. Doctors King and Matt Oliver wrote him
glowing letters of recommendation, with Oliver writing that he was
"very keen and hard-working."

AT Mnene, Dr. Zshiri was happy to have Swango back, and felt that
his performance had indeed improved as a result of his months at
Mpilo. Swango's earlier enthusiasm and cheerful mood, however,
seemed to have evaporated. Perhaps the stimulation of Bulawayo
had soured him on the isolation of the bush—it was in the month he
returned, for example, that Swango asked for the use of a car, saying
he wanted to attend "medical conferences" in Bulawayo. While he
remained affable and friendly toward Zshiri, his habits increasingly
struck the doctors and others at the hospital as peculiar. Dr. Larsson
told Zshiri that something about Swango made him uneasy, and he
didn't want his children to be around him. Although Swango had indicated he was something of a diet and fitness buff, Zshiri couldn't
figure out what he was eating. He never cooked for himself, didn't
eat with others, and seemed to live on popcorn and Coke.
    There were also a few complaints from the nursing staff, nearly
all of whom were black Lutheran nuns, that Dr. Swango was irrita-
ble and rude to them, in some cases refusing to allow them to accompany him on his rounds. This was highly unorthodox; it was
hospital policy that a nurse always be present during doctors'
rounds, to take down instructions for medications and to administer injections, for example. Swango seemed unduly sensitive about
his lab coat; he once flew into a rage after accusing a nurse of touching it. There were even a few murmurings that Swango was racist.
All this was discounted by Zshiri. Still, that a nurse would mention
another doctor to him at all, let alone to complain, was highly unusual. The nursing staff was deferential to a fault, and rarely spoke
to medical doctors unless their opinions were solicited. And while
Swango's long hours and frequent visits to patients seemed laudable, it did seem odd that some of those visits came in the middle of
the night, and that Swango used unattended entrances to the wards.
Nurses and aides would sometimes be startled to find Swango min-
istering to a patient when they weren't aware he was in the building.
    On May 24, 1995, little more than a week after his return from

Bulawayo, Swango came into Zshiri's office to report that one of his patients, Rhoda Mahlamvana, had suddenly "collapsed" and was dead. Swango had prepared a death certificate. Zshiri was startled. Swango had no real explanation for the sudden demise of his patient. Mahlamvana had been admitted to the hospital earlier that month with burns over about 20 percent of her body, but she had responded well to treatment and nothing about her condition seemed life-threatening. Still, death, even sudden and unexplained death, is a fact of life in hospitals. Zshiri accepted Swango's account and didn't make further inquiries.

Then came the incident in which Swango awoke Keneas Mzezewa from his nap and injected him. Mzezewa was paralyzed, unable to speak, yet conscious. When he recovered sufficiently to tell nurses that "Dr. Mike" had given him an injection, Swango denied it. Mzezewa was now terrified of Swango, and begged to be moved from the recovery room. He was afraid to be alone there.

Initially the nurses seemed to believe Swango's claim that Mzezewa must have been hallucinating when he accused him of giving him an injection. But Mzezewa proved surprisingly astute and resourceful at rebutting Swango's claim. He told the nurses that Swango had concealed the syringe in his jacket pocket, but that he'd dropped the needle cap. He retrieved the cap from the floor near the foot of his bed and turned it over to the nurses, pointing out that he had not been scheduled to receive any injections. How, then, could a needle cover have appeared near his bed unless Swango had dropped it, as Mzezewa claimed?

Mzezewa's insistence that he had been fully conscious throughout the episode and was aware of Swango's actions began to make an impression on the nurses, especially after the mysterious death of Mahlamvana. They granted his request to rejoin the other patients. But the nurses were afraid to say anything to Zshiri or Larsson. The situation was too serious, the accusation against Swango too grave, and they assumed the doctors would take Swango's word over theirs.

In the wake of the incident, Mzezewa developed an infection in his lower leg; two weeks later, the leg had to be amputated near the knee, surgery again performed by Dr. Larsson. Mzezewa was convinced that Swango had caused him to lose his leg. He was so fright-

ened by the prospect that Swango might have access to him that he
again insisted he not be left alone during his recovery.

Though the nursing staff began to keep a wary eye on Swango,
there were no unusual incidents, and speculation subsided. Then, in
late June, two deaths in as many days shattered the calm.

On the afternoon of June 26, Katazo Shava was recuperating
from surgery on his leg when Swango arrived at his bedside. The
doctor seemed annoyed to find Shava surrounded by relatives—his
son, his sister, and his nieces and nephews—who were planning to
spend the night at the hospital complex. Swango told them he
needed to be alone with his patient, and drew the curtain around
Shava's bed. The family members left the ward, but remained just
outside the open door. Minutes later, as Shava's son later put it, "my
father cried out like a wild animal. I never heard such a cry from a
man." The family was alarmed, but afraid to interrupt the doctor.
Almost immediately, Swango hurried out, ignoring their questions.
When they reached Shava's bedside, he was crying out, "We won't
go home together because I am going to die." When they asked him
why, he replied, "The doctor has injected me with something and I
think I am going to die." The family thought Shava was delirious,
since he clutched his buttock and kept sobbing and repeating, "I
won't get home. I am going to die."

He was still crying when the afternoon visiting hours ended
and the family members were asked to leave the ward. When they
returned that evening, a nurse told them that Shava was dead.
Swango had signed the death certificate that afternoon, within
hours of administering the shot. The family's complaints were dismissed, since Shava's records didn't indicate that there had been any
injection.

Later that night, at 2:30 A.M. on June 27, Swango, who was on
call that night, woke Zshiri to report that Phillimon Chipoko had
suddenly died. Chipoko was a farmer who had been admitted in late
April; his right foot had been amputated. He had been recovering,
and in any event, sudden death in the wake of a foot amputation is
highly unusual. Swango again signed the death certificate, citing cardiopulmonary arrest as the cause of death.

Chipoko's wife, Yeudzirai, had come to the hospital to visit her
husband, and because the distance from their homestead was so

great, had been sleeping that night on a bench next to her husband's bed, located in the same private ward where Mzezewa had been recovering. Despite his recent amputation, Chipoko had been cheerful and looking forward to his discharge from the hospital. Husband and wife had been discussing plans for their farm plot and the work that would need to be done when he returned.

Yeudzirai later told the nurses that she had been awakened at around eleven P.M. by the sound of the door opening, and saw that "Dr. Mike," whom she'd met earlier that day, was entering. The doctor went straight to her husband, saying nothing to her, and she saw him bend over Phillimon. She was overcome with drowsiness and must have fallen back asleep, for the next thing she remembered was the sound of the door as the doctor left the room. She wasn't sure how much time had elapsed, and thought little of the incident; she assumed Swango was simply being attentive to her husband.

Some time later, she was awakened by the touch of a nurse's aide. "Did anyone tell you that your husband is dead?" the aide asked. Shocked, Yeudzirai turned to Phillimon's motionless body and broke into sobs.

To have two deaths in such a short space was unprecedented at Mnene. Zshiri was alarmed, though nothing yet led him to consider that Swango might somehow be responsible.

In early July, a maternity patient, Virginia Sibanda, began experiencing what she thought were labor contractions and was moved into the labor ward in anticipation of the birth of her child. Nurses kept an eye on her for two days, and then, on the morning of July 7, as the contractions intensified, told her they would have a doctor check her progress, since they expected the baby to be born soon. "Dr. Mike" soon arrived, along with a nurse. He examined Sibanda briefly, noting that she was dilating normally. He smiled and reassured her, saying he anticipated no complications.

Not long after, the nurse called Swango back to the labor ward to check on a newborn baby who, with its mother, was sharing the room with Sibanda. Sibanda didn't pay much attention, but when Swango finished with whatever he was doing to his other patient, he approached her bedside, leaving the nurse with the baby he'd just examined. Without offering any explanation, he began to reexamine Sibanda; she felt his right hand probing her womb and vagina. At the same time, she noticed that he was groping for something with his left hand, either in a T-shirt pocket or in an inside pocket of his medical coat. What she thought was odd was that he wasn't looking at her or the pocket—his head was twisted so he could see the nurse across the room. He began withdrawing a syringe from inside his jacket, but when the nurse looked toward him, he quickly put it back, as though trying to conceal it.

Sibanda watched as Swango moved to a cupboard, withdrew a syringe, filled it from a plastic bag of sugar solution hanging from the wall, then placed it in the outer pocket of his coat. Sibanda noticed that the syringe filled with the sugar solution had a green cap over the needle. Swango spoke briefly to the nurse, then returned to Sibanda's bedside.

Swango again removed a syringe from inside his coat—not the green-topped syringe Sibanda had just seen him fill—and turned his back to the nurse. Sibanda could see that this second syringe was filled with a pinkish liquid. Swango inserted the needle into the intravenous drip attached to Sibanda's left arm. Then he called to the nurse, saying Sibanda was ready to be moved into the surgical theater for delivery. He made no entry in her chart indicating that any substance had been administered to her intravenously, and quickly left the ward without saying anything to Sibanda or looking back.

Within moments Sibanda began to feel violent abdominal pains. The baby began kicking and rocking within the womb. Sibanda screamed. Then she began to feel as though she were on fire. She cried for water, asking that it be poured over her body. Nurses converged, covered her with cold wet towels, and asked her what had happened. "Dr. Mike gave me an injection," she said, still gasping with pain. They quickly moved her to the surgical theater, where Swango was waiting. "What did you inject her with?" asked one of the nurses. Swango emphatically denied giving any injection, saying that Sibanda must have been mistaken. He said he had simply flushed her intravenous tube with a sugar solution.

Though Sibanda felt too weak to push, the pain precipitated strong contractions. With the aid of the nurses, a baby girl was successfully delivered, and Sibanda recovered.

Word of the incident spread through much of the hospital,

Chakarisa applied immediately for a search warrant, which was granted by the police superintendent at about four P.M. About an hour later, he, Dhlakama, and two police detectives reached Mnene, where they met an obviously shaken Zshiri. Zshiri spent about fifteen minutes briefing them on his recent discoveries, then indicated that Swango was on duty in one of the wards. When the group arrived, Swango was chatting with a nurse and looked relaxed. Zshiri called him aside, then led him outdoors, where he introduced him to the police officers and Dr. Dhlakama. Swango seemed calm, neither surprised nor alarmed, and suggested that the group join him in his bungalow next to the hospital.

When they reached Swango's verandah, Chakarisa produced the search warrant, gave Swango a copy, and then, reading from the warrant, said that he and his colleagues were authorized "to look for and locate drugs and syringes that are in the possession of Dr. Swango and under his control, which are on reasonable ground to believe [sic] might afford evidence of the commission of the crime." When they entered, they found the house a mess, with Swango's few clothes strewn about along with some soiled lab coats. The bed was unmade; in the kitchen they found evidence of the popcorn Zshiri had often smelled and empty Coke cans. The detectives found several charts and X rays, which they assumed to pertain to Swango's patients, as well as a list of names on a chart from Mpilo Hospital. But what immediately captured their attention was an extensive array of drugs and medical equipment. Several used syringes still contained fluids. Many of the substances were unfamiliar to Zshiri and Dhlakama. In any event, drugs were supposed to be stored in the hospital's dispensary, not in doctors' residences.

Of the hundreds of medication containers in Swango's house, forty-six had been opened, indicating the possibility they had been administered to patients. Among them were adrenaline, ephedrine, Valium, Xylocaine, Nupercainal—all fatal if injected in sufficient doses—and potassium chloride, which is not only deadly but virtually impossible to identify as a cause of death, since potassium levels are typically elevated post mortem.

As the detectives collected and inventoried the array of drugs, Chakarisa asked Swango if it were true that he had been injecting

though no one mentioned it to Zshiri or Larsson. Some patients now began saying they didn't want to be treated by Swango. One of them, Stephen Mugomeri, who was suffering from a venereal disease, demanded to be discharged, claiming he had suffered a painful reaction after an injection from Swango. His relatives tried to persuade him to stay. Among them was his niece Edith Ngwenya, a nurse's aide who worked with Swango. She was a staunch defender of him in the face of the rumors, which she attributed to some nurses' resentment over his treatment of them. But Mugomeri was adamant. He left the hospital, and died shortly after returning home.

Ngwenya was among the mourners at her uncle's funeral. She herself had been feeling unwell for several days—nausea, vomiting, dizziness, chills—and when she returned to work on the morning of July 17, the day after the funeral, she told Swango that she wasn't feeling well. Swango suggested she lie down, and contacted Zshiri, saying she should be admitted as a patient. Zshiri, of course, knew Ngwenya and was concerned, and he and Swango discussed the symptoms, concluding that she was likely suffering from malaria or possibly typhoid, even though malaria is rare during the winter months of July and August, and typhoid has largely been eradicated. As a precaution, Zshiri prescribed chloroquine and chloramphenicol. Swango reported that Ngwenya was resting comfortably; he said she felt much better.

At 11:25 A.M., Ngwenya was pronounced dead by Swango. He completed the death certificate, citing the cause of death as pneumonia. Zshiri was dumbfounded.

Swango was professionally detached from the other deaths, but he had worked closely with Ngwenya and, to all appearances, had liked her. She had been his strongest defender within the nursing staff. He seemed genuinely upset by her sudden death. Still in mourning over Mugomeri, who had left five children as orphans, Ngwenya's family was distraught and likely to be even more impoverished. They were wary of Swango and upset when he said he wanted to attend the funeral. But then he bought them a coffin. And after attending the funeral, where he seemed genuinely bereaved, he bought groceries for everyone who attended. They were touched by these acts of kindness and generosity. When one of the relatives insisted that Swango be reported to the provincial medical authorities, or at the least to the hospital director, the family overruled him, arguing that the deaths were likely caused by witchcraft by some of the nurses. They argued that it was inconceivable that Swango would have done anything to harm Ngwenya when he was willing to buy her a coffin and attend the funeral.

Two days later, Margaret Zhou was treated by Swango after suffering an incomplete (spontaneous) abortion. The patient, thirty-five years old, was otherwise healthy, and her condition was quickly stabilized with medication. That evening Dr. Larsson performed a routine evacuation of the remaining parts of the fetus, and reported that the operation had been a success. At 7:30 the next morning, July 20, Zhou was found dead.

Alarmed, Dr. Zshiri immediately launched an inquiry, summoning members of the nursing staff to his office. They seemed terrified, but refused to tell him anything. Finally a maternity nurse, Sister Gurajena, told him that she had been in the maternity ward when Virginia Sibanda had "cried for help since the doctor had injected something." The doctor in question, she said, was Dr. Mike. Sibanda was still in the hospital, and Zshiri went immediately to her bedside. Encouraged by the nurse, she told Zshiri what had happened, emphasizing that she had been injected not with the syringe containing sugar solution, but with a syringe that had been concealed in Swango's coat pocket.

Then another nurse, Sister Hove, came forward, and said she believed that Dr. Mike had injected another patient while he was asleep, but that the doctor said the patient was hallucinating. She took Zshiri to Mzezewa's bedside, where Mzezewa narrated the incident, describing in detail how he'd been paralyzed after the injection by Swango, concluding, "I did not understand what happened later but I nearly lost my life." He told Zshiri he was still frightened and wanted to be moved to a different hospital. That afternoon, Zshiri had him transferred to the Mzume Mission Hospital.

Dr. Zshiri had to face the possibility that a killer was at large in his hospital. He "panicked," as he later put it.

THE next day P. C. Chakarisa, a superintendent in the Zimbabwe Republic police, was summoned by the commander of the Midlands district to an emergency meeting in Zvishavane, the nearest town of any size to Mnene. Zvishavane is a dusty place with an aging asbestos mine as the center of economic activity; the police station is a cluster of three tin-roofed, open-air buildings grouped around a small courtyard shaded by a jacaranda tree. When Chakarisa arrived, he met the Midlands medical director, Dr. Davis Dhlakama, Zshiri's superior in the Zimbabwean medical system, and the person ultimately responsible for hiring Swango.

The day before, immediately after interviewing Mzezewa, Zshiri had called Howard Mpofu at Lutheran church headquarters in Bulawayo. Mpofu could hardly believe the reports he heard from Zshiri about the nice young man he'd met at the airport, but he told him to call Dr. Dhlakama immediately. Whereas the U.S. hospital system is decentralized, all medical doctors in Zimbabwe are paid by the state and are indirectly accountable to the minister of health in Harare, who operates through the provincial medical directors such as Dhlakama. Thus, while nominally an employee of the Lutheran church, Swango was paid by the Zimbabwe government and was accountable to Dhlakama.

While shocked by Zshiri's revelations, and concerned that reports of Swango's activities might cause panic among patients, Dhlakama had concluded immediately that the police had to be notified and brought into the case. This was in sharp contrast to the approach adopted at Ohio State. It was also obvious to both Zshiri and Dhlakama that such a situation involving a white American doctor who might be murdering Zimbabweans was politically explosive—and could cost both men their jobs.

At the meeting, Dhlakama looked grim. The medical director quickly briefed Chakarisa: a doctor at Mnene Hospital, Dr. Swango, had allegedly caused a number of deaths "through the administration of noxious substances or drugs." Since the doctor was an American, Dhlakama speculated that he might be using "foreign" drugs unfamiliar to the local doctors, and added that at the very least, there had been reports that he used unsterilized syringes. All the suspicious deaths had been certified by Dr. Swango. Dhlakama felt the police had to move quickly—there had been two deaths in the previous four days, and attempts had apparently been made on the lives of patients still in the hospital.

unauthorized drugs into patients, specifically Sibanda and Mzezewa. In contrast to his earlier statement denying that he had injected Mzezewa at all, Swango said he had injected water into his intravenous tube in order to flush it, a routine procedure. He also acknowledged that he had on occasion used unsterilized needles and had reused the same syringes. Chakarisa was offended by Swango's nonchalance, later characterizing him as "boastful." He and the others were particularly offended by one of Swango's comments to the effect that "as Africa was a jungle, syringes can be used repeatedly without harm." Swango added, by way of example, that in the Congo "injections were used again and again."

At this point, Chakarisa warned Swango that anything he said might be used against him, a statement known in Zimbabwe as a "caution," the equivalent of the U.S. Miranda warning, by which suspects are advised they have the right to remain silent. Swango said he would say nothing further until he consulted a lawyer. Dr. Dhlakama told Swango that his medical privileges would be suspended pending an investigation, and that he was not to enter any of the hospital wards.

The next morning, Swango showed up in Zshiri's office. "What's happening?" Swango asked, obviously upset.

"The staff is concerned" about the sudden outbreak of unexplained deaths, Zshiri said.

"People are against me," Swango countered. "They think I'm killing patients." Zshiri nodded, looking closely at Swango, since that was precisely what people were thinking. Swango looked very earnest, very grave. "It's not true," he said.

Zshiri thought Swango seemed too sincere, almost as though he had rehearsed the line. Earlier, perhaps, Zshiri might have believed him. But now he did not. He told Swango the suspension would have to remain in effect; that the matter was "out of his hands" now that Dhlakama, the provincial medical director, was involved. Swango accepted the news quietly. Zshiri was relieved when Swango left the office. He was under the impression that most Americans carried guns, and he feared Swango might have one.

During the next few days, Police Superintendent Chakarisa moved swiftly to interview the nurses and others at the hospital, including Sibanda. He traveled to Mzume, where Mzezewa was under guard and in isolation. The accounts he heard left Chakarisa with little doubt that he was dealing with a killer. As he later put it, "they gave startling revelations of how the murders were committed and how they discovered the crimes." He had the remains of Margaret Zhou, Swango's most recent victim at Mnene, sent to Bulawayo, where a pathologist removed tissue samples from several organs and sent them to Harare for analysis.

For his part, Zshiri drafted a letter to Dhlakama, a copy of which he sent to Lutheran church headquarters in Bulawayo. Dated July 22, 1995, the letter began "RE: Unexplained deaths, Mnene Designated District Hospital":

"There has been a sudden rise in unexplained deaths in the hospital. This led to a lot of questions and rising [sic] of eyebrows within the Mnene community, hence the coincidental findings and reports given to me by the staff. The matter is already known to you, but still I believe it is more appropriate to put it in writing."

The letter briefly summarized the mysterious deaths of Mahlamvana, Chipoko, Ngwenya, and Zhou. "The two last patients worried every health worker in the hospital. I could tell the staff had something to tell but they could not. I had to probe the sisters in charge of the wards and to my surprise there was a lot told . . .

"I have a lot of written statements from the nurses and I received today, the 23rd July, 0800 hours, after yesterday's proceedings, yet another piece of information about Mr. Katazo Shava, 52 years, male. This patient was in the ward admitted 18 June 1995, died 26 June 1995. Sudden death in the ward. I'm not aware of this death but the sisters have a lot to tell."

This was too much for Zshiri. Writing to Dhlakama, he described his reaction: "I panicked. . . . I felt I could not handle this."

Zshiri was by now under considerable stress. He worried that he might be held accountable, either by the Lutheran church or by the government, for deaths occurring on his watch. He realized as well that Swango was entitled to some sort of due process, although, never having been confronted with such a dire situation, Zshiri wasn't sure what procedures should be followed. At the same time, he didn't want to be viewed as a troublemaker, a whistleblower, someone who might bring scandal upon the church and government. All of this is evident in his concluding passage:

Finally, I would like to take this opportunity to say I am not against Dr. Mike, he is my personal friend, but the authority I was given by the Ministry of Health and the Evangelical Lutheran Church in Zimbabwe I feel it's a must that I take up these issues to you, the responsible authorities, and I have to safeguard the good works of Mnene Hospital as a district hospital. In addition, not a single one of the above patients was directly under my day-to-day care, but as overall in charge as DMO [District Medical Officer]. This is only a report as given to me.

Thank you,
Dr. C. Zshiri
District Medical Officer

IN mid-August Dhlakama received a letter from Swango warning him that "something nasty" was likely to "land" on his desk from Mnene, and that if his suspension remained in effect, "the Mnene doctors and the Mission will have to bear the consequences." Dhlakama angrily replied that he would not respond to such "threats" and that he stood behind the decision to suspend Swango from his position as a doctor at Mnene. Dhlakama phoned Mpofu in Bulawayo to inform him about the letter, telling him he thought the situation with Swango at Mnene was "very unsafe." But Dhlakama did not have the authority to terminate Swango's license to practice medicine in Zimbabwe; that action could be taken only after cumbersome administrative procedures at the Ministry of Health.

So Mpofu agreed that the church would assume responsibility for removing Swango. On October 13, he drove to Mnene and personally handed Swango a letter from the Evangelical Lutheran church formally terminating his employment. Without being specific as to the causes, the letter cited a pending investigation by the Ministry of Health and Child Welfare and added, "Also be advised that the community you have been recruited to serve has since expressed their disgruntlement with you. . . . Your services are terminated."

The letter was signed by S. M. Dube, the secretary-treasurer of the Evangelical Lutheran church in Zimbabwe.

Mpofu was frightened that Swango might react violently, but all Swango said was that the allegations were "unfounded" and that he would be consulting a lawyer. He was given a week to remove his belongings, but several nights later Zshiri noticed that Swango's cottage was dark. Swango had left without saying good-bye.

Though he had left quietly, Swango's letter to the effect that the doctors at Mnene would have to "bear the consequences" left Zshiri and Larsson skittish, fearful that Swango would return to exact his revenge. Zshiri resigned his position at Mnene to pursue additional studies in Harare, citing his fear of Swango. When Larsson's contract expired at the end of the year, he and his family returned to Sweden. No doctors responded to ads seeking to replace them.

The nursing staff, similarly afraid that Swango might return at any time, did its best to care for patients who were not only sick but, in many cases, terrified. Stories of mysterious deaths at Mnene circulated throughout the Mberengwa region, passed from homestead to homestead, village to village. Some said the Mnene nurses were practicing witchcraft. Others spoke of a sinister doctor in a white lab coat. Many heard hearsay accounts of Keneas Mzezewa's and Virginia Sibanda's injections and seizures. Increasingly, people in the bush turned to traditional healers for care. Admissions to the hospital dropped off.

Mpofu, who had greeted Swango with such enthusiasm and had been so happy to recruit a doctor from America, was stunned to find that Swango's legacy might be a mission hospital bereft not only of doctors, but also of patients.

CHAPTER ELEVEN

DAVID COLTART, then thirty-eight, tall, slender, sandy-haired, and articulate, seems at first glance the embodiment of Bulawayo's colonial British heritage, but he is in fact Zimbabwe's most prominent human rights lawyer, a specialty that, under the oppressive regime of Robert Mugabe, has kept him in constant demand. He has often aroused the ire of the dictator. In a 1999 speech defending his government's imprisonment and torture of two journalists, Mugabe cited Coltart by name as "bent on ruining the national unity."

Ironically, Coltart first gained prominence as a civil rights lawyer representing dissident politicians who were being harassed in the early years of Zimbabwean independence, many of them now prominent government officials. He founded Zimbabwe's leading human rights organization, the Bulawayo Legal Projects Center, and his dedication to constitutional government, the rule of law, and the rights of the poor and powerless have earned him a wide following and the admiration of many white and black Zimbabweans. He is easily the best-known lawyer in Bulawayo, and he also attends the Presbyterian church.

So when Swango called Ian Lorimer in August saying he might need a lawyer, Lorimer naturally thought of Coltart. The Lorimers hadn't seen much of Swango since he'd gone back to Mnene, but Abdi Mesbah, the Iranian doctor at the hospital, had reported in something of an I-told-you-so manner that Swango had stopped working at Mnene and "something was amiss." This Mesbah claimed to have heard from a Swedish nurse at Mnene, presumably Larsson's wife, but he knew no details. When Swango himself called the

Lorimers from Mnene, he told them only that "something had gone wrong" and he needed a lawyer. He declined to elaborate, saying he would explain everything when he returned to Bulawayo and saw the Lorimers in person. Ian was curious, but not all that surprised that things hadn't worked out for Swango. He knew how isolated Mnene was, and how different the bush culture.

Swango arrived at Coltart's office on the fourth floor of the Haddon & Sly building in downtown Bulawayo on August 23. The blond young doctor struck Coltart as quiet, almost timid, but idealistic and determined to clear his name. He said that he had been summarily suspended by the provincial minister of health without being told any specific charges or given any opportunity to respond. All he knew, he said, was that he was accused of having given some patients injections that caused "ill effects," and that he was being unfairly blamed for the deaths of a few patients who had died of natural causes. He added that police had come to his house at Mnene armed with a search warrant and had seized a quantity of drugs he kept there.

"Why did you have drugs in your cottage?" Coltart asked, immediately concerned that the case might involve narcotics. Swango replied that since he was coming to "darkest Africa," he had brought a selection of drugs that he thought might be unavailable at the mission hospital.

Coltart was impressed that Swango had gone to such trouble, personally carrying drugs into the country. As a lawyer trained to judge the credibility of witnesses, Coltart found Swango earnest and believable. But he was more impressed by the glowing letters of recommendation Swango produced from Doctors Oliver and King at Mpilo Hospital; Oliver, in particular, was a friend of Coltart's and a fellow member of the Presbyterian church. Coltart knew nothing about Mnene Mission Hospital, but he had heard of some factional feuds within the Evangelical Lutheran church. He thought Swango's troubles might possibly be related; then again, this might be a case of reverse discrimination against a white American doctor. Such situations were common in postindependence Zimbabwe. Coltart thought Swango idealistic and probably naive—someone who didn't understand the local culture and was in turn misunderstood. He thought it would be a terrible precedent if a promising young doctor were unfairly driven from Zimbabwe at a time the country so desperately needed doctors. So Coltart agreed to represent Swango, thus lending his considerable prestige to Swango's cause. Swango seemed relieved and agreed to pay the firm's fees in cash.

In any event, to Coltart the charges seemed vague and far-fetched. The next day he sent a letter to the police in Gweru, demanding to know on what grounds they had searched Swango's residence and to learn the details of any charges they anticipated filing. He complained that his client had been confronted with "unspecified allegations" to the effect that he had "injected patients with the wrong drugs that caused a bad effect." Coltart said he would appreciate "precise details . . . at your earliest convenience."

The police replied on September 9, writing that "precise details will be forthcoming in a matter of days." But nine days later, Coltart received a letter saying that "We are now unable to give details as the docket has been referred to a higher office for action." That "higher office" turned out to be Zimbabwe's director of public prosecution, the equivalent of the attorney general of the United States.

But the evidence was still far from conclusive. Lab results from Margaret Zhou's tissue, which had been sent to Bulawayo and then to Harare for testing, proved inconclusive. The pathologist pointed out that unless someone could indicate what substances were believed to have induced death, he had no way of proceeding—the same problem that had beset pathologists in the United States. Given the lack of physical evidence, the prosecutor's office had ordered the police to continue investigating and postponed any decision to file charges.

None of this was known to Coltart or Swango, and additional letters from Coltart produced no further explanation. As time passed and no charges or evidence materialized, Coltart began to suspect that this might indeed be a political case of antiwhite discrimination against Swango. Coltart knew of other cases—white safari operators were a recent example—in which people were arrested but never charged. In Coltart's view, the practice was one of the worst abuses of the judicial system by the authoritarian Mugabe regime.

Then, in October, Swango had received the letter from the Lutheran church terminating his employment, a letter which also made no reference to any specific charges. Coltart recognized as soon as Swango showed him the letter that Swango's termination was improper under Zimbabwean law. An employer may fire an employee only if the employee violates a code of conduct registered by the employer with the Department of Labor. Mnene Mission Hospital had no such code (few employers in Zimbabwe do). Absent such a code, the Lutheran church was within its rights to suspend Swango, but it had to apply to the Labor Ministry for an order terminating his employment, a procedure that would have given Swango an opportunity to respond.

The possibility that he was a pawn in a larger political drama was a theme Swango mentioned when he met with Ian Lorimer. As he'd promised, Swango offered Lorimer a detailed explanation of what had happened, describing three patients whose deaths had been blamed on him. One, he said, evidently referring to Phillimon Chipoko, was a diabetic who became ill after an amputation on a Friday afternoon. Swango had happened to be on duty that weekend when he died, but the man wasn't his patient. (Chipoko actually died on a Tuesday.) The second, evidently Margaret Zhou, was a woman experiencing severe bleeding after a miscarriage. Again, she was not Swango's patient, but had died while he was on duty. And the third account Swango gave was a highly abridged version of Edith Ngwenya's death. Swango said Ngwenya had worked for him, that he'd visited her socially, and that after she complained of abdominal pain, he'd insisted that she be admitted. But neither he nor Dr. Zshiri had been able to diagnose her illness before she died. Nurses unfairly suspected, he said, that he had given her a drug, which he denied. Because he was a white doctor, he said, he was being made a scapegoat for every death in the hospital.

Swango's account made selective use of the facts, and naturally Lorimer had no way of knowing that he had already told inconsistent versions of the same stories to the nurses (denying any injections) and the police (claiming he had injected water). Lorimer and his colleagues at Mpilo found Swango's account plausible, though Lorimer did think it odd that none of the doctors at Mnene had been able to diagnose Ngwenya. Mike Cotton, another resident at Mpilo, said he'd known two Dutch doctors, a husband-and-wife team, who had worked at Mnene for two years and then left when something went wrong. So there was obviously some precedent for trouble at Mnene. But Lorimer did quiz Swango about the matter.

"Did you do anything you shouldn't have?" he asked on one occasion. Swango emphatically denied it, adding that "no doubt can be cast on my management of patients."

"Did you clash with anyone?" Lorimer asked.

"No, I got along very well with everyone."

Finally, Lorimer asked him, "Were you on drugs?"

"No, of course not," Swango answered, laughing at the suggestion.

Even more persuasive than Swango's denials was the fact that David Coltart had taken on his case. Lorimer, Oliver, and other doctors at Mpilo held Coltart in exceptionally high regard, and given Coltart's reputation for integrity, believed he would not have accepted the case unless he believed Swango was being persecuted.

So when Swango said he'd like to practice medicine again at Mpilo, Lorimer and others on the medical staff were for the most part enthusiastic. Lorimer went to Mpilo's director, Dr. Chaibva, and argued that Swango should be hired despite having been dismissed from Mnene. Mpilo was desperately understaffed, and even if Swango couldn't handle everything, at least the other residents would only have to be on call every fourth night rather than every third. Swango was better than no doctor at all. Dr. Oliver, too, urged Chaibva to hire him.

Finally, Swango himself went to Chaibva and said he would be willing to work without pay if the hospital would provide living quarters. Chaibva asked him what had happened at Mnene, and Swango told him he didn't get along with church officials. But Chaibva said he'd have to get some kind of explanation from Mnene.

The next day, Chaibva called Zshiri, saying that Dr. Swango had volunteered to work at Mpilo, and that the hospital was short of staff. Zshiri was silent, which Chaibva found odd. Finally Zshiri said, "If I were you, I would not employ him."

"Why not?" Chaibva asked.

Again, there was a pause. "It's under investigation," Zshiri said. Chaibva again tried to get an explanation, but Zshiri would say nothing more, repeating only that if it were up to him, he would not hire Swango.*

Despite this admonition, Chaibva made no further inquiries about what had transpired at Mnene; he assumed, as his staff doctors had, that the problems had arisen from disputes over religious doctrine, not medical matters. And in any event, Swango's license to practice medicine was still in effect. Chaibva restored Swango's hospital privileges and Swango took up his duties at Mpilo. He began living in a room that had been used for residents when they stayed at the hospital overnight. It had a private bath and a separate entrance, and it also provided immediate—and discreet—access to the hospital wards at any hour of the day or night. By actually taking up residence in the hospital, Swango could now reach virtually every patient without being noticed by other members of the staff.

In no time, it seemed, Swango resumed his congenial life in Bulawayo—the weekly prayer meetings at the Presbyterian church, the volleyball and table tennis games, the visits to the Lorimers and the Mirtles. He even baby-sat for the Lorimers' infant daughter, Ashleigh. People thought it laudable that he was willing to work without pay at Mpilo. He threw himself into his job, carefully writing down the full names of all his patients so he could greet them by their first names. He became an advocate for patients' rights, arguing, for example, that people were having to wait too long before having operations once their conditions were diagnosed. Though they had been curious when he first arrived, no one now thought it odd that Swango, who could presumably go anywhere and earn a handsome living, was working without pay and living in a room in the hospital.

But word of the mysterious deaths at Mnene, already widespread in the Mberengwa region, inevitably reached a wider audience in Bulawayo. In mid-January a local newspaper, the *Sunday News*, ran an unbylined article with the headline "Expat Doctor 'Experimenting' on Patients"—the first published account of Swango's activities in Africa. The article read:

---

* Zshiri says that Dhlakama told him not to discuss Swango while the matter was under investigation because "they should establish the facts before anyone spoke out."

An expatriate doctor at a hospital in Mberengwa is alleged to have been experimenting with some drugs on patients, resulting in the death of three of them, The Sunday News has learnt.

The doctor, who is white, has since been relieved of his duties and it is reliably understood that he was arrested by members of the Criminal Investigations Department and is still in the country helping police with investigations.

Sources said the doctor was using drugs imported from his country on patients, especially women. Three people died as a result but The Sunday News could not establish whether the deceased were all women. Officers from the CID have carried out their investigations as far as Gweru Central Hospital.

Though there weren't many white doctors in Mberengwa, the article didn't mention names, or even the doctor's nationality, and was both sketchy and inaccurate. It didn't alarm Lorimer and the other doctors at Mpilo, who were already aware of Swango's dismissal, nor were there any follow-up articles.

Then one evening Lorimer's mother phoned him from Harare, where that day she had had lunch with someone who worked in the Ministry of Health. When Mrs. Lorimer mentioned that her son was a resident at Mpilo Hospital, the health official had told her about an American doctor who had interned there who had done "some terrible things" at Mnene Hospital, including administering poisonous injections. Mrs. Lorimer had immediately recognized that the doctor must be Dr. Swango, Ian's friend. "I don't believe it," Lorimer told his mother, dismissing the stories as preposterous rumors. "It's all political, and he's being framed." He insisted that he knew Swango well enough to trust his instincts, and his mother seemed satisfied. Still, her last words to him in the conversation were "Be careful. Beware."

The next day, Lorimer did say something to Swango to the effect that there were rumors he had injected people at Mnene, which was odd since doctors generally don't administer injections. "Did you ever give injections?" Lorimer asked him. "Did you ever experiment with poisons?"

Swango seemed shocked and genuinely puzzled. "No," he said, shaking his head emphatically, adding only that he had occasionally administered intravenous antibiotics because some of the nurses were nervous about doing it.

But the Iranian doctor, Mesbah, was also continuing to raise concerns about what had happened at Mnene, based on secondhand accounts he was hearing from the nursing staff. Finally, Mike Cotton said he'd go to Mnene and investigate himself. When he returned, he said rumors were running rampant. Swango was being blamed for scores of deaths—even of patients who died while Swango was doing his internship at Mpilo. This was obviously preposterous, and it undermined all the claims against him.

Thus, continuing reports about Swango's activities paradoxically seemed to strengthen the sense that he was a victim of antiwhite prejudice. This was reinforced by Swango's demeanor, his enthusiasm for practicing medicine, the care that he bestowed on his patients. The other doctors at Mpilo trusted their own judgment as to medical matters, and those who were white feared that the same prejudice that had apparently been aimed at Swango might easily be turned against them. Thus, other pieces of a puzzle for which the solution would later seem obvious made little or no impression on them—even the sudden rise in unexplained deaths at Mpilo that coincided with Swango's move into the hospital.

One of Lorimer's patients was a man in his late thirties who needed emergency surgery for an incarcerated hernia (a dangerous condition in which the herniated tissue cannot be pushed back into place). The patient was brought into the operating room at two A.M. and Lorimer had completed the surgery two hours later. The procedure posed no complications; indeed, Lorimer thought it had gone exceedingly well. At five A.M. the patient was dead. Swango wasn't involved with the patient, but he was in the hospital that night and, along with Lorimer, expressed bafflement at the sudden death. A postmortem was conducted, but no cause of death could be established.

A few days later, a patient was admitted with burns to the esophagus and stomach; he had swallowed hydrochloric acid in an apparent suicide attempt. He was placed on a fluid diet and, a week later, seemed to be recovering. Lorimer decided that a feeding tube should be inserted through a small incision in the abdomen, just below the stomach. It was a simple operation, and Lorimer had Swango assist him. The surgery was uneventful, and the patient seemed fine. Three days after the tube was inserted, the patient died. Again, no cause of death could be established.

Several other doctors found similar mysterious deaths among their patients, but in the rush of hospital life, and with the hospital so understaffed, no one compared notes or spotted a pattern. But finally Dr. Cotton raised a concern. A fourteen-year-old boy had been admitted to intensive care after suffering an auto accident. Swango was on duty when the teenager was admitted, and treated him. Indeed, trauma injuries were one of Swango's few strong areas of practice, and he'd recently been credited with saving the life of another teenager injured in a similar accident. Cotton subsequently oversaw the boy's progress and thought he was improving rapidly. Then the patient suddenly died.

Given the nature of the rumors from Mnene, it was perhaps inevitable that eventually Swango would be linked to the deaths at Mpilo. "I wonder if Mike was somehow involved," Cotton mused to Lorimer after discussing the mysterious case. But the two concluded it was impossible. Hadn't Swango just saved another teenager in similar circumstances?

Despite the problems at Mnene, the long hours at Mpilo, and his cramped living conditions, Swango himself seemed happier than ever, delighted to be back in Bulawayo. Although he had been dating a black nurse at Mpilo, he now seemed smitten by a thin, dark-haired young woman with two children, LeeAnne Payne, who had recently moved back to Bulawayo to live with her parents after separating from her husband in South Africa. He brought her to services at the Presbyterian church, introduced her to the Lorimers and Mirtles, and spent extended periods of time with her and her young children.

Swango would often speak to the Lorimers about what a difficult time LeeAnne was having. Her husband, he claimed, had been abusive, but her parents were strongly opposed to divorce and didn't approve of her dating Swango. But neither did they seem all that pleased that she had come back to live with them, especially her father, who often complained about the children, Swango said. At one point Swango told Lorimer that he felt so sorry for her, given what she'd been through, that he had offered to pay for some therapy for her. He asked Lorimer for the names of some psychologists or counselors who might be able to help.

Ian Lorimer wasn't sure that LeeAnne felt as strongly about Swango as he did about her. While she was obviously shaken by the apparent failure of her marriage and needed a friend, Lorimer thought that Swango often dominated her in conversation and seemed to want to control her movements—the very kind of relationship-threatening behavior that was discussed at the Lorimers' marriage seminars. LeeAnne mentioned this to the Lorimers on occasion, and also that Swango talked too much, a problem the Lorimers were familiar with. But these seemed minor complaints.

Much as the Lorimers enjoyed the company of Swango, they did find some of his tastes somewhat peculiar, especially for a professed Christian. On one occasion the Lorimers rented the movie *Pulp Fiction*, because Swango said it had been a popular and critical success in America and had revived John Travolta's career. They invited Swango to watch it with them. The film was exceedingly violent and bloody, with a particularly intense sequence of sadomasochistic torture. Within ten minutes, the Lorimers were horrified and wanted to turn off the tape. But Swango was fascinated, insisted on watching, and said afterward that he loved the film.

They ascribed his enthusiasm to the fact that Swango was a film buff. He attended every film festival in Bulawayo. He seemed to know every classic movie, and devoured reviews of new films in *Time* and *Newsweek*. He watched *Twelve Angry Men*, the 1957 film about a murder trial, with the Lorimers and proclaimed it a "brilliant" film, which he'd like to see again. He was also wildly enthusiastic about two films that became available on video while he was in Bulawayo. One was *The Shawshank Redemption*, a critically acclaimed 1994 film in which a young banker is unjustly sent to prison for the murder of his wife and his wife's lover. But his favorite, he often said, was *Four Weddings and a Funeral*, which he described with delight as a "sleeper," a film that Hollywood hadn't expected to do well, but that had taken the movie world by storm. Nominated along with *Shawshank Redemption* for an Academy Award for best picture, the film features Hugh Grant as a young man whose own romance unfolds in the settings of his friends' weddings. But for many viewers, the film's most moving sequence concerned the sudden death and the funeral of another character.

Violence and death often surfaced one way or another in conversations with Swango. One evening Swango gave the Lorimers copies of an article he had clipped from the South African edition of *Reader's Digest* and insisted that they read it. He continued to pester them about it until they said they had. The article, "Stalking Evil," was an excerpt from a book by John Douglas, an FBI agent, who, the article said, did "nothing less than peer into the minds of serial killers and rapists." Douglas had been instrumental in developing psychological profiling as a technique in solving serial crimes, and as part of his work, had interviewed numerous convicted serial killers. As Douglas wrote in the article,

> It used to be that most crimes, particularly violent crimes like homicide, happened between people who knew each other, and resulted from feelings that we can all experience: anger, greed, jealousy, revenge. But these days more and more crimes are being committed by and against strangers. In recent years a dangerous type of violent criminal has become more common—the serial offender. Because their victims are strangers and their motivations are complex, serial killers and rapists are the most difficult to catch of all violent criminals.

The article surveyed a number of murders in which Douglas had been involved. While no clear psychological pattern emerged among the perpetrators, several were above average in intelligence, all but one were white, some were the children of "a domineering mother and physically abusive father," and some had suffered chronic bed-wetting as children. And Douglas insisted that no matter how peculiar they may be, all serial killers establish a pattern that can eventually identify them: "No matter how such a serial killer throws us off his track, he's still going to give us behavioral clues to work with, whether he intends to or not," Douglas wrote. And, he concluded, "I learned that even the smartest, most clever criminals are vulnerable. It doesn't matter how shrewd or experienced they are. And it doesn't even matter if they know about our techniques. They can all be gotten to—it's just a matter of figuring out how."

Ian and Cheryl read the article, found it mildly interesting, and wondered why Swango had gone to such efforts to share it with them.

Swango's reputation at Mpilo was now so solid that on March 4, Dr. Oliver, at David Coltart's request, wrote another glowing letter of recommendation for him, one that could be used in a suit against the Evangelical Lutheran church.

Coltart had still gotten no further explanation from the police. Eight months later, on November 16, he received a letter saying that "the docket had long since been completed" and that Swango should await the decision of the public prosecutor. But no charges were forthcoming, and a December letter went unanswered. Coltart said that Swango himself could bring matters to a head by filing suit against the church, alleging wrongful discharge. While the Lutheran church had told Coltart that under no circumstances would it re-employ Swango, he might be able to collect damages and back pay. Swango was immediately enthusiastic, saying he wanted to go forward with the suit to clear his name.

On the one hand, Swango's reaction was reassuring, since it would have been foolhardy to proceed if there were any truth to the reports from Mnene. On the other hand, Coltart at times wondered why Swango was going to such trouble and expense in an African country that was suffering so many problems and was not, after all, his native land. Before proceeding with the suit, he felt obliged to air these concerns with his client.

"Why bother with this?" he asked Swango when the two met to go over the complaint. "Why not go back to the U.S.? You are a medical doctor. You could practice anywhere."

But Swango insisted he loved Zimbabwe and wanted to stay. And, almost shyly, he suggested a more important reason: he had fallen in love.

FOSTER DONGOZI, a reporter for the Bulawayo *Chronicle,* the local daily newspaper, shared an apartment with his cousin, who happened to be an orderly at Mpilo Hospital. "There's a white expatriate doctor living in the ward," he mentioned one evening. Dongozi found the claim hard to believe. Why would a doctor live in the ward? But his cousin insisted it was true, so Dongozi drove out to the hospital and approached several staff members. No one wanted to talk. So Dongozi asked his cousin to check the report. This time he not only confirmed the story, but added, "It is believed he was chased from Mnene after killing people," a story which he said was circulating widely among the hospital staff. He said the doctor's name was Swan.

Sensing a major story, Dongozi returned to the hospital, again asking staff members if such a doctor was working there. No one would comment, but several gave him cryptic smiles, and one urged him to speak to the hospital superintendent. No one denied anything, and that suggested he was on to something. So Dongozi went to the hospital switchboard and asked the operator to page "Dr. Swan." The operator declined, saying he thought the doctor was out. But just then, a voice said, "Did I hear someone mention my name?"

"Dr. Swan?" Dongozi asked, turning to a young blond man wearing blue corduroy trousers and a white lab coat.

"I'm Dr. Swango," the man replied. "Can I help you?"

By this time several people had gathered in the switchboard room and were curiously looking on. Dongozi stepped out into the corridor and said, "My name is Foster Dongozi, and I'm a reporter for the *Chronicle*." Dongozi noticed that Swango's eye began to twitch. "I understand you are being investigated for a series of deaths at Mnene Hospital."

Swango's whole body began to tremble. He raised his right hand as if to ward off Dongozi, and began to back away. "I can't answer that," he said. "Talk to my lawyer." He began to run down the corridor. "What's his name?" Dongozi shouted after him.

"David Coltart." Swango rounded a corner and disappeared.

The next day Dongozi called on Dr. Chaibva and asked him if Dr. Swango was living in the hospital. "I don't know where he lives," Chaibva answered.

"Is he being investigated for killing people at Mnene?"

"I don't know that." Chaibva was obviously uncomfortable at the questions. "I have heard stories about him, but it's not clear what the stories are."

"Why did you hire him?" Dongozi asked.

Chaibva shrugged. "There's a shortage of doctors."

Dongozi left, unsure whether he had enough for a story. But events quickly overtook him.

That same week, Swango had gone to Chaibva and asked to be paid for his work. Chaibva had said that was out of the question. He was also annoyed, since he thought Swango was reneging on their agreement. In any event, Chaibva didn't have a discretionary fund of that kind. Now the press was asking about Swango, which meant the situation could erupt into a public scandal. Worried about his own potential exposure, Chaibva called the Ministry of Health in Harare.

News that Swango was working at another hospital in Zimbabwe came as a shock to Timothy Stamps, the minister of health and child welfare. "Stop him," Stamps ordered Chaibva. He told him to terminate Swango's employment immediately and remove him from the hospital's premises. He told Chaibva what had really happened at Mnene, which left Chaibva in stunned disbelief.

Chaibva summoned Swango to his office. "Your services are no longer required," he announced, and told him to vacate the hospital. Swango seemed resigned to the news. He shrugged and said, "Okay," then left the office without seeking any further explanation.

The following Sunday, March 24, 1996, the *Sunday News* ran a huge front-page headline: "Ministry Dismisses Doctor." The story began:

> HARARE—The Ministry of Health and Child Welfare is investigating an American expatriate doctor for allegedly fatally injecting five patients at a district hospital in the Midlands province.
>
> Dispelling fears that the expatriate doctor was now operating at Mpilo Central Hospital in Bulawayo, the Minister of Health and Child Welfare, Dr. Timothy Stamps, said the doctor had since been dismissed.
>
> He said the doctor only worked for a week at Mpilo where, due to an acute shortage of medical practitioners, he had been employed after being dismissed by the ministry in October last year.
>
> The American doctor has been accused of deliber-

ately and unlawfully experimenting with patients at
Mnene District Hospital in Mberengwa, by injecting them
with unknown chemical substances which allegedly led to
the death of five patients at the hospital.

The article was much more extensive and accurate than the
brief January account in the same newspaper; it alleged that the doctor had "sneaked into patients' wards at night," that "nurses actually
saw him give the injections," and that a "cocktail of drugs" was discovered by police at the doctor's house in Mnene. Still, the article
did not name the doctor.

Dongozi was upset that the *Chronicle*'s sister publication had
beaten him to the story. "We've been scooped," his editor complained.

CHAPTER TWELVE

L YNETTE O'HARE excused herself from the guests at her champagne brunch to answer the phone. Born in British Burma, O'Hare had moved to Rhodesia as a child. Tall, with erect posture, she had a dignified manner, impeccable manners, and an accent that all spoke of her colonial British background and her training at the London Academy of Music and Dramatic Art. She'd had the servants get out her best crystal and silver for the occasion, a farewell party for her daughter, Paulette, who, at age twenty-seven, was leaving home and, like many other white Zimbabweans in recent years, moving to England.

"Paulette," O'Hare called, "it's for you."

Despite the festive trappings that morning in late March 1996, O'Hare was depressed that her only daughter was moving so far away. Her husband had died in 1990, and his hunting trophies, including the head of a water buffalo, hung on the walls. She'd become a certified public accountant—though her real loves were drama and speech—and she had taken a job at National Foods to support herself and their daughter. Now that Paulette was leaving, O'Hare would be left without close relatives in Bulawayo.

Not that she was likely be alone with time on her hands. She had two servants, Mary Chimwe and Elizabeth Keredo, who lived in a cottage next to the swimming pool and were in the house most of the day, as well as a gardener who maintained the collection of flowering vines and plants in the walled gardens that surrounded her spacious house in Malindela, an attractive suburb just south of the Bulawayo Golf Club. O'Hare not only had her job, but was prominent in Bulawayo's influential Rotary Club and the Presbyterian church (though she was contemplating conversion to Catholicism). She also gave private voice lessons. Still, she'd miss Paulette and her youthful circle of friends, who so often enlivened gatherings at the house.

When Paulette returned from taking the call, she seemed delighted. "It's an American chap I know from Bible study," she told her mother. "Why don't you take him in?" Indeed, every Tuesday evening the Bible group joined hands to pray for one cause or another, and just the week before, Paulette had asked everyone to pray "that someone nice would come to live with Mum." Paulette had pretty much convinced her mother that the solution to her anticipated loneliness was to find a suitable lodger, and now a possibility had presented itself.

The gardener admitted Michael Swango through the front gates a few days later, on March 31, 1996, and O'Hare met him at the door. She noticed a tic, or squint, that seemed to affect his right eye. She looked around to see what kind of car he drove, but there was none in sight. He introduced himself as Michael Swan.

O'Hare invited him into the parlor, where the two sat down and Keredo served them tea. O'Hare was immediately reassured when "Swan" told her he was a doctor, a profession that was not only eminently respectable but would assure her of steady rental payments. He said he had been working at Mpilo Hospital, and had come from America to help "uplift" the Africans, "to do his part for humanity." She asked him his age, and he teasingly replied, "How old do you think I am?"

"Thirty-five," O'Hare guessed.

"Oh no," he answered, in mock indignation. "I'm twenty-seven."

"That's Paulette's age," O'Hare exclaimed, delighted that she would have someone her daughter's age around the house.

It seemed that in no time "Swan" had ferreted out O'Hare's interest in military history, something that even some of her friends in Bulawayo didn't know about. He told her his father had had a military career, and then mentioned several books in the field he'd read. O'Hare was captivated. She proudly showed him her own extensive library, each book carefully shelved and catalogued. He exclaimed

over her works of English literature, and told her that he loved
everything English. That, too, delighted O'Hare, an unabashed An-
glophile.

Terms of Swango's lodging were quickly reached. O'Hare
would provide a room, breakfast, and lunch. Lizzie Keredo and
Mary Chimwe would clean, provide linens, do the laundry, and cook
for him. In return, he would pay Z$800 per month. He would also
be responsible for buying his own meat for the evening meal.
O'Hare gave him a choice of bedrooms, and he picked the one that
had been Paulette's, at the rear of the house. O'Hare found him
charming, delightful, articulate, and well-read. She could hardly believe her good fortune. It seemed that Paulette's prayers had indeed
been answered.

Swango arrived the next day with two metal trunks, a large duffel bag, and a backpack. Keredo and Chimwe had moved Paulette's
furniture out of the room Swango had chosen, but now he changed
his mind, saying he preferred the room at the front of the house, directly adjacent to O'Hare's corner bedroom. The two women were
annoyed, because they had to shift the heavy furniture again and
Swango neither offered to help nor even thanked them when they
had finished. Indeed, O'Hare's servants took an almost instant dislike to Swango, a feeling that hardened as he proceeded to give them
orders, act rude and unfriendly, and never express any appreciation
for their efforts.

But none of this was apparent to O'Hare, who was so pleased
with her new lodger that she began inviting him to share dinner
with her. They would discuss books—both turned out to be avid
fans of political novelist Allen Drury, author of *Advise and
Consent*—and current events, which they would typically discuss
after watching the evening news while sipping a cocktail, often prepared by Swango. One evening Swango brought LeeAnne to the
house, introducing her to O'Hare as his girlfriend. O'Hare found
LeeAnne attractive and pleasant, though obviously lonely, because
of her failed marriage.

O'Hare did notice, however, that Swango never seemed to be
at work at the hospital, or anywhere else for that matter. Keredo
and Chimwe reported that he spent most of his days in the house.

"Are you taking a leave?" she asked one evening.

"No," he replied. "I'm waiting for my work permit to come through."

This sounded plausible to O'Hare, who like many white Zimbabweans had been appalled by the decline in administrative efficiency since independence. She gave the matter little further thought, assuming the permit would arrive in due course. She hadn't noticed the article in the *Sunday News,* which appeared the same day as the brunch.

Another reason that Swango was at home so often was that LeeAnne had curtailed their visits and outings. Her husband was coming from South Africa to visit the children, and she said she thought it best if Swango wasn't around when he arrived. When he told Lorimer this news, Swango seemed incredulous. He couldn't believe that LeeAnne would banish him in favor of her husband, who'd been so abusive to her. Though he was upset, he remained confident that LeeAnne would come to her senses (as he saw it) and resume their relationship as soon as the husband left. But during the visit, LeeAnne phoned to tell Swango that she and her husband might reconcile, as her parents hoped they would do. Although she didn't mention it, it is also possible that she or her parents had seen the *Sunday News* article and connected it to Swango. Whatever the cause, she said she couldn't see Swango again, and broke off the relationship.

When O'Hare saw Swango that evening, he was ashen and shaken. He could talk of nothing but LeeAnne, and seemed desperate. He even asked O'Hare to phone LeeAnne to tell her she "was doing the wrong thing." But O'Hare demurred, feeling it would be pointless to get in the middle of what was obviously a tangled domestic situation. Besides, she didn't even know LeeAnne, having met her on only the one occasion. Swango seemed bitterly disappointed, as though O'Hare had let him down, and retreated to his room.

There he remained for eight days. He stopped shaving and looked increasingly gaunt and haggard. His curtains were drawn. He refused to emerge for meals, demanding that one of the servants bring them to him on a tray. When they knocked on his door, he opened it only slightly before wordlessly taking the tray and slamming the door shut. He refused to allow Keredo and Chimwe to clean the room, answering their knocks with a surly "Who is it?" and "What do you want?" Finally he told them, "Don't worry about me. I'm only worried about my girlfriend." If he encountered O'Hare when he emerged to use the bathroom, he'd immediately retreat, or rush to the bathroom and close the door. When O'Hare's nephew, Duncan, visited from South Africa, she insisted that Swango come out to meet him. He did so briefly, seemed hostile, and immediately returned to his room. When the Kerrs, other friends whom she wanted Swango to meet, came for drinks, Swango refused to greet them.

O'Hare was so worried about Swango that when she had to leave for a visit to South Africa, she feared he might attempt suicide. She called a local organization, the Samaritans, spoke to a psychologist named "Dave," and asked him to phone Swango in her absence.

But Lizzie Keredo took a more wary view of Swango. She told O'Hare that she was growing frightened of him and that he had treated her and Mary Chimwe rudely. Once he threw a tantrum, saying he didn't like the smell of floor polish. He continued to lock the two women out of his room so they couldn't clean, asking "Why are you so curious? What do you want to see?" Swango insisted on the same breakfast every morning: two fried eggs, four slices of toast, and a full kilogram of fried bacon. He was furious if he was served less than a kilogram of bacon, which Keredo thought was an exorbitant and costly amount. He also ran up electricity bills, always using a space heater while he bathed and frequently using it in his bedroom as well. (Few homes in Bulawayo have central heating.) When O'Hare complained about the high electricity bills, Swango denied using the heater. Keredo and Chimwe were too frightened to contradict him, though they knew he was lying. Even more ominous, Lizzie had recently mentioned to her boyfriend that they were living with an American doctor, and the boyfriend had asked, "Is he the one who killed people at Mnene?" Shocked, she replied that no, he worked at Mpilo. But the question had made her wonder.

When Keredo mentioned this to her employer, it reminded O'Hare of the brief article about an unnamed American expatriate doctor who was "experimenting" on patients. O'Hare had noticed the original, January article, but had given it little thought since then. Now it dawned on her that she was living with a white expatriate doctor who had worked at Mnene, and how many others fitting the description were there likely to be? "I think he's the doctor from Mnene Mission Hospital," Lizzie Keredo told her.

Somewhat alarmed, O'Hare got on the phone to Ian Lorimer, whom she knew from church and as a friend of Paulette's. She also knew that Swango and LeeAnne had been socializing with Lorimer and his wife. "Ian," she began, "[Swango] is behaving very peculiarly." She explained that he'd been virtually locked in his room since breaking up with LeeAnne. Then she mentioned the article in the newspaper. "Is he this expatriate?"

"He is," Lorimer confirmed, but then he quickly reassured O'Hare. "It's all a put-up job." He explained that the nurses at Mnene, evidently jealous of Swango's authority, had been spreading false rumors that he was killing patients. This struck a chord with O'Hare, who is of the belief that, as she put it, "jealousy is part of the African nature. One has to be very careful." She had read of a recent episode in Harare in which a white anesthetist had been accused of experimenting on patients; the case was widely viewed as one of discrimination against white doctors. But what clinched the matter for O'Hare was that Lorimer told her that David Coltart was representing Swango, and that he was suing Mnene Hospital. O'Hare thought the world of Coltart. It was inconceivable he'd represent someone unless he had a good case. Now she assumed that she knew why the newspaper hadn't printed Swango's name: it wouldn't dare to if he was represented by Coltart.

Immensely relieved, O'Hare nonetheless took advantage of the conversation to get a message to Swango through Lorimer. "He's upsetting my domestics," she said. "I wish you'd say something to him."

The next day, having spoken to Lorimer, Swango emerged from his isolation to join O'Hare at breakfast. He had showered and shaved. "I understand you're worried," he said reassuringly. When she explained that she was indeed upset by his recent isolation and state of mind, and then had read the newspaper article, he offered much the same explanation that Lorimer had. The nurses at Mnene had grown jealous, he said. That same morning, he apologized to Lizzie Keredo and Mary Chimwe. O'Hare felt her heart go out to this poor, young, idealistic doctor who was being persecuted, and she chastised Keredo for her dark suspicions. "If you were educated," O'Hare told her dismissively, "you would understand."

IN Newton West, a Bulawayo suburb south and west of O'Hare's house, life lately hadn't been easy for Joanna Daly. Recently separated from her husband, Steve, she was trying to keep divorce proceedings amicable, but he had taken up with another woman, a situation made all the more painful by his proximity. He was living in the servants' cottage on the property, while Joanna and the four children, all boys, ages two through eight, remained in the spacious ranch house with its kidney-shaped pool. With the often boisterous young children on her hands, Joanna couldn't think of getting a job outside the home, so she had begun a dressmaking business in the former sun room. She could no longer afford the maids who once occupied the cottage, and had only a part-time gardener and handyman to help around the house. Her days seemed an unending sequence of cooking, laundry, and sewing, and she was barely making ends meet.

Though Daly was attractive—slender, soft-spoken, with light reddish-brown hair—the idea that she might meet another man or go out on a date seemed remote to her. She hardly ever got out of the house except to drive the children to school, and by nightfall she was usually too tired, even if she could have afforded a babysitter. So she was floored when Karen Kerr, Steve's sister, invited her to dinner late in June 1996, saying that there was a "nice man" she wanted Joanna to meet.

Joanna told herself that she didn't want to meet another man and certainly had no intention of remarrying. Still, she did her hair, put on makeup, and wore her most attractive clothing to the Kerrs' dinner. And much to her surprise, she immediately found the man in question good-looking and charming. He was a doctor. He had apologized for his earlier rudeness in failing to greet the Kerrs, and through O'Hare's persistence, they had since become friendly. The Kerrs, too, embraced Swango's version of what had happened at Mnene. They told Joanna he had been persecuted while working there, unfairly blamed for the deaths of several patients. Indeed, when they introduced her to Michael Swango, they joked that his nickname was "Dr. Death."

Swango seemed instantly attracted to Joanna. Showing the
same unerring instinct he had with O'Hare, he quickly discovered
that both her father and uncle were career officers in the British
military, and then told her all about his own military upbringing: his
father served as a colonel in the Army in Vietnam; the family had
moved frequently; his father was authoritarian and was absent from
the home for long periods. All of this Joanna could relate to. Her
own father had been harsh and domineering, often belittling her
achievements, scoffing at notions of women's rights. He had made
her feel that her only option in life was to marry, have children, and
be a housewife, which was what she had done. As she put it, "I'm
used to being dictated to." But she needed to say very little. Swango
kept up a monologue throughout the evening, and never allowed his
attention to stray. Her head was spinning from the attention.

The next day, Swango phoned her at home, and Joanna invited
him over that afternoon for a cup of tea. Her estranged husband
happened to be in the house when he called, which Joanna men
tioned, and Swango said he didn't want to have to deal with him.
But she assured him that Steve wouldn't be present when Swango
arrived. Overhearing the conversation, her husband did go into
a jealous tirade, and Joanna later suspected him of spying on
Swango's arrival.

Swango came for tea and stayed for hours. He asked Joanna
how old she was, and when she said she'd be twenty-eight in November, told her he was the same age. He talked about what a committed Christian he was, citing his attendance at the Presbyterian
church, at Bible study, and at the Lorimers' marriage seminar. He
even showed her a pamphlet on Christian marriage that he'd been
studying. Daly was a bit nervous about such sudden talk of marriage, but she was impressed by his seeming earnestness and de-
cency. By the end of the afternoon, she felt all but overwhelmed by
the handsome, attentive young doctor who had so suddenly bright-
ened her otherwise bleak life.

Soon Swango was spending nearly every day at Daly's house.
She'd pick him up at Lynette O'Hare's in the morning when she
drove two of the boys to school, and take him back when she picked
them up at the end of the school day. Often he would regale her
with stories, especially of Mrs. O'Hare, whom he ridiculed as a

fussy English aristocrat, always worrying that he was touching her things. He told Daly he was convinced O'Hare had commissioned the servants to spy on him.

Swango would plan excursions for the two of them and the children—picnics, for example, or outings to a game park. He was a fitness buff and would sometimes go jogging in a West Virginia Mountaineers sweatshirt. He wouldn't eat sugar and fretted about getting enough fiber in his diet. Increasingly often, Joanna would prepare dinner for him, and he would stay with her for most of the evening. He told her how much he'd loved *Four Weddings and a Funeral,* and when she said she had a VCR, he got a copy of the tape and they watched it together. Swango seemed especially to enjoy the part where the Hugh Grant character leaves his prospective bride at the altar in order to marry his real love, Andie MacDowell. Daly came to realize that death and marriage were Swango's favorite topics.

Swango continued his volleyball, table tennis, and badminton games, usually without Daly, but the two socialized with the Lorimers, or visited the Kerrs or other friends of Joanna. One afternoon Swango took her to meet his landlady, and O'Hare served them tea by the pool behind the house. But Joanna felt somewhat intimidated by O'Hare, whom she deemed to come from a higher social class than her own, and on the many other occasions when she picked Swango up or dropped him off at the house, she stayed in the car or remained outside the gate.

Although Swango was talkative and sociable, most days he preferred to work alone in Daly's living room while she worked on her sewing. He always seemed to be scribbling in notebooks, doing some kind of writing, but he made it clear that he didn't want Daly to pry into his activities. Given how upset he was that O'Hare's maids were spying on him, Daly respected his privacy. She wouldn't go so far as to say she was in love with him, let alone that she would marry him, but the relationship blossomed into romance. Although Swango never spent any money on her or bought her gifts, neither had other men in her life, and she recognized that as a missionary doctor, he was unlikely to have much money. After the emotional trough she had been in with her husband, she was flattered by Swango's affection and attention. While he never asked her in so many words to marry him, he often discussed the subject, saying how much he would like to be married and leaving little doubt that she was his choice for a wife. Daly felt better about herself than she had in years.

Acquiescent by habit, she didn't ask Swango many questions. As he'd been with everyone else in Bulawayo, he was vague about his birthplace, his schooling, where he'd worked in the United States—any geographic reference that might be traced. He attributed his lack of a medical job to reverse racism, but otherwise said little about Mnene or Mpilo. Still, as the weeks went by and their lives settled into something of a comfortable routine, Daly learned a good deal about him; more, probably, than had anyone else in Bulawayo. He often talked about his father, a man he seemed to resent bitterly. He said Virgil had had a brilliant military career, but ended up dying an alcoholic. He told her that his father had kept a famous photograph of a Viet Cong soldier on his knees with a gun held to his head—the Pulitzer Prize–winning photograph Virgil had shown him years before. He also told her how, when he and his brothers were young children, his father would make them march in formation, salute, and execute his commands whenever visitors came to the Swango home. He said it was something he had always hated. When Daly said she didn't think it sounded so terrible, he angrily retorted, "I don't think it's right."

Swango rarely mentioned his brothers, except for his older half brother, who, he said, also despised their father and was the only one of their siblings he got along with. Nor did he refer to any friends, with one exception. He spoke often of "Bertie Joe," a Southern name, he said, belonging to his best friend. Bertie Joe was a medical specialist who traveled a lot, Swango told Daly—a description that fits Bert Gee, the respiratory therapist in Atlanta with whom Swango often stayed after he left Stony Brook. But he never used Gee's real name, so Daly could never have contacted him, had it occurred to her to do so. Swango described Bertie Joe as a "big, powerful guy" who was always very protective of him. If there was any trouble, Swango said, Bertie Joe would just pull out his big revolver. Joanna laughed at the image, thinking that this must be what life was like in America, where everyone carried guns.

Swango often returned to the subject of his family. He said that

he dreaded family vacations, when he and his brothers would be in-
stalled in the backseat for what seemed like endless drives across
middle America. He said their parents ignored them, sitting in the
front seat, mostly in silence, smoking. He said he never detected
any warmth in his parents' marriage, and that they rarely saw each
other, even during the increasingly rare periods when Virgil was at
home. Swango spoke with much more affection about Muriel, who
he said had read to him as a child, typed all his school papers for
him, and held a semblance of a family together. Still, he described
his home life as a lonely one, from which he often sought refuge in
books at the public library. He wistfully described a Christmas
break when he spent every day alone at the library.

Indeed, he remained an avid reader, especially of crime and detective novels, which he read constantly when he wasn't busy with
his own writing. Sometimes he tried to tell Daly the plots, but they
sounded twisted and sordid to her, and she told him she wasn't interested. But one day Swango seemed unusually excited, and said he
wanted to write a book himself that he thought might be a best-
seller. He insisted on telling her the idea. "Someone is in town," he
began, "and there's a serial killer at large. Then someone else kills in
the same way. Everyone thinks this person is the serial killer—but
they're wrong! They relax, and ten years go by. Then the serial killer
kills again—just for fun." Daly wasn't sure she ever quite understood the plot, but Swango seemed so excited that she bought him a
large book of blank paper so he could begin writing the novel.

Then there was his fascination with Ted Bundy. When Swango
heard that a miniseries on Bundy's life was going to air on Zimbabwean television, he insisted on watching and taping it on Daly's
VCR. Swango was riveted to the screen. He told Daly that he loved
Bundy.

"You mean you loved the show."

"No, I love Bundy," he said. "He was a genius."

Swango took the tape and played it for the Lorimers. He called
particular attention to the program's description of Bundy's mental
state, which suggested that the "normal" Bundy was unable to recognize the "abnormal" state that coexisted in his mind.

He showed a similar interest in Jim Jones, the charismatic religious leader of the People's Temple whose nearly one thousand fol-

lowers committed mass suicide in 1978 by poisoning themselves in Guyana.

If these incidents struck Daly as somewhat macabre, as they did, they hardly seemed cause for concern. Many people were fascinated by people like Bundy and Jones, she assumed, or there wouldn't be miniseries about them. And Swango's interest in murder was more than overshadowed by his sense of humor, his kindness, and his encouragement. She especially liked the way he could converse with her pet green parrot, comically imitating the bird's voice. At the same time, he said he felt bad for the parrot being confined in a cage, saying no one should be cooped up like that. He was also affectionate toward Daly's part-Siamese cat, though he told her an odd anecdote about a cat he had once owned. He said he'd left the cat alone for a month with a supply of food, and the cat had thrived. "But what about the litter box?" exclaimed Daly, aghast at the idea of the filth, knowing that cats abhor an unclean litter box. Swango only shrugged, and seemed amused by her reaction.

Swango also seemed concerned for the rights of minorities. One day he criticized the city of Los Angeles, where alcohol commissioners were allegedly harassing gay bars. He staunchly defended the rights of homosexuals. Daly was surprised at his view, saying that she thought homosexuality was "wrong" and that in conservative Zimbabwe, most straight men would like to shoot gay men. Swango insisted that she was wrong, spent a good deal of time explaining homosexuality to her, and eventually persuaded her to change her views on the matter.

He was even more forceful on the subject of women's rights, an unusual stance in Zimbabwe. He insisted that it was ridiculous for women to assume they could only aspire to be housewives. He encouraged Cheryl Lorimer to pursue an interest in psychology. And at his urging, Joanna began reading some of Swango's medical texts, which she found surprisingly absorbing. Swango told her he thought she might have an aptitude for medicine. He urged her to go back to school, finish the equivalent of a high school degree, and study medicine. She was thrilled by the suggestion. No man had ever before suggested she was intelligent or encouraged any intellectual pursuits, let alone told her that she might have the ability to become a medical doctor.

At times like this, Daly thought she might be in love with Swango. But at the same time, she knew on some level that the relationship might not last. She was well aware there were things that Swango wouldn't share with her, that kept him at a distance, such as his pent-up anger or frustration. He went through mood swings, which she could tell from his handwriting: when he was cheerful and ebullient, his handwriting was open and rounded; when he seemed depressed, it became cramped and slanted, almost as though it were someone else's. When he was in a dark mood, Daly couldn't reach him; she found it better to leave him alone, writing furiously in his notebooks.

There was also the possibility that he might soon find work and leave Zimbabwe altogether, even though he said he loved the country and wanted to stay in Bulawayo. She knew he was filling out applications for medical jobs in places like South Africa and Zambia; he mentioned a trauma unit in Johannesburg that he was especially interested in. Daly took out a post box in both their names so that he would have a mailing address to use on his job applications.

Swango never said much to Daly about what had happened at Mnene, or why he was having trouble finding medical work in Bulawayo, which was suffering from such a shortage of doctors. Like the Kerrs, who had introduced him to her, she was vaguely aware that he had been falsely accused of malpractice of some sort, and that he was suing the Lutheran church. But she didn't press him for any further explanation and he didn't volunteer any.

One day, however, she had what she considered a peculiar call from Karen Kerr, who asked her how things were going with Michael. Joanna said they were fine. "Just be careful," Kerr said.

"Why?" Daly asked, surprised.

"You know he had another girlfriend, and she dumped him," Kerr said ominously.

"Why? Is there anything else?"

But Kerr said she couldn't say any more. Daly mentioned this to Swango, and it seemed to irritate him. "Everyone is gossiping about me," he complained. He seemed to want to go out less and less.

Then, in late July, the *Sunday News* ran another article: "Whereabouts of Fired U.S. Doctor Unknown." The article said police were "mum" on the whereabouts of "an American doctor who is alleged to have caused the deaths of five patients at Mnene Hospital." It added,

> The American doctor is alleged to have administered fatal injections to five patients at the district hospital, resulting in their deaths.
>
> Five nurses from the hospital were summoned to Zvishavane to help with the investigations.

Swango's name still wasn't mentioned, but Joanna knew it was he, and she raised the subject of the continuing press coverage. "People just don't write all these stories out of nothing," she told him. "You must have done something."

Swango seemed shocked and annoyed at her suggestion. "No, no," he insisted. "They're just causing trouble. It's a nuisance. People are always hassling me."

"Are you sure?" she persisted. "You're not lying, are you?"

"No, no, no," he repeated, shaking his head emphatically.

Although she had questioned him, Daly didn't doubt Swango. She trusted her intuition and her feelings, which told her he couldn't be guilty of murder, or a danger to anyone else.

The first week of August, all four of Daly's children fell ill with nausea, vomiting, and diarrhea. She blamed the illness on the local water supply, which had been causing problems in the wake of a severe drought. She was getting them into her car to take them to the doctor when her husband emerged from the cottage and asked where they were going. She said the boys were sick. "Why don't you have your doctor boyfriend take care of them?" he asked in an insinuating tone. This infuriated her. She had never considered having Swango treat them. He wasn't a proper doctor, as she saw it, since he wasn't practicing, and in any event he wasn't a pediatrician. The children's doctor sent them home, saying they probably had a stomach virus.

Though her hands were full with the sick children, Joanna still felt obliged to cook Swango's dinner that evening. She'd promised him fried chicken, as close as she could get to commercial Kentucky Fried Chicken, which he'd often said was his favorite food. Swango arrived that afternoon in an unusually good mood, asking after the children and offering to fix her a cup of tea. She was surprised. He'd never offered to prepare anything for her before. "That would be nice," she said, grateful for the kind gesture.

Swango brought Daly the tea, and she sat down and drank at least half of it, perhaps more. Then she went into the kitchen to begin preparing dinner. But after about ten minutes, she suffered a sudden attack of nausea. "Excuse me," she said to Swango as she rushed to the bathroom and vomited. Then she lay down on the bed, weak and disoriented.

But all she could think about was Swango's dinner. Conditioned over the years by her father and husband, she felt it her duty to fix a meal, no matter how ill she felt. She struggled to her feet, returned to the kitchen, and fried the chicken. She managed to get the food to the table, then sat down, saying she couldn't possibly eat herself. Swango paused before eating and looked at her with a searching gaze. Finally he said, "I can't believe you're doing this for me."

Weak and nauseated, drenched with perspiration, Joanna did her best to stay at the table as Swango ate. But finally she said, "If you don't mind, I think I'll lie down." She returned to her bedroom, and felt as though she blacked out. She remembered nothing more of that night. She spent the next day in bed, and took several days to recover. Though she had never before felt so violently ill, she assumed she had come down with the same bug that had afflicted the children.

LYNETTE O'HARE couldn't get over the change in Swango since he had met Joanna Daly—he seemed as he had been when she'd first met him, sunny and talkative. She fussed over him and tried to encourage him in his medical career despite the persecution she believed he was suffering. She introduced him to "nice people" she thought he'd enjoy, including Judith Todd, a prominent human rights activist, and a Catholic priest she held in high regard. He spoke to a class of children at the Catholic school about what it was like to be a doctor. It seemed Swango made a favorable impression on everyone he met. He wrote O'Hare's daughter regularly, usually two to three times a week, lavishing praise on her and filling his letters with quotations from the Bible. He struck up a friendship with the Samaritan who had called him when Mrs. O'Hare feared he might attempt suicide.

Swango continued to seek work as a doctor, but seemed to be growing discouraged. He applied for a position at the mental hospital, but its director, though lamenting what a waste it was that someone with Swango's skills was unemployed, said she could do nothing as long as the Ministry of Health maintained his suspension. Even though he was suing the Lutheran church, O'Hare thought Swango should be more aggressive at vindicating himself. "Why don't you go to the American embassy in Harare?" she urged him. "Surely you have rights as an American citizen." But he argued that such a trip would be pointless, since he wasn't formally accused of any wrongdoing. O'Hare was also busy with a Rotary campaign to eradicate polio; she urged Swango to volunteer at one of the stations where parents were bringing their children for inoculations. But Swango adamantly refused, saying "no doctor will go near me" given the accusations against him.

O'Hare was nonetheless grateful to have a doctor in the house, since her own health had been declining precipitously. Though she had always had a strong constitution, she had been experiencing recurring bouts of severe nausea, vomiting, and diarrhea, some of which kept her in bed for days. But Swango reassured her, telling her the symptoms were just a bad bout of the flu. Each time she fell ill, he gave her some medication, and seemed solicitous and concerned about her welfare.

While O'Hare was convalescing, she and Swango would watch TV and continue their conversations. He was passionately interested in anything having to do with O. J. Simpson, who had been acquitted the previous October of murdering his wife, and spoke often of how much he admired him. He seemed thrilled at the verdict, which puzzled O'Hare. "Do you actually think he's innocent?" she asked him.

He stared at her in disbelief. "Of course not," he snapped.

He seemed almost as fascinated by the story of English serial killer John Reginald Christie, who was convicted of murdering eight people, including his wife and a baby, over ten years ending in 1953. But before Christie was caught, another man, Timothy Evans, whose wife and child were among Christie's victims, had been tried, convicted, and hanged for their murders. Evans was posthumously pardoned in 1966. Swango told O'Hare the whole story, and seemed especially to savor the fact that Christie had been able to deflect blame onto an innocent man. (This same notion, that the wrong man might be accused of serial murder, figured in the suspense thriller he told Joanna he was writing.) Swango often spoke of the incompetence of the police and other members of the medical profession.

And Swango exhorted O'Hare—as well as everyone at the Bible study class—to watch the TV miniseries on Ted Bundy, professing his admiration for the handsome law student and exulting that no one had suspected him for so long. O'Hare had never heard of Bundy, but at Swango's insistence, she watched the program. Under the circumstances, O'Hare found Swango's enthusiasm peculiar.

"In view of what you're suspected of, I wouldn't go around talking about serial killers," she warned him after watching the show.

Given his faithful attendance at the Presbyterian church and his friendship with the Lorimers, she was also surprised by the irreverence of some of his comments. He often mocked participants in the Bible study class, especially Rosie Malcolm, the woman with the "ginger hair" he had once shown a romantic interest in, and would comment sarcastically, "Guess what we prayed about today?"

"Why do you go?" O'Hare finally interjected.

"I like to mix with nice people," he replied.

On another occasion, Swango seemed so contemptuous of religion that O'Hare asked, "What do you believe in?"

"I believe in God," he replied.

"Do you believe in Christ?"

He didn't reply.

But O'Hare drew nothing of significance from these conversations, which were isolated puzzling notes in a generally cordial relationship. She trusted her young lodger so much that she turned her car over to him. He would take her to work in the morning, pick her up for lunch, and return to take her home at the end of the day. That gave him unlimited mobility, and freed him from having to depend on Joanna or other friends for rides. Only the servants, Lizzie Keredo and Mary Chimwe, remained suspicious. One afternoon Keredo was washing O'Hare's car, as Swango stood watching.

"Are you sure it's clean?" he said as she finished.

"Yes, I am," she replied, annoyed at the insinuation.

"Well, maybe I should wipe it with a white cloth," he said. "In jail, the security officers wipe everything with a white cloth to see if it's clean."

"How would you know what they do in jail?" Keredo shot back.

Swango looked momentarily flustered, then explained that jail was just like the Army, and they'd done the same thing when he was in the Army. But Keredo was suspicious.

One day Swango offered Keredo and Chimwe some empty plastic vials, and asked if they wanted them. They said they did, but then thought the vials had a strange smell, so they threw them away. Another time, Keredo suspected that Swango had tampered with the peanut butter she kept in the kitchen in her cottage. It was a new jar, but it had been opened and an indentation suggested something had been pushed into it. She was afraid to eat it.

If Swango was at home when she needed to clean, he would stand in the room and make Keredo vacuum around him. When he left, he always carried a duffel bag slung over his shoulder, which made her wonder whether he had something he didn't want her to see. But her "madame" would hear nothing of these suspicions.

Then one day Keredo came to O'Hare and insisted that she come into Swango's room. They all had considered it odd that Swango insisted on so much bacon and four slices of toast for breakfast every morning. Now Keredo pointed to a closet shelf and said, "I'm worried." There, neatly wrapped and arranged, were dozens of bacon sandwiches. O'Hare was upset. When Swango returned that evening, she told him a fib, that the cat had come across the sandwiches in his closet. "That is unwholesome in our climate," she lectured him. "It will attract ants, if not worse. Please put the sandwiches in this plastic box and put it in the refrigerator."

But a few weeks later, Keredo came to her again with a triumphant look on her face. "Come look," she said, and led O'Hare into Swango's room.

This time she opened the bureau drawer. Wrapped with minute precision, concealed in the center of the drawer, were more bacon sandwiches. O'Hare was alarmed. Obviously, Swango suffered from some sort of food-hoarding syndrome. "I'm frightened," Keredo said. "No doctor would hide food in such a way." She insisted that

she and Chimwe begin sleeping in the other bedroom, next to
O'Hare's, with their door open. If he asked why, they would tell
Swango they had come into the house from their cottage because
they were suffering from colds.

Swango did seem upset at their presence, scoffing at the explanation and asking them every day when they planned to return to
the cottage. But they felt their vigilance was vindicated. O'Hare
slept with her bedroom door ajar so the cat could go in and out during the night. On several evenings, Keredo heard Swango open his
door and come into the hallway. He would stand motionless, peer-
ing into O'Hare's room. Each time, Keredo made a sound to indicate she was awake, and he quickly returned to his room.

O'Hare began to notice odd things around the house: a few
souvenirs and books were missing; small amounts of money vanished; the liquor bottles were nearly empty. She began to worry
about what he was doing with the car; sometimes he was out until
four A.M., and would come creeping into the house in a way that
frightened the servants. Then one day, when Swango was supposed
to pick her up for lunch at home, he failed to show up, stranding her
at the office. When he arrived that evening, she was angry. "Where
were you?" she demanded.

"Do you think I was trying to make a getaway to Botswana?"
he asked in a mocking tone, offering no other explanation. O'Hare
was suddenly alarmed. Such a possibility had never even crossed her
mind. Had he tried to flee? If so, was there something to those stories from Mnene? These suspicions hardened when the *Chronicle*
ran a brief news item two days later, "Doctor Tried to Escape":

> An American doctor accused of causing the deaths of
> five patients at Mnene Hospital in Mberengwa, reportedly
> tried to leave the country for Botswana, but was appar-
> ently stopped, police sources claimed.
> They said the doctor was believed to be still in Bul-
> awayo, but his exact whereabouts were not known. . . .

In the wake of the incident, O'Hare terminated Swango's car
privileges, a decision he greeted with what she considered a cold,
hostile stare.

Then a fax arrived for Swango from a medical school in Pretoria, South Africa, which O'Hare retrieved from the machine. "Because you are forty-two, we cannot accept you for the course," the letter began. It was addressed to Michael Swango, not "Swan," the name by which O'Hare knew him. O'Hare was startled. He had told her he was twenty-seven, her daughter's age. That evening she asked him about his name and age. Without any hesitation, he explained that Swango was pronounced "Swan" in America to avoid ethnic prejudice. (Swango is an Anglicized name of Swedish origin, according to family members.) As for his age, the school must have misread his résumé. "The '68 in my birthdate looks like '53," he said. That all sounded plausible when he said it, but the more she thought about it, the less sense it made. When she mentioned the discrepancies to Keredo, the maid again led O'Hare into Swango's room, where she opened the cupboard and showed her Swango's Zimbabwe work permit. The birthdate on it was not 1968. It was 1954. He was actually forty-one.

O'Hare wondered if Swango's strange symptoms might indicate post-traumatic stress disorder. Was he perhaps a Vietnam War veteran? She decided to phone his former girlfriend, whom she still knew only as LeeAnne. She'd wondered at the time why she'd broken off the relationship, and thought the reason might shed some light on the recent strange events. She retrieved LeeAnne's phone number, which she'd saved from the time Swango had asked her to call and tell LeeAnne she was making a mistake in breaking off with Swango.

O'Hare told LeeAnne that she was Swango's landlady and reminded her that they had met when Swango brought her to the house, adding, "I know you've broken up." She didn't want to sound alarmist, so O'Hare said only that she'd begun to feel "uneasy" about Swango. "Were you uneasy as well?"

"I can't say," LeeAnne replied.

"Is he possibly older than he claims?" O'Hare continued.

Not that she knew of, LeeAnne said. "I saw a document, a driver's permit, that said he was twenty-eight."

But LeeAnne hardly seemed talkative or forthcoming, so O'Hare got directly to what was really worrying her. "Do you think I'm in any danger? Am I quite safe with him in the house?"

"I don't want to answer," LeeAnne replied, which was hardly reassuring.

"Why not?"

LeeAnne hesitated, as if she might say more. But then she said, "You know what he's accused of," and hung up.

O'Hare suddenly felt weak and lightheaded. There must be something to the Mnene charges after all. She had to find a way to get Swango out of the house without alarming or angering him. She immediately called her cousin in South Africa.

"I'm scared," she said. "I want to get rid of him." She and her cousin worked out a scheme in which the cousin would send a fax to the effect that her son would be teaching at the university in Bulawayo and would need a place to live, both a bedroom and an office. The fax arrived. O'Hare took it and nervously presented it to Swango when he returned that evening. She said that under the circumstances, she'd have to give him two weeks' notice.

"Fine," he said. "I'm running out of money anyway. I don't know how much longer I can afford the rent." He even mentioned that he might leave for work in Zambia, which lies north of Zimbabwe. O'Hare was immensely relieved that he had taken the news so calmly and didn't ask any questions about her flimsy cover story.

The next day, Thursday, August 8, 1996, when O'Hare returned from work, Keredo met her at the gate. "Mike has done something," she said breathlessly. "He's too happy. He's been singing, and playing your CD player." This annoyed O'Hare, because Swango had been expressly asked not to use the CD player.

When she entered the house, tapes and CDs were strewn about the lounge. She knocked on Swango's door. "Mike, I believe you've been playing my CD," she said when he opened it. "You know that's my private property."

"Since when?" he replied, and slammed the door.

O'Hare immediately phoned her lawyer and told him everything—the Mnene allegations, the bizarre behavior, the missing money, and the unauthorized use of her tapes and CDs. "Get him out today," her lawyer said. "I'll come out to help."

She went back to Swango's room and knocked again. This time she said, "Mike, I want you to leave tonight."

He seemed resigned to her decision. It looked as though he

had already cleaned out his room. "I suppose you'll refund the rent money," he said curtly, and she wrote him a check for the balance. Then she told him she was changing the locks and hiring a security guard.

"Do whatever you want," he said.

When he later emerged from the room, carrying his bags, a neighbor had arrived. O'Hare hoped there wouldn't be a scene. But to her surprise, he now seemed as charming as ever. He smiled and shook O'Hare's hand, bidding her farewell.

"I hope you're not going to talk about me," he said. "And then I won't talk about you."

"What do you mean by that?" O'Hare asked indignantly. "What could you possibly say?"

"That you've gone raving mad."

With that he left, slamming the door behind him.

The next morning, O'Hare discovered what had evidently put Swango in such a good mood the previous day. She tried to start her car, but the motor quickly sputtered and died. She tried several times, but the car wouldn't start. On Sunday, she had the car towed to a service station. It didn't take long to diagnose the problem. "Your tank is full of sugar," the mechanic said.

Furious, O'Hare went directly to the police, accusing Swango of sabotaging her car.

ON August 9, the day after Swango left O'Hare's place, Joanna Daly drove him to Gweru for a hearing in his lawsuit against the Lutheran church. Since the day before, he'd seemed on edge. He was especially worried that reporters might hound him at the hearing, and he told Joanna that under no circumstances did he want to talk to the press. Nor did he want Joanna to witness the proceedings. He told her to wait in the car.

David Coltart and his firm continued to represent Swango, not only in the suit against the church, but in the administrative proceedings that had begun in Harare to suspend his license to practice medicine. But Coltart's enthusiasm for Swango had begun to cool. Judith Todd, his fellow civil rights lawyer, had mentioned at church that O'Hare was "unhappy" with Swango. Though she hadn't been able to provide any details, this had caused Coltart some concern, since he respected O'Hare. Partly because of growing doubts about Swango, he sent an associate to handle the hearing, which was held at the Midlands Labour Relations Office before an administrative officer.

The lawyers expected the church to reveal the evidence it had regarding Swango's involvement in the mysterious deaths at Mnene, which might also shed some light on where the criminal investigation was headed. But any concern Swango might have felt about this possibility quickly evaporated. In keeping with its strategy of attracting as little attention as possible to the Mnene deaths, the church surprised Swango's lawyers by relying entirely on a technical procedural defense. It argued that it couldn't be sued for wrongfully dismissing Swango, since he was actually employed by the Ministry of Health, which paid his salary. Thus the church lawyers sidestepped the actual cause of Swango's dismissal.

While no ruling was made, Swango was elated. There had been no reporters at the proceeding, and no mention of his alleged crimes. The hearing officer had given the church's argument short shrift, even noting in passing that six other labor complaints against the church were pending from Mnene. Joanna now felt justified in her belief that Swango had been unjustly dismissed.

But Swango's euphoria proved short-lived. Several days later, Joanna answered the phone, then called to Swango and said the police wanted to speak to him. He turned pale and told her to say he was out. The police called several more times, and each time she said Swango wasn't there. Finally he called the police and asked what they wanted. They were vague, saying they wanted to interview him in person. He agreed to appear at the police station on August 28.

In the next few days Swango seemed increasingly on edge. His squint and eye twitch became more pronounced. The *Chronicle* had reported on July 28 that "investigations [at Mnene] were at an advanced stage and officers would be questioning the last group of people soon." Soon after the calls from the police, Swango told Joanna that he thought he might take a vacation. He felt he needed to get away after the stress of the court hearing, and said he'd like to visit the national park at Nyanga, a wild, mountainous region on Zimbabwe's northeast border with Mozambique, where he said he had friends. Numerous hiking trails cross the border in the wilderness area, and many local people walk across the border without observing any immigration or customs formalities.

Joanna had mixed feelings about Swango's impending departure. She thought it a bit abrupt. After leaving O'Hare's, Swango had agreed to house-sit for a family he knew from church, and several weeks remained before their return. He asked Joanna if she'd check the house every day while he was gone. Though she agreed, it was an unwelcome addition to her daily chores. He also hadn't asked her to accompany him on his vacation, and although she probably couldn't have left the children in any event, the omission had hurt her feelings. Moreover, she was growing a little tired of having him around the house all day, of having to cook for him, talk with him, follow his directions; of being constantly fearful that she might be violating his privacy. And he had never taken her to dinner, paid for a movie, or given her a present.

Swango also wrote to Coltart to tell him of his plans. He said that he'd been contacted by the police, and "an officer wanted to speak to me. He agreed to delay my coming in until August 28. I have a strong suspicion" as to what this was about, the letter continued, but "I will be gone for a few days," and would be "back on the 28th."

He sent two cards to the Lorimers, one wishing Ian good luck on some upcoming medical exams, another wishing Cheryl a happy birthday on August 27. He took two trunks and dropped them off at the Mirtles' house, asking Cheryl's parents if they'd mind keeping them for him until he returned and found another place to live.

On August 14 Joanna drove Swango to the Blue Arrow bus terminal in downtown Bulawayo. Blue Arrow operates long-distance buses to major cities in Zimbabwe, South Africa, and neighboring countries. He had packed carefully, leaving one box of belongings with her, carrying only his duffel bag and backpack. He told her he would be gone for two weeks.

He kissed her, asked her to collect any mail for him, said he would be in touch with her, and vanished into the bus station.

AUGUST 28 came and went. Swango did not keep his appointment at the police station. Joanna began to worry when he didn't return.

She told the police he was with friends in Nyanga, but he had never told her their names, and she had no way to reach him. It dawned on her that he was gone, and that she'd never see him again.

When Swango didn't show up for his police interview and Coltart hadn't heard from him, his misgivings increased. He phoned the U.S. Embassy in Harare to ask about Swango, and was stunned by what he was told: Swango was wanted for murder in the U.S.*

Ironically, Coltart won the Lutheran church case for Swango. In early October, the labor relations hearing officer ruled that Swango had indeed been wrongfully discharged by the Lutheran church, and awarded him Z$35,000 in damages. The award wasn't collected, nor were Coltart's bills paid.

After several weeks, Joanna tore up the mail she was keeping for Swango and went through the box of things he'd left behind. She found only two things of interest. One was a bottle of blond hair dye. She was surprised that he had evidently been dying his hair. The other was a supply of Ant-Kil, a brand of ant poison. How odd, she thought. Why would Swango have a supply of ant killer? She put the Ant-Kil with her household supplies and threw everything else away.

EVEN after the sugar was removed from the gas tank, O'Hare's car continued to have problems. No one seemed able to locate the trouble. Finally a mechanic discovered crystallized sugar in the carburetor.

O'Hare's health problems persisted. In addition to the occasional nausea and headaches, she felt weak, and had a nagging cough, which a doctor thought was chronic bronchitis. She mentioned her symptoms one day to Mike Cotton, one of the doctors who had worked with Swango at Mpilo. Cotton told her he thought she should have a hair sample tested. "Why?" she asked. He explained that given her symptoms—recurrent bronchitis is a side effect of arsenic poisoning—and the nature of the accusations against Swango, he thought it would be a good idea. O'Hare was shocked.

---

* Of course, while under investigation for murder, Swango had not been charged. Thus the embassy statement was inaccurate.

"Surely he didn't do anything to me," she insisted, but she agreed to the test. The hair sample was sent to a laboratory in South Africa, which found a concentration of arsenic that was more than twelve times the norm. O'Hare had to go on long-term disability from her job.

The Lorimers and the Mirtles heard of O'Hare's plight, and also learned that books and other objects had disappeared from her house. Ted Mirtle called her and mentioned the trunks Swango had left with them, saying he would bring them over to her house. Perhaps her missing items might be found there.

O'Hare opened the trunks and went through Swango's belongings. She was shocked by what she discovered. There were about ten hospital gowns from Mpilo, all of them rank and filthy. There were a kidney-shaped hospital dish and a used syringe. There were numerous newspaper clippings about the O. J. Simpson murder case and the Christie serial killings in Britain. There was a cardboard hospital form with a list of names written on it. O'Hare noticed the name "Edith," which she recognized from newspaper accounts as one of Swango's alleged victims. There were some Mensa puzzle books. There were books about murder and the supernatural. In one book Swango had underlined a sentence, "The British are arrogant." Swango had written "Yes!" in the margin, which O'Hare took as a personal affront. And there were books, including the anthologies *High Risk* and *High Risk 2: Writings on Sex, Death, and Subversion*. Glancing at some of the pages made O'Hare feel faint. Several passages were highlighted in yellow marker. They were violent, scatological sexual descriptions that O'Hare found revolting. But most upsetting to O'Hare was makeup that had belonged to her daughter, Paulette, as well as a pair of Paulette's panties.

Tucked between the pages of one of the books was a piece of paper. On it Swango had carefully handwritten a poem by W. H. Auden. O'Hare was initially puzzled, but then she recognized the poem as the funeral oration in *Four Weddings and a Funeral*:

> *Stop all the clocks, cut off the telephone,*
> *Prevent the dog from barking with a juicy bone,*
> *Silence the pianos and with muffled drum*
> *Bring out the coffin, let the mourners come.*

Let aeroplanes circle moaning overhead
Scribbling on the sky the message He Is Dead,
Put crepe bows round the white necks of the public doves,
Let the traffic policemen wear black cotton gloves.

He was my North, my South, my East and West,
My working week and my Sunday rest,
My noon, my midnight, my talk, my song;
I thought that love would last for ever: I was wrong.

The stars are not wanted now: put out every one;
Pack up the moon and dismantle the sun;
Pour away the ocean and sweep up the wood;
For nothing now can ever come to any good.

CHAPTER THIRTEEN

O<small>N</small> J<small>UNE</small> 27, 1997, an immigration official at O'Hare International Airport in Chicago took the American passport of a man arriving from Johannesburg via London. He was en route to Portland, Oregon, and then, on the same day, to Dhahran, Saudi Arabia. The immigration official entered the name on the passport, Michael J. Swango, and the passport number into a computer. When the results appeared, he asked Swango to step into a private room.

Swango was arrested on federal charges of fraud. The outstanding warrant for his arrest had shown up on the INS computer. The next day, he was transferred by a federal marshal to the Metropolitan Detention Center in Brooklyn, New York, the federal prison primarily serving the Eastern District of New York, which covers Long Island.

Since leaving Zimbabwe nearly ten months before, Swango had already obtained two new positions as a physician. The first was at University Teaching Hospital in Lusaka, the capital of Zambia, the African nation which lies to the north of Zimbabwe and east of Angola. He had obtained a temporary medical license from the Zambian government and had been treating patients for over two months when Zimbabwe authorities issued an alert on him to other southern African nations, including South Africa, Namibia, Botswana, and Zambia. Zambian authorities promptly fired Swango from the hospital on November 19, 1996, and suspended his medical license.

Swango protested the action by letter, saying he had left Zimbabwe because the medical system there was in turmoil and he was

being harassed by government authorities and had never been given
an opportunity to contest the charges. But as in South Dakota, he
didn't stay to pursue the appeal. By the time hospital officials
replied, Swango had again vanished.

Swango next surfaced in Johannesburg, South Africa.
Through a medical placement firm there, he quickly secured a position at a hospital in Saudi Arabia, far from the scrutiny of U.S. or
southern African investigators. There was only one snag: he had to
obtain a Saudi visa through a consulate located in the United
States. Saudi Arabia only issues visas to foreigners in the country
of their citizenship. Swango argued strenuously that it was absurd
to make him fly all the way back to America rather than travel directly from Africa to Riyadh. But Saudi officials would not make
an exception. Since the Saudi royal family, which ran the hospital
that had hired Swango, had often used a medical placement firm in
Oregon to obtain physicians for its hospitals, it was arranged for
Swango to pick up his visa there, then travel that same day to
Saudi Arabia.

Though his reluctance to return to America suggests that
Swango was aware that a warrant had been issued for his arrest, and
that he might be picked up while going through customs and immigration, he nonetheless traveled under his real name, using his own
passport. Perhaps he felt he had no choice, since the medical diploma
he had used to secure his job was in the name Michael Swango. Or
perhaps he simply couldn't forge or obtain a new passport in the
short time before his scheduled departure. Of course, he could have
turned down the job offer and sought nonmedical employment. But
access to hospital patients appears to have become a compulsion,
something he would take extraordinary risks to maintain.

Swango's arrest attracted little public attention. An indictment
charging him with "willfully making a materially false, fictitious or
fraudulent statement and representation" to gain admittance to the
New York veterans hospital, a "matter within the jurisdiction of a department or agency of the United States," was filed on July 3, but it
wasn't unsealed and made public until July 25. The hitherto somno-
lent FBI investigation now went into high gear, and an assistant U.S.
attorney for the Eastern District of New York, Cecilia Gardner, was
assigned to handle the case. A brief New York *Daily News* article on

July 26 reported that Swango had been "nabbed" in Chicago. When Elsie Harris, Barron Harris's widow, heard the news, she could hardly believe it, and burst into tears. She thought everyone had forgotten about Swango, even though in her heart, she was convinced Swango was responsible for her husband's death.*

In September she traveled to federal district court in Uniondale, Long Island, for Swango's arraignment. She noticed that he had lost weight but seemed calm, polite and respectful. She was hoping he might offer some explanation, or say something to her. But he avoided her eye and didn't acknowledge her presence.

IN Quincy, Dennis Cashman, the judge who had found Swango guilty of poisoning his coworkers eleven years earlier, heard about Swango's arrest from a *Newsday* reporter who called, and then from Nancy Watson, the official at the AMA in Chicago who had rejected Swango's application while he was in South Dakota. The judge was amazed and dismayed that Swango had surfaced yet again, en route to still another job as a physician.

This time he picked up the phone and called me.

I have known Dennis Cashman nearly all my life. I was born and grew up in Quincy, Illinois. Cashman's parents were friends of my parents. I was on a swimming team with one of his sisters, and while Dennis was several years older than we were, I knew him as the city golf champion and an outstanding athlete.

My parents still live in Quincy, and I have other friends there, so I usually visit at least twice a year. Over the years I have come to appreciate much about Quincy that I took for granted while I lived there: the beautiful architecture, much of it dating from Quincy's heyday in the late nineteenth century; the wide, tree-lined streets and numerous parks; the well-maintained though mostly modest homes; local pride in the school system; and the friendly goodwill that greets me no matter how far I've traveled or how long I've been gone. But given the town's relative isolation (St. Louis is over two hours away) and its population of just over 40,000, I was at first

---

* Elsie Harris and relatives of two other patients who died sued Swango, the Veterans Administration, and University Medical Center at Stony Brook for wrongful death. Andrew Siben, a lawyer for the plaintiffs, said the cases were dismissed because they could not prove that Swango had caused the deaths.

skeptical when Dennis Cashman told me he thought he had been
caught up in a story of national significance.

Cashman told me that he'd just learned that a Michael Swango
had been arrested at O'Hare. He said Swango had grown up in
Quincy and had been the valedictorian of his high school class. I
had to think for a moment, but the name Swango was familiar to me
from campaign signs that used to dot local lawns when Michael's
grandfather ran for Adams County recorder of deeds. Cashman
confirmed that it was the same family. I didn't know Swango, nor
had I ever met him, as far as I can recall. Though he was just three
years younger than I, and would have been in high school at the
same time, I attended the public Quincy High School, and there
was little contact with students at the private Catholic high school.
I didn't remember the poisoning charges that had rocked Quincy
back in 1985.

I asked Judge Cashman why Swango had been arrested.
"They've got him on a minor charge," he said. But the real issue, he
said, was far more serious. Two years earlier, an FBI agent from the
bureau's Springfield, Illinois, office, John R. McAtee, Jr., had visited
Cashman in his chambers and said the Bureau was trying to develop
a psychological profile of Swango as it continued its search for him.
McAtee said the Bureau had recently intervened to have Swango
fired from a job dealing with the water system of a large Southern
metropolitan area (evidently he meant Atlanta) because of fears he
might try to poison the water supply there. Cashman found this
startling enough, but then the agent told him the FBI had now connected Swango to numerous possible homicides. The bureau was
"reasonably confident," he said, that Swango had killed sixty people.

"Did you say six?" Judge Cashman asked in disbelief.

"No, sixty," McAtee replied.

The number of Swango's alleged victims, would, if proved,
rank him among the most prolific and successful serial killers in
American history. But Cashman was equally disturbed by the conduct of members of the medical profession. He briefly recounted to
me Swango's employment history, pointing out that doctors and
administrators had entrusted patients to a man they knew to be a
convicted felon. The medical profession seemed blind to the possibility that one of its own could be a serial murderer. "It's outra-

geous that he has been allowed to go on," Judge Cashman said. "It's a national scandal."

I, too, was stunned by the possibility that someone from my hometown could be a prolific serial killer, and that he had been able to move from one hospital to another. How could such a thing have happened? What could possibly explain the mind of a doctor who took an oath to help people, but instead killed them, seemingly at random? Or was it possible that, as Swango always maintained, he was a victim of a bizarre series of coincidences and a miscarriage of justice?

My nearly two-year-long search for answers took me back to Quincy, to Ohio, Virginia, South Dakota, and Long Island, and finally to Africa. It was only as I stood in a remote field in Zimbabwe, face-to-face with one of Swango's victims, that I became convinced of his guilt. That Keneas Mzezewa would tell substantially the same story as Rena Cooper, a woman he had never met or heard of, who spoke a different language, and who lived a hemisphere away, could not be coincidence. At the same time, the full horror of Swango's story sank in. For Swango had preyed on the trust and hopes of sick, helpless people. Mzezewa, who is now impoverished and unable to till his modest plot of ground because he has only one leg, had rolled over and pulled his pants down to make it easier for Swango to inject him. Like all Swango's victims, he had looked to "Dr. Mike" to save him.

MICHAEL SWANGO has consistently refused to be examined by a psychiatrist or clinical psychologist. He has maintained that there is no reason why he should be examined, since he has done nothing wrong. Or perhaps he is intelligent and knowledgeable enough to have a pretty good idea what a psychiatrist would find.

To better understand someone like Swango, I contacted Dr. Jeffrey Smalldon, a clinical and forensic psychologist whose specialty is psychopathology, and more specifically, serial killers. He has consulted in about 120 death penalty cases, and has interviewed numerous serial murderers, including John Wayne Gacy. As it happens, Dr. Smalldon lives in Columbus, Ohio, and while he has no association with the Ohio State medical school or hospitals, he was familiar with Swango from local news accounts. During the spring of 1999, I shared with him nearly everything I had learned about Swango's early life and upbringing, his relationships with family members, girlfriends, and others, and the charges and suspicions he amassed during his medical career.

When we spoke, Dr. Smalldon cautioned me that no diagnosis, however useful, can entirely explain an extreme case such as Swango's. "Any single explanation will ultimately come up way short," he said. "Antisocial, narcissistic—there's still a large amount of unexplained variance and large unanswered questions."

Still, in many ways Swango seems a textbook case of a psychopath who exhibits extreme narcissistic tendencies. Though the term "psychopath" isn't currently in formal diagnostic use, the label is still widely used by both professionals and laypeople. A psychopath is generally understood to be someone who lacks a capacity for empathy and may exhibit aggressive, perverted, criminal, or amoral behavior. The psychopath tends to be highly self-absorbed. The condition is usually classified as an extreme and dangerous variation of narcissistic personality disorder, narcissism being the excessive love of self. But it is not a form of insanity; psychopaths are fully aware of their actions and of the actions' consequences, and can distinguish right from wrong.

Dr. Smalldon emphasized that he could not diagnose someone he'd never met. But he said that almost immediately after reading the materials I gave him, he "was struck by the incredible narcissism, which is often the most prominent personality feature of a lot of these people [serial killers]. Swango seems to have that sense of entitlement, a preoccupation with control and manipulation." Swango was a narcissist in some relatively obvious ways, such as his obsession with physical fitness and control over his body's appearance, and in the control he exerted over his girlfriends. But the ultimate expression of a narcissistic preoccupation is control over life and death.

Serial killers typically betray a fascination with the military and law enforcement, careers in which people are armed, and they often fantasize about violence and disasters in which they emerge as heroes. Serial killer David Berkowitz, the so-called Son of Sam, aspired to be a fireman. He later told an interviewer, "I wanted to die while saving lives, battling a blaze. This is why I wanted to become a fireman, helping people, rescuing them, and being a hero, or possibly dying in the blaze." *

It is significant that Swango indicated in his high school yearbook that he wanted to be a state trooper, and that he later enlisted in the Marines. His fascination with what might be called armed careers was also manifested in the arsenal found in Quincy when police searched his apartment; in his obsession with disasters; in his work as a paramedic, when he came to the scene of accidents even when he was off duty; and in fantasies in which he would arrive on the scene of disasters and have control over the fate of the victims. All these were situations in which he had control over the lives of others. The narcissistic psychopath is not motivated by empathetic concern for the victims or by desire to help them, but by a grandiose sense of self.

There are numerous theories suggesting a biological, genetic predisposition toward psychopathology, and this may have played a role in Swango's development. But narcissism, in the classic Freudian view, is an attempt to compensate for early, profound feelings of being unloved and undervalued. Swango experienced an absent, detached father, and a mother, who, however devoted, had difficulty expressing love and affection. The father who is either physically or emotionally absent figures in the history of most male psychopaths, and is a common feature in the profiles used to detect serial killers.

Swango spoke often of his absent father, glorifying Virgil's career in Vietnam while expressing his own anguish at being all but abandoned. Yet his fascination with disasters, with killing, and with weapons echoed similar interests he perceived in his father, as when he learned that Virgil also kept scrapbooks of disasters. "It is almost too simplistic to say that Swango is trying to close the gap between himself and his dad," Dr. Smalldon noted.

In Swango's case, the problem may have been compounded by Muriel's focus on him, to the exclusion of her other children, as "special," as "gifted," as someone deserving of a private school edu-

---

* D. Abrahamson, *Confessions of Son of Sam* (New York: Columbia University Press, 1985), as quoted in J. Reid Meloy, *The Psychopathic Mind* (New York: Jason Aronson, 1988), p. 113.

cation. "In someone who seems as narcissistic as Swango," Dr. Smalldon said, "you find a pattern of overvaluing by one or both parents. Everything they do is superior and special. His mother's inability to absorb that Michael wouldn't graduate with his class, and the need to keep up the front that he was special and brilliant, is significant. He may have lost the ability to evaluate his own self-worth by any realistic standard."

Severe narcissists often demonstrate their grandiose sense of self by deceiving others. They experience both exhilaration at their own superiority and contempt for their victims when they successfully put something over on another. Their activities may range from relatively innocuous lies, to, in extreme cases, serious crimes, committed largely for the thrill of eluding detection. Paradoxically, the thrill and sense of superiority may be enhanced by taking risks that actually increase the likelihood of getting caught.

Swango seems an extreme example of the grandiose personality in action. He lied constantly, sometimes for seemingly rational reasons, such as concealing his past in order to get a job, but often, it seems, simply to get away with something. He lied about his military record, telling Quincy College he received a Bronze Star and a Purple Heart, and saying his mother was dead. He was a good liar, able to deceive even trained psychiatrists at Stony Brook, which no doubt stoked his own sense of importance. His claims that he didn't give Rena Cooper an injection, that he wasn't even in her room; that he didn't give Mzezewa an injection, even as Mzezewa pointed to him as the doctor who had injected him with a paralyzing drug, must have been intensely thrilling.

Dr. Smalldon said he was "struck by the gratuitous falsification, the idea of putting one over just for its own sake, just because you can get away with something. There's a sense of power in this." Noting Swango's bizarre comments about violence, sex, and death in Quincy, his open admiration for serial killers like Ted Bundy, his calling attention to articles about serial killers and to movies such as *The Silence of the Lambs,* Dr. Smalldon said that "he continually drew attention to himself in ways that are hard to understand except in terms of the thrill of going right to the edge."

Another revealing clue to Swango's psychopathic mind was his reaction to criticism. He bridled when teased and belittled in medical school. Dr. Smalldon suggested that the incident in which

Swango botched his cadaver and was criticized and mocked would
have been experienced by him as an extreme humiliation. He may
have begun killing in retaliation. Swango's failure to graduate with
his SIU medical school class was so humiliating he couldn't bring
himself to tell his mother or show up at the dinner where he would
have to face his relatives. He subjected himself to the self-pun-
ishment of push-ups when criticized by residents at Ohio State, and
his apparent crime spree there began right after his performance as
an intern was criticized by a faculty member. He seems to have poisoned his fellow paramedics after he was mocked for not being assigned to the primary ambulance. He appears to have begun
poisoning at least two of his girlfriends, Kristin Kinney and Joanna
Daly, and his landlady, Lynette O'Hare, immediately after they
questioned his innocence. And he erupted in rage when Sharon
Cooper commented that he had put on a few pounds.

While some of the criticisms he encountered may seem trivial,
"a cardinal feature of the severe narcissistic personality is that they
cannot brook criticism or challenge of any kind," Dr. Smalldon said.
"He was criticized in med school. He couldn't take it. He was thin-
skinned. He was extraordinarily self-absorbed. The narcissistic
theme is very strong." The extreme narcissistic psychopath almost
invariably attributes criticism or a challenge to persecution, as did
Swango in his many claims to be the victim of a "miscarriage of justice."

Besides enjoying the thrill of controlling life and death and getting away with it, serial killers feel no empathy for the victims, so
complete is their absorption in themselves. When Swango poisoned
his victims short of the point of death, he very well may have felt
they deserved the punishment he meted out. But a serial killer who
chooses his victims at random has no motive in any rational sense.
The thrill of killing and getting away with it simply has no deterrent
in the form of empathy for the victim. Precisely why this would be
the case—why some people utterly fail to develop a capacity for
emotional bonding or identification with another human being—is
a subject of much debate among psychologists. Some Freudians
have suggested that a child who fails to undergo an Oedipal transfer
to either parent risks losing the capacity for empathy, and other
researchers have suggested biological causes. Psychopathic serial
killers invariably lack any capacity for empathy.

This deficit may have been most evident in Swango's numerous callous remarks about death, in his delight in being the doctor to inform relatives of the death of a loved one, in his failure to express any remorse after people died while in his care, and especially in his curious lack of emotional reaction to the death of Kristin Kinney. Yet many people found Swango charming, attractive, and personable; numerous women dated him, and at least three loved him. But this seeming paradox is also common in the psychopath.

As Dr. Smalldon explained, "I would imagine him [Swango] as profoundly deficient in his ability to connect emotionally with other people, but probably very adept at exhibiting counterfeit displays of emotion when he'd perceive a purpose in doing so"—for example, to maintain a relationship that provided sexual gratification. "The psychopathic personality is often described as the mask of sanity. It's superficial. These people seem to have the normal emotional equipment. But it doesn't run deep. They pantomime it. They don't feel it. It appears Swango was obviously very good at crafting a social persona that would serve his interests."

Another telltale clue in Swango's behavior is his peculiar relationship to food: eating the entire chocolate cream pie his mother baked for him; hoarding the cream cheese pastries at the hospital in South Dakota; and especially, obsessively wrapping and storing the bacon sandwiches he prepared at Lynette O'Hare's house. Such obsessions are usually characterized as aspects of an attachment disorder, an attempt to overcome the deep insecurity fostered by the failure to bond with a parent.

It is, of course, easier to describe a psychopath than it is to explain one. No doubt many people grow up with an absent father and an emotionally distant mother, aspire to be a policeman or a Marine, have a controlling personality, and even hoard food. Mercifully few are psychopaths. As Dr. Smalldon cautioned, nothing entirely explains someone as aberrant as Swango. His good looks, his charm, his intelligence—our very inability to predict or explain his psychopathology—are part of what makes him so frightening.

NEARLY all those who came into contact with Swango and were duped by him defended themselves by pointing out that he was such a skilled psychopathic liar that they could not have been expected to detect his deception, and that his behavior is so aberrant that the possibility of similar occurrences is remote. It would be comforting to believe this to be the case, but all indications are to the contrary.

The disturbing fact is that serial killing, while mercifully infrequent, is on the rise and is largely a contemporary phenomenon. While isolated examples surface in the nineteenth century—Jack the Ripper is a notorious example—serial murderers have proliferated since the 1950s, especially in America. Over half the known instances of serial killing in America since 1795 have occurred since 1970, when the rate soared exponentially. It increased tenfold in the 1970s alone. There seems to be little doubt among experts that serial killing is a socially influenced phenomenon, and that one instance with its attendant publicity encourages emulation, especially on the part of grandiose, narcissistic personalities determined to generate a blaze of publicity for themselves.

Swango is the first alleged serial killer in this century to have emerged in the guise of a physician. (Two other known physician cases, Dr. Thomas Neill Cream in Britain and Dr. H. H. Holmes, thought to be the first serial killer in America, committed their murders in the late nineteenth century.) But serial killers within the health care field, while they remain relatively few, have been increasing at an alarming rate. Even since Swango's arrest, there have been two examples that received national publicity: Orville Majors, a nurse in the intensive care unit of a hospital in Indiana, and Efren Saldivar, a respiratory therapist in Los Angeles. Serial killings were discovered in hospitals in Ann Arbor in 1975 and in San Antonio in 1981. Some killers have defended their murders in a hospital setting as mercy killings, but relatively few of these claims stand up to scrutiny. Others seem to be random acts of serial murder. From the point of view of a determined serial killer, a hospital is almost the ideal setting, since murder can so easily be camouflaged as natural death.

A chilling counterpart to Swango emerged in 1987, when a medical examiner in Cincinnati smelled cyanide in the stomach cavity of a man believed to have died from injuries suffered in a motorcycle accident. The cyanide poison was traced to a quiet thirty-five-year-old nurse's aide at Drake Memorial Hospital named Donald Harvey. When confronted, Harvey admitted to poisoning the accident victim and to a killing spree that spanned sixteen years and four hospitals, including the Veterans Administration hospital in Cincinnati, where he worked for nearly ten years. He admitted to fifty-two murders and eventually pleaded guilty to twenty-five Ohio murders and nine in Kentucky in return for being spared the death penalty. He was sentenced to multiple consecutive life sentences, and will be ninety-five before he is eligible for parole.

As in many such cases, it is hard to know precisely how many victims Harvey actually killed. Henry Lee Lucas, the itinerant killer who had so excited Swango, was convicted of eleven murders and confessed to nearly six hundred. But in 1998 his death sentence was commuted to life in prison by Texas governor George W. Bush after the state officials concluded that Lucas's claims were a bizarre hoax and that he was responsible for, at most, three deaths. In Harvey's case, investigators felt they could prove only one instance, and it is common for a grandiose personality to exaggerate. But there seems little doubt that Harvey ranks among the nation's most prolific serial killers. Harvey kept a written list of his victims, and cited a litany of the methods he had used to kill them: pressing a plastic bag and wet towel over the mouth and nose; sprinkling rat poison in a patient's dessert; adding arsenic and cyanide to orange juice; injecting cyanide into an intravenous tube; injecting cyanide into a patient's buttocks.

Harvey confessed that he didn't always poison people to kill. Fearful that his lover was cheating on him, Harvey slipped small doses of arsenic into the man's food so that he would become sick and have to stay home. When a tenant quarreled with his lover over utility bills, he put arsenic in the topping on a piece of pie he gave her.

Harvey's arrest and confession shocked people who knew him. He was religious, polite, and a reliable employee. A family friend told the press: "He was such a good boy. He was such a good Christian man. No finer fellow ever lived." But Harvey had a troubled childhood and had attempted suicide on several occasions, he later said, to try to stop himself from killing.

In a 1991 interview with a reporter from *The Columbus Dispatch,* Harvey revealed many of the characteristics typical of a psychopathic, narcissistic personality:

"Why did you kill?"
"Well, people controlled me for 18 years, and then I

controlled my own destiny. I controlled other people's
lives, whether they lived or died. I had that power to control."

"What right did you have to decide that?"

"After I didn't get caught for the first 15, I thought it
was my right. I appointed myself judge, prosecutor and
jury. So I played God."

Harvey also described the thrill he experienced when he es-
caped detection: "I felt a feeling of power. I was able to pull one
over on the doctors. I had plenty of common sense. It made me feel
smart that the pathologist couldn't catch me, plus to show that doctors are prone to mistakes."

In the wake of Harvey's confession, and a public uproar in
Cincinnati, it emerged that Veterans Administration police had
stopped Harvey in 1985 and searched his gym bag. In it they discovered a .38-caliber revolver, needles and syringes, books on the occult, a cocaine spoon, and various medical texts. Harvey was fined
$50 for carrying a firearm on federal property and was allowed
to resign quietly rather than be fired. Nothing was said to state
authorities or prospective employers. No investigation was conducted by the VA hospital into Harvey's contacts with patients.
After Harvey's arrest, former VA police officer John Berter charged
that "they just wanted to get rid of him and push their problem off
on someone else." After the Harvey incident, Berter was fired
himself, he claimed because he was a whistle-blower. The hospital
said his claims about Harvey were nothing but speculation, and
said Berter was dismissed because he had abused its sick leave
policy.

After Harvey left the VA hospital, he moved to Drake Memorial Hospital. VA officials made no effort to monitor his subsequent
employment or warn Drake officials. Harvey pleaded guilty to
killing twenty-one people at Drake.

GIVEN the rise in serial killings generally, and in hospitals specifically, it seems inevitable that more Swangos will surface, and it thus
seems all the more critical that criminal physicians be monitored
and prevented from having access to patients. When Judge Cashman spoke to AMA officials after learning of Swango's arrest, he

demanded to know how Swango could have been hired at two university teaching hospitals after being convicted of poisoning. He
was assured that whatever the explanation, it couldn't happen again,
because a new national monitoring system had gone into effect in
1990: the National Practitioner Data Bank. But how then, Cashman
wondered, could Swango have been accepted at SUNY–Stony
Brook in 1993?

Neither at Stony Brook nor at South Dakota, of course, had
officials checked with the data bank. Such a step was optional under
the Wyden legislation, in any event, nor is it obvious that the data
bank would have reported anything on Swango, since there's no indication that anyone reported Swango to the data bank in the first
place. When I called the data bank to find out if it had any information on Swango, I was told indignantly that any such information—
even whether his name appeared in the data bank—was confidential.

Dr. Salem, who accepted Swango's application in South
Dakota, insisted to me that he was familiar with the data bank and
its operations, but that medical residents were exempt from its requirements. But others, including administrators at Stony Brook,
seemed to be only vaguely aware of its existence; some had never
heard of it.

My suspicions about the ineffectiveness of the much-touted
data bank were confirmed when I spoke to Alan S. Levine, an inspector with the U.S. Department of Health and Human Services.
HHS conducted a study of hospital compliance with the reporting
requirement in the Wyden bill over a three-year period, from September 1, 1990, when the data bank began operation, to December
31, 1993. According to the HHS report, a copy of which I obtained,
"About 75 percent of all hospitals in the United States never reported an adverse action to the Data Bank." In other words, three-
quarters of the nation's hospitals over a three-year period either
took no disciplinary action against any physician—something that
strains credulity—or failed to report to the data bank when they
did, as required by law. In the case of South Dakota, an astounding
93.2 percent of the state's hospitals failed to report any action. This
compared with 51.7 percent in New Jersey, the state with the highest rate of compliance. The notion that the rate of medical malpractice would be so much higher in New Jersey than in South Dakota

also strains credulity. Finally, in 1989, it was predicted by the U.S. Office of Management and Budget that the data bank would be required to process 5,000 hospital reports a year. The actual average was only 1,000 per year.

The HHS report concluded that "our review suggests a sufficient basis for concern about the hospitals' response to the Data Bank reporting requirements. The wide variation in reporting rates from state to state is in itself troubling."

The AMA, offered an opportunity to comment on the HHS findings, attacked the methodology and the conclusions and continued to wage its rearguard action against any federal monitoring or reporting on incompetent or criminal physicians. "The AMA's review . . . concludes that the report falls far short of its purported goal. . . . Our review has revealed important gaps in both accuracy and completeness of data, creating a misleading picture." Furthermore, the AMA asserted, "it is universally recognized that punitive measures against physicians do not prevent adverse events from occurring and overall is [sic] not an effective patient safety/quality improvement measure." The association insisted it was "premature" to even discuss strengthening the reporting requirements.

Even without the glaring Swango example, it is perfectly plain that the data bank is not protecting the public. I will not even address the broader and more complex issues raised by entrusting physicians to police themselves through the peer review process, or by the widespread failure of state medical boards to enforce statutory standards; the solution at the federal level cries out for some obvious reforms. The government must:

- Require hospitals to check with the data bank before granting hospital privileges to any physician, whether licensed or unlicensed, whether an experienced practitioner, intern, resident, or medical student.
- Require hospitals to report any adverse action against a physician, not just action resulting from a peer review process, and at the very least including all criminal charges and their dispositions.
- Provide meaningful penalties for failure to comply, such as a significant fine, and provide HHS with an adequate

enforcement capability. Public Citizen's Health Research Group, in commenting on the HHS study, noted that "the current penalty . . . for noncompliance by hospitals may be insufficient to deter violations of the law. . . . We are unaware of any instance since the Data Bank's inception in which a hospital was penalized for failing to submit records."

- Make information in the data bank available to the general public. It is paid for by our tax dollars.

In short, the performance of the data bank to date, and its failure to warn of a Swango in our midst, is, as Judge Cashman put it, a "national scandal."

AT times, Judge Cashman feels that it may be his life's mission to monitor Swango's career, and not just because the FBI has warned him that Swango might come after him after he's again released from prison. Cashman's ire is in large part directed at the medical profession. In his view, hospital administrators and doctors were so concerned about potential liability that they refused to acknowledge evidence of numerous wrongful deaths, and thus became Swango's unlikely allies. In particular, Ohio State "did nothing," Cashman told me. "He should have been prosecuted in Ohio. No one would cooperate. There is an unwritten rule in the medical profession: Inept doctors do not get reported. Just get them out of town."

Even the most cursory glance at the medical profession's treatment of Swango appears to support Cashman's assertion. Swango performed poorly at SIU and was the subject of investigations both there and at Ohio State. Each institution made it possible for him to procure a licence to practice medicine in its state, and did nothing that prevented him from being hired in South Dakota and New York, let alone in foreign countries. Ohio State doctors actually *recommended* that Swango be licensed. Their myopia seems little short of astonishing. Repeatedly, doctors at respected hospitals and medical schools were willing to believe a fellow physician, even when they knew him to be a criminal. In some cases, they went so far as to recommend that he be hired elsewhere. How could a felon convicted of poisoning, or even of a less sensational form of battery, be granted an interview, let alone obtain a position?

"Most doctors I know are fine, upstanding people," Judge Cashman said as we discussed this question. But, he added, some consider themselves to be members of an elite, and treat one another accordingly. The loyalty among physicians makes police officers' famous "blue wall of silence" seem porous by comparison. This loyalty, and the corresponding distrust of outsiders, have only been intensified by decades of personal liability and medical-malpractice litigation that has left doctors, as a group, feeling beleaguered, unappreciated, suspicious, and fearful of outside regulation. Many physicians, often with some justification, have come to view lawyers—and indeed, the entire legal system—with distrust, if not outright hostility. In such a climate, some physicians seem willing to take the word of almost any doctor rather than accept the rulings of the courts.

As she pondered the Swango case, Cecilia Gardner, the assistant U.S. attorney in charge of it, faced a quandary. It was she who had thought of obtaining a warrant on fraud charges; she and the FBI now believed they had a murderer in custody, but the only crime they could prove against him was making a false statement. Under federal sentencing guidelines, perjury doesn't carry a mandatory prison term. Gardner was convinced that as soon as Swango was out of custody, he would again find a position as a physician, probably in a foreign country. She either had to give the FBI time to develop a stronger murder case by delaying the trial, or she had to strengthen the government's case by expanding the charges.

Gardner moved on both fronts. Since Swango had had access to drugs deemed narcotics—"controlled substances," within the federal criminal code—she amended the indictment to include charges of fraudulent access to and distribution of controlled substances. Conviction on these counts carried a maximum prison term of three years. She also persuaded Swango's lawyer, Randi Chavis, a court-appointed public defender, to agree to delay proceedings while Gardner traveled to Africa to seek evidence of similar "bad acts." Such evidence would be admissible to prove that Swango's actions on Long Island were part of a consistent pattern.

Gardner traveled to Zimbabwe in the fall of 1997; there she gathered evidence of the fraudulent representations Swango had made to the Lutheran church and to the health ministries of Zimbabwe and Zambia. These included a forged letter, dated May 19, 1994, from an executive vice president of the Federation of State Medical Boards, saying that Swango was "in good standing" with the federation. The document was notarized by Swango's friend Bert Gee, as were all Swango's application documents. Swango also said he'd been working as a "chemical soil analyst" with "Gee Enterprises," which Gee later said meant Swango had "turned the soil" for a worm farm he maintained in his basement.

The résumé Swango used to obtain employment in Saudi Arabia maintained that from 1990 to 1995 he was an "emergency room physician" in the United States in "large urban inner-city hospitals" and that he was a physician with the U.S. government from 1984 to 1990, which includes the time when he was actually in prison. His employment application said he had never been convicted of a criminal offense, and his "solemn declaration" to the Zimbabwe Health Professions Council stated that he had "never been debarred from practice on the grounds of professional misconduct."

Rather than face a trial that would include an extended inquiry into his activities in Africa, on March 16, 1998, Swango agreed to plead guilty and accept a prison sentence of forty-two months. But even after his plea, he tried to deceive the federal probation officer preparing his presentencing report. Though he was required to disclose all previous employment, he did not mention that he had worked at Aticoal in Virginia, where workers had come down with symptoms of poisoning, and at Photocircuits outside Atlanta, where he had access to the city's water supply.

On June 12, Swango appeared in the federal courthouse in Uniondale, Long Island, for sentencing. He was wearing glasses, and his hair was cut short, not nearly as blond as it had been in Africa. He still looked younger than his forty-three years, though he could hardly have passed for a twenty-eight-year-old. There were few spectators. No friends or family members appeared. He took notes throughout the proceeding, as he had at his trial in Quincy thirteen years before. He conferred frequently with Chavis, his lawyer.

Chavis said that despite Swango's guilty plea, her client wanted to lodge an "emphatic denial" of any poisoning deaths. She added that he denied having "any poison-making abilities."

Judge Jacob Mishler pronounced the agreed-upon prison sentence of forty-two months, stipulating that while in prison Swango "shall not engage in any duties that directly or indirectly require the preparation or delivery of foods or dispensation of medication or pharmaceuticals."

The judge asked Swango if he had anything to say. "I'm very, very sorry, Your Honor," he replied, and then remained silent.

THERE was no glimmer of satisfaction on Swango's face as he left the courtroom, escorted by two federal marshals. But on some level he must have felt a sense of triumph, for despite the guilty plea, despite the dire hints of trouble in Africa, he had again evaded murder charges.

Cecilia Gardner resigned from the Justice Department shortly after Swango's plea. Despite her efforts at delay, the FBI had failed to complete its investigation and was nowhere close to a provable murder case. The obstacles the Bureau faced were formidable. The deaths at SIU and Ohio State linked to Swango were now so old, and so much evidence had decayed, or been lost or destroyed, that the likelihood of finding admissible physical evidence was remote. Morgan, the prosecutor in Ohio, had tried and failed to do so more than ten years earlier. Officials in South Dakota and on Long Island had already rushed to proclaim that they had found no evidence of suspicious deaths of patients under Swango's care, which hardly enhanced the possibility of finding evidence there. That left Africa. Zimbabwean officials conceded that the country lacked the technology and expertise to test for the sophisticated substances likely to have been used by Swango on his victims. In any event, even had Zimbabwe sought Swango's extradition under a recently completed treaty between the two countries, the United States doesn't extradite its citizens to foreign countries that, like Zimbabwe, have the death penalty (even though the U.S. may impose the death penalty itself).

The FBI concluded that it had to find physical evidence of at least one American murder to make a case against Swango. If they could, they could then introduce evidence of Swango's activities in Africa to show a pattern of serial murder, much as Gardner had used evidence from Africa to establish a pattern of fraud. To that end, agents reexamined the records of every patient Swango treated at the Northport VA Hospital, his most recent U.S. employer, looking for symptoms consistent with the kinds of poisons already linked to Swango—among them arsenic, nicotine, ricin, potassium chloride, and succinylcholine. The process was tedious and lengthy, but despite the hasty reassurances issued by Stony Brook officials, their suspicions were strongly aroused by some of the evidence.

Eventually, three bodies were exhumed on Long Island. In addition, autopsy remains were preserved from two potential victims, including Barron Harris, who had lapsed into a coma then died, after an injection by Swango. One of those exhumed was Dominic Buffalino, the retired Grumman employee. Tissue and hair samples were collected and sent to the FBI laboratory in Washington, D.C., for analysis. Agents also obtained a sample of Kristin Kinney's hair from the lock saved by her mother.

Tests to determine the presence of poisons are labor-intensive and time-consuming. Even the suspected Long Island victims had been dead for over five years, and many potentially lethal substances decay and disappear in that length of time. But only a few months after Swango's sentencing, Andrew Buffalino, Dominic's brother, heard from one of the federal investigators, who said he didn't want to call Teresa, Dominic's widow, because his news might upset her.

"Was Dominic a smoker, by any chance?" he asked.

"No," Andrew replied. "He quit smoking more than fifteen years ago. Why?"

The investigator told him that test results showed an "extreme" level of nicotine in his brother's body—a level consistent with nicotine poisoning.

EPILOGUE

MICHAEL SWANGO, after eight months at a federal prison in Florence, Colorado, entered the Sheridan Federal Correctional Institution in Oregon, a medium-security prison fifty miles southwest of Portland, on February 10, 1999. Following publication of this book and related publicity, including a feature on ABC's *20/20* seen by other inmates, Swango was moved to a maximum-security facility in Colorado, ostensibly for his own safety. There is no parole in the federal system. But with credit for the seventeen months he had already spent in prison, including the time he was held in Brooklyn, and with credit for good behavior, Swango was scheduled for release on July 15, 2000. He would be forty-five years old, with the possibility of a long medical career ahead of him.

Not long after Swango entered Sheridan, I wrote to him to request an interview for this book. Scott Holencik, a prison spokesman, called to tell me that Swango had emphatically declined my request, and that it would be a waste of my time to pursue the matter.

"What did he say?" I asked.

"You don't want to know," Holencik replied. I said that, on the contrary, I did want to know.

"Trust me, you don't want to know," he insisted.

As is often the case with suspected serial killers, it is impossible to say with any certainty how many victims Swango has claimed. He began working as a paramedic even before he entered SIU medical school in 1979, and except for the time he was in prison in Illinois, had access to potential victims in an emergency or hospital setting almost continuously until his arrest at O'Hare airport in

1997. My own investigation found circumstantial evidence that links him to the deaths of five patients at SIU, five at Ohio State, and five at the VA Hospital in Northport, Long Island, for a total of fifteen in the United States. In Africa, he became either more prolific or more reckless or both. The evidence suggests that in the three years he spent there, he killed five people at Mnene and fifteen at Mpilo, for a total of twenty in Africa, or thirty-five in total. At least four of his intended victims survived. Given my limited access to patient records, and the efforts of the hospitals involved to minimize the possibility of murder on their premises, it seems highly probable that the actual total is higher. For example, I included no deaths from hospitals in Sioux Falls, although some patients died there while in Swango's care. The FBI may well suspect sixty murders, as an agent told Judge Cashman in 1995.

If proven, these numbers alone would make Swango one of the top serial killers in American history, possibly the most prolific. The only person for whom reliable data suggest a larger number is Donald Harvey, the Ohio nurse's aide, who confessed to fifty-two. The next highest total belongs to John Wayne Gacy, who is believed to have killed thirty-three young men. Swango's hero, Ted Bundy, is estimated to have killed nineteen.

Swango also poisoned people nonfatally. In addition to the five victims in Quincy, evidence links him to three poisonings at Ohio State, three at the placement office in Virginia, and two at Aticoal, to his landlady Lynette O'Hare, and to his girlfriends Kristin Kinney and Joanna Daly, as well as Daly's four children, for a total of twenty poisoning victims.

If, indeed, Swango was responsible for so many deaths, then, given the evidence of his psychopathology, it is all but certain that such a pattern of killing and poisoning would resume if he is released from prison. At Swango's sentencing, Judge Mishler ordered that he remain under supervision for three years after his release, and that he receive psychiatric counseling, but Mishler noted that "if the patient doesn't want it, it won't do any good." In any event, there is no known effective treatment for the severe psychopath. To deter Swango from manufacturing or harboring poisons or weapons, the judge also provided for periodic, random searches of Swango's living quarters during his supervised release. Ominously,

Swango protested this aspect of his sentence, and appealed on the ground that it is unconstitutional.

The FBI feared that Swango would flee the country immediately after release, rendering all efforts to monitor or control him futile. Only conviction on a murder charge would secure the mimimum sentence likely to protect the public: life imprisonment. (The federal code specifically cites murder by poison as a crime punishable by "death or imprisonment for life.")

With encouraging test results from Dominic Buffalino in hand, FBI agents, other federal investigators, and pathologists traveled to Zimbabwe in late 1998. They exhumed the bodies of four of Swango's victims at Mnene: Mahlamvana, Chipoko, Ngwenya, and Shava. They returned to the United States with tissue and hair samples, as well as samples from Margaret Zhou that had been saved by Zimbabwean authorities.

While the critical physical evidence that had so long eluded investigators appeared to be falling in place, proving murder beyond a reasonable doubt still seemed less than certain. The earlier FBI record in the Swango case had hardly been stellar. The Bureau repeatedly lost track of Swango—in Florida through what seems sheer disorganization—and allowed him to elude prosecution for years. By the time it occurred to Cecilia Gardner to pursue him on lesser fraud charges, Swango had fled the country. Nor was a thorough investigation of suspicious deaths at the Northport VA hospital undertaken until after Swango's arrest at O'Hare, when evidence had had four more years to disappear or grow stale. But the FBI no doubt deserves credit for its more recent work on Long Island and under difficult conditions in Zimbabwe, as well as for its sophisticated lab work.

Despite this success, the FBI had no potential U.S. case in which an eyewitness saw Swango give an injection to a patient who died and in whom subsequent tests found physical evidence of poisoning. No one saw Swango inject Buffalino or any of the other suspected victims on Long Island apart from Barron Harris. Though the Buffalino family was told that Dominic's body had elevated levels of nicotine, they weren't immediately shown the official autopsy results. Then investigators seemed to back away from nicotine as the likely poison. (In fact, test results indicated a lethal dose of a drug called epinephrine, a form of adrenaline readily available in hospitals. In moderate doses it is used to stimulate a failing heart but in higher concentrations can be fatal, causing the heart to go into overdrive.)

Though Elsie Harris saw Swango give an injection to her husband, Barron Harris lingered in a coma for thirty-seven days, making it extremely difficult to prove that the injection she saw was the immediate cause of his death. Only in Africa were there numerous potential eyewitnesses. Even though test results there could have been contaminated because the corpses were not embalmed and, buried in simple cloth shrouds, were exposed to the earth, Swango could be extradited to Zimbabwe. The extradition treaty between Zimbabwe and the United States was ratified in late 1999.

Still, given the overwhelming amount of consistent, circumstantial evidence from numerous possible victims, from multiple hospitals and locations, it seemed highly likely that Swango would face a murder charge before the end of his prison term. A grand jury was convened for that purpose in the spring of 2000.

MURIEL SWANGO, Michael's mother, who had set such store by her bright, talented third-born child, knew nothing of his fate. Despite Michael's occasional references to his mother being dead, she was alive in a nursing home in Palmyra, Missouri, a hamlet across the Mississippi River from Quincy. Michael never visited her or, so far as nursing home officials knew, made any attempt to contact her. Her condition steadily deteriorated. She didn't recognize the last relative who visited her, one of Michael's cousins, who found Muriel lying in the fetal position, unable to feed herself and unable, or unwilling, to speak.

Muriel died in the autumn of 1999 at the age of seventy-eight. There was no ceremony and no announcement.

Only Michael's half brother, Richard Kerkering, visited him in prison. Swango asked to be assigned to a prison in Oregon so he could be near Richard, who retired from his accounting practice in Florida and now lives in the Portland area. But after Swango was transferred to Colorado, the visits from Richard ceased.

Swango's brother Bob has read avidly on the subject of the psychopathic mind and serial killers. He and his brother John have spoken on the phone about Michael, and agreed that Michael is fully capable of murder.

●   ●   ●

AT Ohio State University in Columbus, Dr. Manuel Tzagournis remained vice president for health services after Swango's apprehension. Tzagournis, both through a spokesman and his secretary, repeatedly declined comment on all aspects of this book. In late 1999, Tzagournis resigned his administrative post, saying "this is a good time to make the change." To mark the occasion, the university trustees named the OSU medical school research facility after him. He remained a practicing physician and faculty member at the medical school.

Michael Whitcomb, the hospital medical director and the doctor in charge of the Swango investigation, took a leave of absence and then left Ohio State. He became dean of the University of Missouri school of medicine in Columbia in 1986 and then, in 1988, became dean of the medical school at the University of Washington in Seattle.

In 1990 Dr. Whitcomb resigned after an employee claimed he plied her with liquor, left with her in his car, and, after suffering a flat tire, sexually assaulted her, first on the ground outside the car and later in a public park. She filed a criminal complaint, but evidence suggested that the sexual activity was consensual, and the King County prosecutor declined to file charges. At the time of his resignation, Whitcomb said the charges were "false and unfair" but conceded, "This is conduct I consider unbecoming for anyone." He acknowledged he had had a drinking problem for several years, but said he had stopped drinking and was undergoing counseling.

Despite the controversy in Seattle, and despite the problems that had surfaced while Whitcomb was still at Ohio State, Tzagournis rehired Whitcomb as director of the Institute of Health Policy Studies; he returned to Ohio State in 1992. He resigned two years later.

After working briefly for the AMA in Chicago, Whitcomb became senior vice president for medical education at the Association of American Medical Colleges in Washington, D.C. Reached there in 1998, Whitcomb said, "I have no interest in talking to anyone about this [Swango]. It's been poorly reported and there have been many inaccuracies."

Dr. Joseph Goodman, who initially handled the hospital's investigation of Swango, was promoted from assistant to associate professor of surgery and remained on the faculty, specializing in neurosurgery. Goodman did not respond to repeated phone calls.

•   •   •

ROBERT HOLDER, the Ohio assistant attorney general who handled
the Swango investigation, became an associate to Tzagournis in
charge of legal affairs, retaining the post after Tzagournis's resignation. When I reached him at his office early in my research for this
book, he defended the university's investigation of Swango and the
decision to allow him to complete his internship. "Naturally, our review was criticized after the fact," he said. But "you don't come to a
meeting thinking someone is a complicated psychopathic killer."
He emphasized that at the time, no one knew of any blemish on
Swango's character. "This complaint was taken very seriously and
was considered by a distinguished group" that "did a more extensive
review than my subsequent experience tells me that a lot of places
would do." He added that "the concern of the group at the time was
to be evenhanded," and he denied that concern over potential liability was a factor. Still, he acknowledged that with benefit of hindsight, "we could have done better—there's no doubt about that."
He said the university and the hospital had heeded the recommendations in the Meeks report and that steps have since been taken to
improve relations between the police force and the hospital.

But of the three most important recommendations contained in
the Meeks report, none was implemented. In 1999, thirteen years after
the report was issued, there was no security office that reported to a
hospital administrator staffed "with persons trained as investigators
and capable of handling medically-related investigations," as Meeks
recommended. Nor was a "statement of principles" formally implemented to govern police presence in the hospital in an effort to ease
tensions between law enforcement and hospital personnel.

Following publication of this book, *The Columbus Dispatch* did
its own inquiry, confirming that the important Meeks recommendations had not been implemented. "The people I talk to say it's worse
than it was before," former OSU police chief Peter Herdt told the
Dispatch. And the director of hospital security, Robert Meyers, told
the paper, "Doctors are doctors. . . . believe me, I know. They're like
fighter pilots—you can't tell them much."

Meeks also recommended that Ohio State take steps to improve relations with the press. Initially, Ohio State's director of
communications, Malcolm Baroway, who also dealt with the press

during the original Swango affair, offered to help with my research and make others at OSU available. But little assistance was forthcoming, and doctors and other staff later told me they had been discouraged from talking. I arranged all of my interviews independently of the OSU public relations office. After David Crawford, a spokesman for the hospital, demanded that all questions be in writing and then refused even to disclose the number of beds in the Ohio State Hospitals, I called Baroway to complain. "Frankly, we're just not very interested in helping you," Baroway replied.

It is one thing to try to thwart a journalist. But Cecilia Gardner, the former assistant U.S. attorney in charge of the Swango case, told me that her repeated calls to Holder went unreturned—the only instance she could think of in her career of another lawyer's failing to return a call from the U.S. Department of Justice.

Nor did Holder return my calls after our initial conversation. Baroway told me Holder was "tired" of talking about Swango and would not be calling me back.

UNLIKE some of those who exonerated Swango, Jan Dickson, the chief of nursing who brought Swango to top OSU hospital administrators' attention, left the university in 1985, shortly after the Swango investigation was concluded, after her position was eliminated in a reorganization. She became chief of nursing at Baptist Medical Center in Little Rock. "The doctors did not want to believe," she told me recently. "They were in denial."

Donald Boyanowski, the acting OSU hospital executive director who thought the police should have been called, was replaced in 1985 and joined a hospital in Newark, Ohio. He was more blunt than Dickson. "Jan and I were ostracized" at OSU for raising concerns about Swango.

Boyanowski and Dickson were married in 1988. They retired and moved to Dickson's family farm in northeast Missouri, which coincidentally is not far from Quincy. Dickson, who was afraid to walk her dog alone in Columbus while Swango was there, still worried that if Swango was released, he would return to the Quincy area.

ED MORGAN remained an assistant prosecuting attorney in Columbus. After more than a decade, he was still bitter about his inability to prosecute Swango and the behavior he encountered at OSU. "I was frustrated," Morgan told me. "It was incredibly frustrating. If we had been contacted, there was a lot of evidence that would have been available. Instead, the evidence had disappeared. You have to have physical evidence. The circumstantial was not enough. It was shocking to me that this was not referred to me earlier."

The doctors and administrators at the university hospitals "greatly resented the intrusion of law enforcement in their affairs," Morgan said. "From day one they resented us. They never really co-operated, or it was grudging cooperation. They didn't trust us. They were petrified of lawsuits. When they realized they had an errant doctor, they [simply] didn't renew his contract and let him slip away." In short, he said, "They covered it up, that's what it was."

Every year, Morgan and Tzagournis attended a New Year's Day party at the home of a mutual friend. In the thirteen such occasions since he issued his report on Swango, Morgan said, Tzagournis barely spoke to him.

AMONG other university medical personnel who dealt with Swango, Dr. John Murphy, the faculty member who defended Swango at SIU and saved him from dismissal, continued as a pathologist in Springfield and remained on the SIU faculty. Having taken Murphy's course that covered toxicology, Swango wrote him from prison after his conviction in Quincy asking Murphy to help him disprove the charges. But by then Murphy had changed his views about Swango, and realized he had made a terrible mistake in defending him. He didn't reply to Swango's letter.

"To be honest, I feel very bad," Murphy told me. Rosenthal and Swango's other critics, he conceded, "were much more correct" about Swango. "I was wrong about him. I was duped."

Dr. Anthony Salem, who recommended Swango's admission to the University of South Dakota residency program, left Sioux Falls in 1998 for reasons unrelated to Swango and is now a physician at the Veterans Administration hospital in Las Vegas. "I bungled it, no question" he said. "But I wasn't the only one who bungled it."

Dr. Robert Talley, who warned SUNY–Stony Brook that Swango might be among their residents, remained dean of the medical school at the University of South Dakota. He declined to comment on any aspect of this book.

Dr. Alan Miller, the former director of admissions for the residency program at SUNY–Stony Brook, remained on the faculty as a part-time professor of psychiatry. At the time he was asked to step down as director of the psychiatric residency program, residents protested that he was unfairly made the fall guy; they wrote a letter of protest to the dean and asked Miller to speak at their graduation. Dr. Miller was also forthright about what happened. Admitting Swango was "a conspicuous oversight," he said, "and I take responsibility for it." Still, he said, it pains him to think that after a long and illustrious career, this is how he will be remembered. "In my professional life, this is the worst single episode," he told me.

After he resigned his post as dean at SUNY–Stony Brook, Jordan Cohen accepted a position as head of the Association of American Medical Colleges in Washington, D.C., the same organization that handles applications for residencies. Cohen said at the time that he saw the new position as a "once-in-a-lifetime opportunity to be of service, nationally, to academic medicine." Ironically, he was working there with Dr. Whitcomb, which meant that two of the doctors involved in Swango's career were overseeing the application process of all medical school residents in America.

AL AND SHARON COOPER, Kristin's parents, moved to an attractive new condominium development in Yorktown, Virginia, with their cat and dog. Al fully recovered from his heart surgery. Sharon said that after Kristin's death, and especially after she learned of his past, she feared Swango, but now would be happy to confront him face-to-face. "I don't care if he tries to kill me," she told me when I visited their home. "He can't take anything more precious away from me than he already has." After repeated inquiries, the Coopers were finally told by the FBI that Kristin's hair sample had tested positive for the presence of a toxic substance. The sample also indicated that Kristin had been poisoned over a lengthy period of time.

Sharon Cooper has agonized over the thought that if she had acted sooner to warn people about Swango, others might be alive today. After she learned of Barron Harris's death on Long Island, she called Elsie Harris, and both women wept. Harris tried to reassure her, saying that Sharon had done everything that could have been expected, probably more than most people would have done. "I was grateful to talk to Mrs. Harris," Cooper told me, but whatever happens to Swango now, "we feel we have been given a lifetime sentence. All I want from Michael is an admission of guilt for what he's done and his willingness to take the consequences. My main interest is to make sure, or to try to help, to see that he is not back in circulation."

RENA COOPER, the woman whose paralysis and brush with death at Ohio State Hospitals in 1984 launched the first serious investigation of Swango, was still living in Columbus at the time of Swango's sentencing. She was eighty-four years old, lived alone on $737 a month in Social Security, and complained to me that she was subsisting at the "poverty level." Her mind seemed alert and she said she clearly remembered the terrifying events in the hospital. "You know, they said we were crazy," she told me with some indignation, referring to herself and her hospital roommate, Iwonia Utz. She told me that there was no doubt in her mind that Swango was the person who injected something into her IV tube. "It was Swango himself," she said emphatically. "I'd seen him before, on his rounds." She maintained that she never identified her attacker as a female, or as wearing a yellow pharmacy coat.

Cooper filed suit against the hospital in 1986. Advised by her lawyer that it was the best she could hope for, she settled the case in 1989 for a mere $8,500, an outcome that prompted her to write a letter to the judge. On lavender stationery adorned with small flowers and bees, she wrote:

> I did not know that life was so cheap in the eyes of some people.
> I have nothing against O.S.U. hospital, nor do I have any hatred for young Swango.
> I do feel that he is asking for help but no one seems to hear him screaming. I hope before it goes too much further young Swango will get the help he is asking for and needs.
>
> Sincerely,
> [signed] Mrs. Delbert Cooper, Sr.
> Rena E. Cooper

2000

NOTES ON SOURCES

I WROTE MICHAEL SWANGO three times in the course of my work on this book, once while he was in the Metropolitan Detention Center in Brooklyn after his arrest, and twice after he had pleaded guilty and was transferred to Sheridan, Oregon. He declined each of my requests for an interview. In my last letter, I offered him the opportunity to write his own statement, which I would include in the book. He declined.

As I told Swango, "At times I feel I have visited, spoken to, or tried to speak to virtually everyone who has known you." Much of the information in this book is based on hundreds of interviews with participants in the story, conducted from September 1997, when I first spoke to Judge Cashman, until May 1999.

Most of these were on-the-record interviews. In researching most of my previous works, I had to conduct many interviews on a not-for-attribution basis because sources feared retaliation in the form of damage to their careers and professional lives. With respect to the present book, fear of retaliation was a factor primarily for sources at Ohio State. But some sources expressed a different and more potent fear: that Swango would exact retribution by poisoning them or their families.

Because of these concerns, some people refused to talk. A few interviews were conducted on a not-for-attribution basis and in one instance, that of the person who alerted Dean Talley to Swango's presence on Long Island, I deleted a name. For others, the decision to speak to a journalist required an unusual level of personal courage and dedication to the truth. While I think it highly unlikely that Swango would seek revenge—it has not been his modus operandi to do so—I decided it would be unfair to protect some sources by withholding their names and not do the same for others. I have thus taken the unusual step of not listing the people I interviewed, not even the many who spoke on the record.

All quotations of dialogue and descriptions of states of mind were carefully reported and whenever possible, verified with multiple participants. Usually, where I have attributed a state of mind to someone, that person has expressed it directly, in an interview or in contemporaneous notes; in rare instances, the person in question revealed his or her state of mind to someone else. Quotations come from the speaker, from someone who heard the remark, or from transcripts and notes of conversations.

The major events of this story span approximately fifteen years, and participants' memories of some events, especially those occurring in the mid-1980s, have naturally faded over time. Some of these incidents, however, were so shocking and unusual that they seemed to lodge quite clearly in witnesses' and participants' memories, and many people were able to provide remarkably detailed accounts. Fortunately, the events at Ohio State in 1984 and 1985 and in Quincy, Illinois, in 1985 were the subject of numerous interviews and written reports shortly after they occurred. Most of the relevant dialogue comes from those earlier written records; in cases where later recollections differed, I have generally deferred to the earliest accounts. Particularly useful were the voluminous trial records in Quincy and the Meeks and Morgan reports in Ohio. In other cases, the text refers to notes and diaries kept by participants, which provided insights into their thoughts and comments at the time of the events in question.

These materials made possible an unusually detailed account of events that happened some time ago. But readers should bear in mind that remembered conversations are rarely an exact reproduction of the words actually spoken. Multiple witnesses to an event often provide at least slightly different accounts of what they saw and heard. This is apparent in the discrepancies between the Meeks and Morgan reports, which described some of the same events. In a few instances I discovered that both reports, while consistent, were nonetheless wrong. In nearly every case I was able to harmonize conflicting accounts, and that version appears in the text.

An exception is the varying accounts Dr. Whitcomb gave of his pivotal interview with Swango soon after Rena Cooper suffered her respiratory arrest at Ohio State. Did Swango say he was in the room because Cooper asked for her slippers, as Whitcomb told Meeks, or because he was going to draw blood, as Whitcomb later told police?

In another discrepancy, Rena Cooper insisted in an interview with me that she was never interviewed by Dr. Whitcomb, who was in charge of the hospital's investigation. During the Meeks investigation, however, Dr. Whitcomb said he interviewed Cooper. Meeks concluded, however, "it is not clear to us whether Dr. Whitcomb separately spoke with [Cooper] or simply relied upon Dr. Goodman's interview."

In each of these instances, Dr. Whitcomb could presumably clarify these inconsistencies, but he declined to be interviewed.

Spellings of African names are English transliterations of the Shona and Ndebele languages. The spellings are based, whenever possible, on police records. However, in many cases different spellings are in widespread use.

Published accounts on which I relied are usually mentioned in the text. Following is a bibliography of the principal written source material. Several books are included for general background on the psychology of murderers.

BOOKS

Abrahamsen, D. *Confessions of Son of Sam.* New York: Columbia University Press, 1985.

Capote, Truman. *In Cold Blood.* New York: Random House, 1966.

Douglas, John E. *Journey into Darkness.* New York: Pocket Books, 1997.

———. *Mind Hunter: Inside the FBI's Elite Serial Crime Unit.* New York: Pocket Books, 1996.

Hickey, Eric W. *Serial Murderers and Their Victims.* Pacific Grove, California: Brooks/Cole Publishing, 1991.

Lane, Brian, and Wilfred Gregg. *The Encyclopedia of Serial Killers.* London: Headline Press, 1992.

Linedecker, Clifford, and William A. Burt. *Nurses Who Kill.* New York: Pinnacle Books, 1990.

Mailer, Norman. *The Executioner's Song.* Boston: Little Brown, 1979.

Meloy, J. Reid. *The Psychopathic Mind: Origins, Dynamics, and Treatment.* New York: Jason Aronson, 1988.

Ressler, Robert K. *I Have Lived in the Monster: Inside the Minds of the World's Most Notorious Serial Killers.* New York: St. Martin's, 1998.

———. *Whoever Fights Monsters.* New York: St. Martin's, 1994.

Rule, Ann. *The Stranger Beside Me.* New York: New American Library, 1996.

Sullivan, Terry. *Killer Clown: The John Wayne Gacy Murders.* New York: Pinnacle Books, 1999.

ARTICLES

On Swango's father:

McGauley, John. "Swango: We Could Have Left as Winners," *Quincy* (Ill.) *Herald-Whig,* Sept. 20, 1979.

Swango, John Virgil. "The Year of the Rat: Free World Assistance in Vietnam," Agency for International Development, 1972.

On Swango at Ohio State:

Associated Press. "Girlfriend Says Swango Innocent," *The Plain Dealer* (Cleveland), Aug. 20, 1985.

Barry, Steve. "Seizure Witness Voices Fear of Dr. Swango," *The Columbus* (Oh.) *Dispatch,* Feb. 20, 1985.

Durant, Susan. "Swango's Reaction to Death Rapped," *Columbus* (Oh.) *Citizen-Journal,* Feb. 7, 1985.

Meeks, James E. "Report to the President Regarding Incidents in the Ohio State University Hospitals Related to the Internship of Dr. Michael Swango and the University Handling of Those Incidents," 1985.

Morgan, Edward. "Report to the Prosecuting Attorney, Franklin County, Ohio," 1986.

Sharkey, Mary Anne. "Swango Probe Botched, OSU Says," *The Plain Dealer* (Cleveland), April 3, 1985.

———— and Gary Webb. "OSU Faces State Probe on Swango," *The Plain Dealer* (Cleveland), Feb. 10, 1985.

Webb, Gary, and Mary Anne Sharkey. "Medic Probed in OSU Deaths," *The Plain Dealer* (Cleveland), Jan. 31, 1985.

————. "OSU Covered Up, Poison Prober Says," *The Plain Dealer* (Cleveland), Feb. 1, 1985.

On Swango in Quincy:

Cullumber, Jim, and Michael Snellen, "Cashman Finds Swango Guilty," *Quincy* (Ill.) *Herald-Whig,* May 3, 1985.

Hagan, John F. "Swango Guilty of Poisonings," *The Plain Dealer* (Cleveland), May 4, 1985.

Skaugen, Cindy, "Swango's Associates Saw a Studious Loner Under Stress," *The State Journal-Register* (Springfield, Ill.), Feb. 10, 1985.

Thrasher, Donald K., producer, "A Trail of Poison," *20/20,* Feb. 13, 1986.

On Swango in Virginia:

Berens, Michael. "Swango Is Suspect in New Poisonings," *The Columbus* (Oh.) *Dispatch,* June 8, 1989.

Dewitt, Dan. "Newport News Probing Poisonings," *Newport News* (Va.) *Daily Press,* June 9, 1989.

Ruth, Robert. "Co-worker's Tip to Police Started New Swango Probe," *The Columbus* (Oh.) *Dispatch,* June 10, 1989.

On Swango in South Dakota:

Associated Press. "Swango: 'I'm a Good Doctor,' " Sioux Falls *Argus Leader,* Dec. 7, 1992.

Gutch, Charley F. and Noel Ann English. "Review of Events of Admission of Dr. M. Swango," University of South Dakota, 1992.

Walker, Carson. "Fighting the Memories," Sioux Falls *Argus Leader,* Dec. 13, 1992.

———. "Medical Resident Suspended," Sioux Falls *Argus Leader,* Dec. 1, 1992.

———. "USD Dismisses Swango," Sioux Falls *Argus Leader,* Dec. 3, 1992.

———. "USD Knew of Swango's Past," Sioux Falls *Argus Leader,* Dec. 2, 1992.

On Swango on Long Island:

Slackman, Michael. "Poison in His Past," *Newsday* (N.Y.), Oct. 20, 1993.

Smith, Estelle Lander and Michele Salcedo. "Swango Patient Dies at VA," *Newsday* (N.Y.), Nov. 9, 1993.

Yan, Ellen. "Trail of Poison?" *Newsday* (N.Y.), Sept. 14, 1997.

On Swango in Africa:

Dongozi, Foster, "Bodies of Five Mberengwa Villagers Exhumed," *Bulawayo Chronicle,* Nov. 21, 1998.

———. Maid Relates Swango's Strange Behaviour," *Bulawayo Chronicle,* Nov. 25, 1998.

Ziana. "Ministry Dismisses Doctor," *Bulawayo Sunday News,* Mar. 24, 1996.

On Donald Harvey:

Clark, Paul and David Wells. Gannett News Service, Aug. 27, 1987.
Wells, David. Gannett News Service, Sept. 19, 1987.

On the National Practitioner Data Bank and the Wyden legislation:

Adler, Robert S. "Stalking the Rogue Physician," *American Business Law Journal,* winter 1991.

Brown, June Gibbs, Inspector General, "Hospital Reporting to the National Practitioner Data Bank," U.S. Department of Health and Human Services, February 1995.

Budetti, Peter. "Title IV, Public Law 99-660: Background and Implications," *Federation of State Medical Boards Bulletin,* Dec. 1987.

Iglehart, John K. "Health Policy Report," *New England Journal of Medicine,* April 9, 1987.

Jost, Timothy. "The Necessary and Proper Role of Regulation to Assure the Quality of Health Care," *Houston Law Review,* May 1988.

St. Paul Fire & Marine Insurance Co., "Physician and Surgeon's Update 1985: a Special Report," 1985.

House Subcommittee on Health and the Environment, "Hearings on a Bill to Encourage Good Faith Professional Review Activities of Health Care Entities," March 18 and July 15, 1986.

ACKNOWLEDGMENTS

I AM DEEPLY GRATEFUL for the efforts of my two research assistants on this book, J. R. Romanko in the United States and Foster Dongozi in Zimbabwe. J.R., did extensive research and interviewing and tracked down scores of sources and participants, many of whom had married, changed their names, and moved to distant locations. This alone was a daunting and time-consuming process. He endured a freak snowstorm that closed the Sioux Falls airport, rendering service above and beyond the call of duty. He was also an indefatigable fact-checker. I will miss our work together.

To say the chapters on Africa would not have been possible without the assistance of Foster is no exaggeration. He speaks Shona, Ndebele, and English and served as an interpreter and a guide. I would never have reached Swango's victims and witnesses in the Mnene area without the assistance of Foster and local police. He proved a resourceful and hardworking journalist.

Alice Mayhew, my editor at Simon & Schuster, as she has been for all my books, guided this book from its inception and provided critical support at just the right times in the sometimes daunting reporting and writing process. I am lucky to have the benefit of her wisdom and friendship. Carolyn Reidy, president and publisher of the trade division, was immediately enthusiastic when I proposed this book, and David Rosenthal, vice president and publisher of the hardcover division, was also a strong supporter. I am grateful to them both. My thanks also to Ana DeBevoise, Emily Remes, Layla Hearth, and Jolanta Benal.

My agent, Amanda Urban, encouraged me to pursue this story and made it possible for me to do so. I am grateful for her encouragement and advice.

Steve Swartz, editor and president of *SmartMoney*, provided a professional home for my work and was a valuable sounding board throughout the reporting and writing. I am grateful for his advice and friendship. Julie Allen assisted me in myriad indispensable ways, always with efficiency and good cheer.

I first wrote about Michael Swango in the November 24, 1997, issue of *The New Yorker.* My editor there, John Bennett, encouraged me to pursue the story the moment I mentioned it to him, and provided valuable guidance. He also encouraged me to pursue the many unanswered questions remaining after the story appeared. Tina Brown, then the editor of *The New Yorker,* assigned the story and gave me her unqualified support. Amy Tübke-Davidson was an outstanding fact-checker and researcher.

I am also grateful to Tamar Galed and Jana Drvota at the Ohio State University Archives and to Ron Ackerman in Springfield, Illinois.

Dan Isenschmid, chief toxicologist at the Wayne County (Michigan) Medical Examiners Office, provided valuable guidance on the subject of poisons.

As usual in writing a book, I counted on the patience and love of my friends and family to see me through, even when I must have seemed preoccupied and unavailable. My parents, Ben and Mary Jane Stewart, in addition to deserving my gratitude for all they have done for me, also helped with my research, since they live in Quincy and know many of the participants there. My sister, Jane Holden; her husband, John; my nieces Lindsey, Laura, and Margaret and nephew Jack; my brother, Michael; and his wife, Anna, all provided support and encouragement as well as memorable family gatherings.

Elizabeth McNamara rendered valuable legal counsel as well as friendship. Kate McNamara, now eight years old, inspires and delights me. My thanks, too, to Barbara Noble for her friendship and encouragement.

James Swartz, my godson, and Langley Grace Wallace, my goddaughter, were born during the writing of this book, and I look forward to the day when they can read their names. I am grateful for the friendship of their parents, Steve and Tina Swartz and Monica Langley and Roger Wallace.

Among my friends, I wish to thank Jim Gauer, Joel Goldsmith, Edward Flanagan, Didier Malaquin, Gene Stone, Arthur Lubow, Jeffrey Khaner, Jane Berentson, James Cramer, Jill Abramson, Jane Mayer, Neil Westreich, Laurie Cohen, and George Hodgman.

Benjamin Weil provided daily sustenance and encouragement, read the manuscript, and offered astute editorial suggestions. I will always be in his debt. I am grateful, too, to his parents, Daphne and Richard Weil, who have made me feel a part of their family.

INDEX

admission procedures reviewed at,
187–88, 189
media and, 184–85, 188–89, 192, 193,
217
residency suspension and, 185,
189–202
resurfacing of Swango's past at,
181–88
Swango's acceptance in residency
program of, 171–75, 177–78, 298
Southern Illinois University (SIU)
medical school, 21–24, 28–35,
47–57, 139, 206, 300
acceptance criteria of, 28
cadaver dissection at, 23
curricula of, 29–34
mandate of, 22
rotations at, 29–31, 48–52
Student Progress Committee of, 31,
50–53
testing regimen of, 22–23
Southern Illinois University medical
school, students at.
black humor of, 33–34
Swango as seen by, 21–22, 23–24,
28–29, 30–32, 33–34, 47, 48, 54
Swango's expulsion urged by, 50–52
Springfield, Ill., 29
Springfield (Ill.) *State Journal-Register*
54
"Stalking Evil" (Douglas), 253–54
Stamps, Timothy, 256
state medical licensing boards:
peer review and, 163–64, 167, 299
see also Illinois Department of
Professional Regulation; Ohio
State Medical Board
Stony Brook, State University of New
York at (SUNY–Stony Brook),
medical school, 204–21, 313
media and, 218
medical school accountability and,
219–20
residency suspension and, 217–18
resurfacing of Swango's past at,
217–21
Swango's interviews and acceptance
at, 205–6, 292, 298
wrongful death lawsuit brought
against, 287n
Stossel, John, 153–54, 183
Strubhart, John, 38

succinylcholine, 304
SUNY–Stony Brook, *see* Stony Brook,
State University of New York at,
medical school
Supreme Court, U.S., 163
suspicious deaths:
author's tally of, 305–6
of Barrick, 61–65, 76, 77, 79, 120,
146, 149
of Buffalino, 209, 219, 304, 307–8
of Chipoko, 232–33, 240, 246,
307
of DeLong, 70, 72, 75, 79, 140,
145–46, 149, 150
FBI's tally of, 288, 306
of Harris, 214–16, 218–19, 287, 304,
308, 313
of McGee, 70, 72, 75, 79, 144,
145
of Mahlamvana, 231, 240, 307
at Mnene Mission hospital, *see*
Mnene Mission hospital,
suspicious deaths at
at Mpilo Hospital, 250–51
of Mugomeri, 235
of Ngwenya, 235–36, 240, 246, 283,
307
OSU Hospitals monetary
settlements for, 144–45
of Pereny, 85, 147, 149–50
of Popko, 85
of Shava, 232, 240, 307
of Walter, 70, 72, 76, 79, 116, 146,
149
of Warner, 84–85, 146–47, 149–50
of Zhou, 236, 240, 245, 246, 307
suspicious deaths investigations, *see*
Mnene Mission hospital,
suspicious deaths investigation at;
Ohio State University Hospitals,
suspicious deaths investigation at
Swango, Bob (brother), 35–36, 38, 39,
40, 43, 44, 105, 131, 228, 267–68,
308
antiwar politics of, 24, 42, 44–45
father's relationship with, 37, 44–45
Michael and, 36, 37, 45, 139
Swango, John (brother), 24, 35, 37, 39,
40, 44, 131, 139, 176, 228, 267–68,
308
Swango, John Harvey (grandfather),
36, 288

Unmisig, Brent, 93, 95, 97, 98, 101, 132
   poisoning of, 98–99, 100, 131, 133,
      135
Utz, Iwonia, 65–67, 73, 77
   as witness to Cooper's paralyzing
      injection, 66–67, 75, 76, 82,
      127–28, 145, 147, 314

Vahle, Chet, 131–32, 136, 141–42
Valery, Thomas, 218
Vann, John Paul, 41
Vara, Thomas, 85–86
Veterans Administration hospital
   (Cincinnati), 296, 297
Viet Cong, 41
Vietnam War:
   John V. Swango in, 36, 37, 40, 41–43,
      45, 46, 142, 190–91, 291
   media coverage of, 41
   "pacification" projects in, 41–42
   protest against, 21, 24, 42, 44–45, 46
   veterans of, 36, 40, 45–46, 139,
      190–91
Vogt, Bruce, 174, 175, 188

Wacaser, Lyle, 32–33, 47, 48, 50
Waco massacre, 201–2
Walden, Scott, 159–60
Walls, Effie, 33
Walter, Rein, 70, 72, 76, 79, 116, 146,
   149
Warner, Charlotte, 84–85, 146–47,
   149–50
Washington Post, 167
Watson, Nancy, 182, 287
Waxman, Henry, 166–67
Weaver, Diann, 226

Webb, Gary, 116, 117, 163–64
Whitcomb, Michael, 75, 78, 80, 81,
   88–89, 107, 309, 313
   Meeks inquiry and, 126
   and OSU Hospitals Cooper inquiry,
      81–83, 88, 111–12, 113, 121, 126,
      146, 147, 148–49, 150, 309
William and Mary, College of, 221
Wipf, Linda, 185, 193, 201
Wolfe, John W., 71, 118
women's rights, Swango on, 269
World Apart, A, 15
Wyden, Ron, 165–68, 298

Zambia, 285–86
   Ministry of Health of, 302
Zawodniak, Mark, 31–34
Zhou, Margaret, 236, 240, 245, 246,
   307
Zimbabwe:
   antiwhite discrimination in, 244, 245,
      246, 250, 263, 267
   centralized medical system of, 237
   civil war in, 14, 15
   HIV rate in, 14
   Ministry of Health of, 237, 249, 256,
      273, 280, 302
   postindependence problems of, 14,
      15
Zimbabwe Health Professions Council,
   302
Zshiri, Christopher, 16–17, 225–26,
   230–42
   and Mnene suspicious deaths
      investigation, 236–41, 247–48
   resignation of, 242
Zvishavane, Zimbabwe, 237

ABOUT THE AUTHOR

James B. Stewart is the author of *Follow the Story, Blood Sport,* and *Den of Thieves.* A former editor of *The Wall Street Journal,* Stewart won a Pulitzer Prize in 1988 for his reporting on the stock market crash and insider trading. He is a regular contributor to *The New Yorker* and *SmartMoney.*